# AIIMS Protocols in Neonatology

Additional Protocols

Third Edition

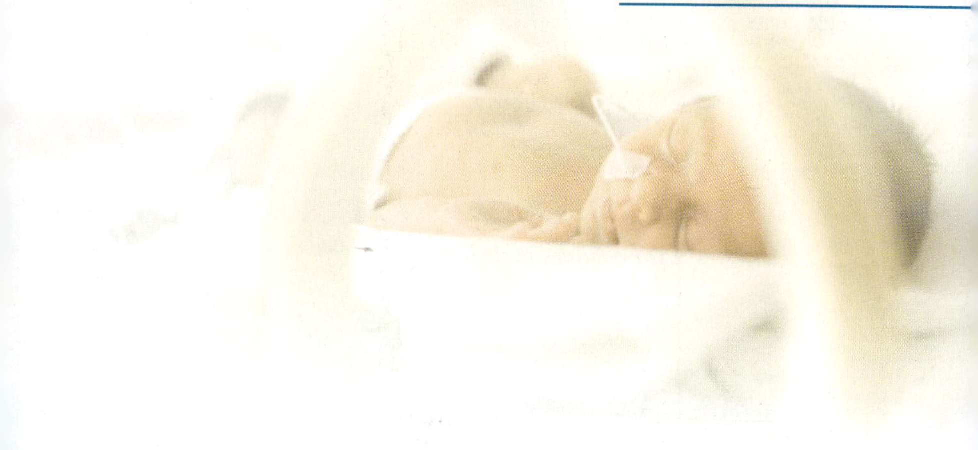

*The volumes in the set*

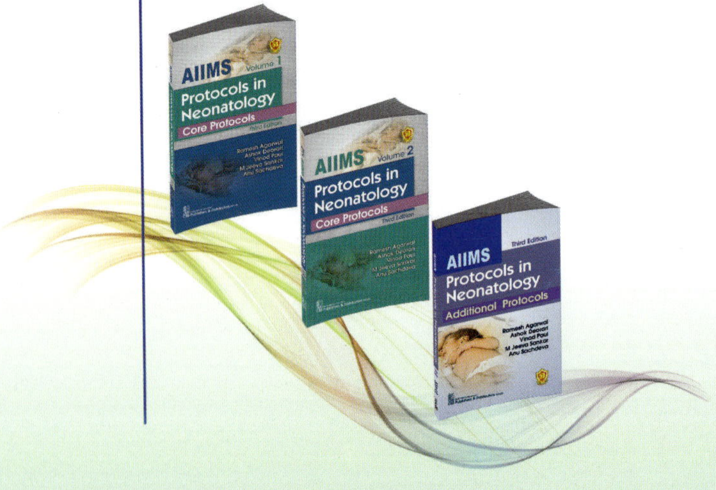

# AIIMS Protocols in Neonatology

## Additional Protocols

**Third Edition**

**Ramesh Agarwal**
MD DM (Neonatology)
Professor*

**Ashok Deorari**
MD FAMS
Principal and Dean, Himalayan Institute of Medical Sciences
Swami Rama Himalayan University, Dehradun
Former Professor and Head*

**Vinod K Paul**
MD PhD DNB FAMS FIAP FNNF
Member, NITI Aayog, Government of India
Former Professor and Head*

**M Jeeva Sankar**
MD DM
Additional Professor*

**Anu Sachdeva**
MD DM
Additional Professor*

***Department of Pediatrics**
WHO Collaborating Centre for Education and Research in Newborn Care
All India Institute of Medical Sciences, New Delhi, India
www.newbornwhocc.org
[PDFs of the protocols are available online: www.newbornwhocc.org]

CBSPD
**CBS Publishers & Distributors** Pvt Ltd
New Delhi • Bengaluru • Chennai • Kochi • Kolkata • Lucknow • Mumbai
Hyderabad • Jharkhand • Nagpur • Patna • Pune • Uttarakhand

*Disclaimer*

Science and technology are constantly changing fields. New research and experience broaden the scope of information and knowledge. The authors have tried their best in giving information available to them while preparing the material for this book. Although all efforts have been made to ensure optimum accuracy of the material, yet it is quite possible some errors might have been left uncorrected. The publisher, the printer and the authors will not be held responsible for any inadvertent errors, omissions or inaccuracies.

The protocols are context-specific, and readers are advised to modify and adapt the protocols for their settings.

**AIIMS Protocols in Neonatology**

Additional Protocols

Third Edition

**ISBN:** 978-93-5466-885-2



**Third Edition: 2024**

*Reprint:* 2025, 2026, **2027**

First Edition 2015

Second Edition 2019



Published by Satish Kumar Jain and produced by Varun Jain for

**CBS Publishers & Distributors** Pvt Ltd

4819/XI Prahlad Street, 24 Ansari Road, Daryaganj, New Delhi 110 002, India
Ph: 011-23289259, 23266838 Website: www.cbspd.com e-mail: delhi@cbspd.com

Corporate Office: 204 FIE, Industrial Area, Patparganj, Delhi 110 092, India
Ph: 011-4934 4934 Fax: 011-4934 4935 e-mail: publishing@cbspd.com; publicity@cbspd.com

*Branches*

- **Bengaluru:** Seema House 2975, 17th Cross, KR Road, Banasankari 2nd Stage, Bengaluru 560 070, Karnataka, India
  Ph: +91-80-26771678/79 Fax: +91-80-26771680 e-mail: bangalore@cbspd.com
- **Chennai:** 18/8B, Subbaraya Street, Shenoy Nagar, Chennai 600 030, Tamil Nadu, India
  Ph: +91-44-42032115, 45022115 e-mail: chennai@cbspd.com
- **Kochi:** 42/1325, 1326, Power House Road, Opposite KSEB, Ernakulum Kochi 682 018, Kerala, India
  Ph: +91-484-4059061-65 Fax: +91-484-4059065 e-mail: kochi@cbspd.com
- **Kolkata:** 147, Hind Ceramics Compound, 1st Floor, Nilgunj Road, Belghoria, Kolkata 700 056, West Bengal, India
  Ph: +91-33-25633055/56 e-mail: kolkata@cbspd.com
- **Lucknow:** Basement, Khushnuma Complex, 7 Meerabai Marg (behind Jawahar Bhawan), Lucknow 226 001, UP, India
  Ph: +91-522-4000032 e-mail: tiwari.lucknow@cbspd.com
- **Mumbai:** PWD Shed, Gala no 25/26, Ramchandra Bhatt Marg, Next to JJ Hospital Gate no. 2, Opp. Union Bank of India, Noorbaug, Mumbai 400 009, Maharashtra, India
  Ph: +91-22-66661880/89 e-mail: mumbai@cbspd.com

*Representatives*

- **Gujarat** • **Hyderabad** • **Jharkhand** • **Nagpur** • **Patna** • **Pune** • **Uttarakhand**

*For trade terms please contact* customercare@cbspd.com
*For general enquiries please contact* info@cbspd.com

*Printed at:* HT Media Ltd, Greater Noida, UP, India

*to*
*Newborn Infants*

# Contributors

**Aathira Ravindranath** DM
Consultant Pediatric
Gastroenterologist
Apollo BGS Hospital, Mysuru
aathira.r@gmail.com

**Abin Sheref Mohammed** MBBS
Junior Resident
Department of Pediatrics
All India Institute of Medical Sciences
New Delhi
Abinsheref.1997@gmail.com

**Aditi Sinha** PhD
Additional Professor
Department of Pediatrics
All India Institute of Medical Sciences
New Delhi
aditisinhaaiims@gmail.com

**Akash Sharma**
Consultant Neonatologist and
Pediatrician
In-charge NICU, Surya Hospitals
Jaipur, drakash.jpr@gmail.com

**Akash Singhal** MD
Senior Resident
Department of Neonatology
All India Institute of Medical Sciences
New Delhi

**Alec Reginald Errol Correa** DM
Medical Geneticist
Lifecell International
Pune
aleccorrea88@hotmail.com

**Alisha Gupta** MCh
Ex-Senior Resident
Department of Pediatric Surgery
All India Institute of Medical Sciences
New Delhi
doc.alishagupta@gmail.com

**Amanpreet Sethi** DM
Assistant Professor
Department of Pediatrics
Guru Gobind Singh Medical College
Faridkot, Punjab
sethi.amanpreet702@gmail.com

**Amit Upadhyay** DM
Consultant Neonatologist
Nutema Hospital, Meerut
au.llrm@gmail.com

**Anapti Anil** MD
Senior Resident
Department of Obstetrics and
Gynaecology
All India Institute of Medical Sciences
New Delhi, anapti.garg9@gmail.com

**Anjan Kumar Dhua** MCh
Additional Professor
Department of Pediatric Surgery
All India Institute of Medical Sciences
anjandhua@hotmail.com

**Ankit Meena** DM
Senior Resident
Department of Pediatrics
All India Institute of Medical Sciences
New Delhi
ankit.aiims.meena@gmail.com

**Ankita** MBBS
Junior Resident
Department of Pediatrics
All India Institute of Medical Sciences
New Delhi
ankiagar23@gmail.com

**Ankit Verma** MD
Assistant Professor
Department of Pediatrics
All India Institute of Medical Sciences
New Delhi
ankitverma0486@gmail.com

**Ankitha Ravishankar** MBBS
Junior Resident
Department of Pediatrics
All India Institute of Medical Sciences
New Delhi
ankitha.ravishankar@gmail.com

**Anubhuti Rana** MD
Assistant Professor
Department of Obstetrics and Gynaecology
All India Institute of Medical Sciences
New Delhi, anubhuti_rana@yahoo.com

**Aparna Chandrasekaran** DM
Chief Neonatologist
Krishna Institute of Medical Sciences (KIMS), Cuddles
Kondapur, Hyderabad
appubanu@gmail.com

**Aparna K Sharma** MD
Professor
Department of Obstetrics and Gynaecology
All India Institute of Medical Sciences
New Delhi
kaparnasharma@gmail.com

**Arunambika Chinnappan** MD
Senior Resident
Department of Neonatology
All India Institute of Medical Sciences
Bhubaneswar
arunambika.chinnappan@gmail.com

**Arun Sasi** DM
Consultant Neonatologist
Royal Children's Hospital, Melbourne
Mercy Hospital for Women, Melbourne
Adjunct Clinical Lecturer
Department of Obstetrics and Gynecology
University of Melbourne
Melbourne, Australia

**Arvind Bagga** MD
Director and Sr Consultant
Department of Pediatric Nephrology
Indraprastha Apollo Hospitals
New Delhi, arvindbagga@hotmail.com

**Ashish Jain** DM
Associate Professor and Head
Department of Neonatology
Maulana Azad Medical College
New Delhi
neoashish2008@gmail.com

**Ashutosh Kapoor** DM
Consultant Neonatologist and Pediatrician
In-charge NICU
Chandan Hospital, Lucknow
ashukap22@gmail.com

**Biswaroop Chakrabarty** DM
Additional Professor
Department of Pediatrics
All India Institute of Medical Sciences
New Delhi
biswaroopchakrabarty@gmail.com

**Chandrakumar Natarajan** DM
Senior Consultant and Head
Department of Neonatology
KKCTH Hospital
Nungambakkam, Chennai
drchandrakumar@gmail.com

**Deena Thomas** DM
Consultant Neonatologist
Muthoot Hospital
Kozhencherry, Kerala
deenathomas87@gmail.com

**Deepak Chawla** DM
Professor
Government Medical College and Hospital, Chandigarh
drdeepakchawla@gmail.com

**Deepika Kainth** DM
Assistant Professor
All India Institute of Medical Sciences
New Delhi
aiims.deepika@gmail.com

**Delona Treesa Joseph** MBBS
Senior Resident
Department of Pediatric Surgery
All India Institute of Medical Sciences
New Delhi, delonatreeza@gmail.com

**Deula Candida D'Cruz** MD
Senior Resident
Department of Pediatrics
All India Institute of Medical Sciences
New Delhi
deulacandidadcruz@gmail.com

**Devi S Saranya** MD
Senior Resident
Division of Genetics
Department of Pediatrics
All India Institute of Medical Sciences
New Delhi, devisaranyas92@gmail.com

**Dhinakaran Raman** DM
Consultant Neonatologist
Prashanth Hospital
Velachery, Chennai
dhina.mmc@gmail.com

**Dilip Kumar** MBBS
Junior Resident
Department of Pediatrics
All India Institute of Medical Sciences
New Delhi

**Girish Gururaj** DM
Apollo Hospital, Mysuru

**Gitanjali Jain** MD
Senior Resident
Department of Neonatology
All India Institute of Medical Sciences
New Delhi
gitanjali_jain@yahoo.co.in

**Haleemath Afrah** MBBS
Junior Resident
Department of Pediatrics
All India Institute of Medical Sciences
New Delhi, helloafrah@gmail.com

**Harshita Nori** MD
Senior Resident
Department of Neonatology
All India Institute of Medical Sciences
New Delhi, harshita.nori@gmail.com

**Jagjit Singh Dalal** DM
Senior Professor and Head
Department of Neonatology
Pandit BD Sharma PGIMS
Rohtak, jagjit.dr@gmail.com

**Kajal Jain** PhD
Scientist, Division of Neonatology
Department of Pediatrics
All India Institute of Medical Sciences
New Delhi, kajaljain12@gmail.com

**Kamal Arora** DM
Professor
Division of Neonatology
Department of Pediatrics
Dayanand Medical College and
Hospital, Ludhiana
dockamalpaeds@yahoo.com

**Kapil Sikka** MS
Professor
Department of Otorhinolaryngology
and Head–Neck Surgery
All India Institute of Medical Sciences
New Delhi
kapil_sikka@yahoo.com

**Krishna Mohan Gulla** MD, FNB (PICU) DM
Resident
Division of Pediatric Pulmonology
and Intensive Care
All India Institute of Medical Sciences
New Delhi
mohangulla35@gmail.com

**Lalit Takia** DM
Assistant Professor
Department of Pediatrics
All India Institute of Medical Sciences
New Delhi, lalitpgims@gmail.com

**Likhita P** MBBS
Junior Resident
Department of Pediatrics
All India Institute of Medical
Sciences, New Delhi
likhu13@gmail.com

**Lumchio Levis Murry** MSc (Nursing)
Associate Professor
All India Institute of Medical Sciences
New Delhi, levis.murry@gmail.com

**Madhulika Kabra** MD
Professor
All India Institute of Medical Sciences
New Delhi
madhulikakabra@hotmail.com

**Madhumati Bose**
Certified Neonatal Oro-Motor
Assessment Scale
Consultant on Autism for State
Initiative on Disabilities (SID), Kerala;
Honorary Consultant
All India Institute of Medical Sciences
Holy Family Hospital, New Delhi
madhumatibose@gmail.com

**Mahesh V** DM (Pediatric Nephrology)
Assistant Professor
Department of Pediatrics
All India Institute of Medical Sciences
Mangalagiri, Andhra Pradesh
vmaahi46@gmail.com

**Manas Upadhyay** DM
Consultant Neonatologist
Cuttack, Odisha
manl013456@gmail.com

**Manisha Jana** MD, FRCR
Professor
All India Institute of Medical Sciences
New Delhi
manishajana@gmail.com

**Manju Saksena** PhD
Physician Scientist
All India Institute of Medical Sciences
New Delhi
manjusaksena@gmail.com

**Mayank Priyadarshi** DM
Assistant Professor
Department of Neonatology
All India Institute of Medical Sciences
Rishikesh, Uttarakhand
priyadarshi.aiims@gmail.com

**Mehak Sehgal** MCh (Pediatric Surgery)
Ex-Senior Resident
All India Institute of Medical Sciences
New Delhi
mehak.sehgal91@gmail.com

**Mohammad Tousifullah** DM
Consultant Neonatologist
Jaswant Rai Speciality Hospital
Meerut, drmdtousif@gmail.com

**Mudit Agarwal** MBBS
Junior Resident
Department of Pediatrics
All India Institute of Medical Sciences
New Delhi
mudit.agarwal07@gmail.com

**Mukul Kumar Mangla** DM
Senior Medical Officer
Safadarjung Hospital and VMMC
New Delhi
drmanglamukul@yahoo.com

**Narendra Kumar Bagri** MD
Additional Professor
Division of Pediatric Rheumatology
and Clinical Immunology
Department of Pediatrics
All India Institute of Medical Sciences
New Delhi
drnarendrabagri@gmail.com

**Neerja Gupta** DM
Additional Professor
Division of Genetics
Department of Pediatrics
All India Institute of Medical Sciences
New Delhi, neerja17aiims@gmail.com

**Nidhi Garg** MD
Senior Resident
Department of Neonatology
All India Institute of Medical Sciences
New Delhi
ng5620@gmail.com

**Parminder Singh Rooprai** MD
Senior Resident
Department of Neonatology
All India Institute of Medical Sciences
New Delhi
param_rules@yahoo.co.in

**Pavneet Kaur** MD
Junior Resident
Department of Pediatrics
All India Institute of Medical Sciences
New Delhi
dr.pavneetkaurthind@gmail.com

**Poonam Coshic** MBBS, MBA (Healthcare Administration)
Chief Medical Officer
Blood Bank (H)
All India Institute of Medical Sciences
New Delhi
poonamcoshic@gmail.com

**Pradeep Kumar Sharma** DM
Senior Consultant
Deep Hospital, Ludhiana
psaiims@yahoo.co.in

**Prashant Jauhari** DM
Additional Professor
Department of Pediatrics
All India Institute of Medical Sciences
New Delhi
pjauhari0@gmail.com

**Pratima Anand** DM
Neonatologist
Department of Neonatology
Lady Hardinge Medical College and Associated Hospitals
New Delhi
anandpratima@gmail.com

**Pragya Tyagi** MASLP
Audiologist
Department of Otorhinolaryngology and Head–Neck Surgery
All India Institute of Medical Sciences
New Delhi
pragyatyagi@hotmail.com

**Praveen George Paul** MD, DM
Senior Resident
Department of Pediatric Endocrinology
All India Institute of Medical Sciences
New Delhi
praveenpaul388@gmail.com

**Priyanka Gupta** MD, DM
Senior Resident
Department of Pediatric Endocrinology
All India Institute of Medical Sciences
New Delhi
prigupta552@gmail.com

**Priyanka Khandelwal** DM (Pediatric Nephrology), International Pediatric Nephrology Fellow
Department of Pediatrics
Great Ormond Street Hospital for Children
London,
drpriyanka8588@gmail.com

**Priyanka Singh** MD
Senior Resident
Department of Neonatology
All India Institute of Medical Sciences
New Delhi
priyanka09singh@gmail.com

**Puneet Kumar Choudhary** DM
Senior Resident
Department of Pediatrics
All India Institute of Medical Sciences
New Delhi
shinepuneet@gmail.com

**Purna Chandra Guggilum** DM
Senior Resident
Department of Pediatrics
All India Institute of Medical Sciences
New Delhi
chandra.puri12@gmail.com

**Rahul Kumar** MBBS
Junior Resident
Department of Pediatrics
All India Institute of Medical Sciences
New Delhi
mailtorahulkumarsuman@gmail.com

**Raja Ashok Koganti** DM (Neonatology)
Consultant Neonatologist
Ankura Hospital for Women and Children, Vijayawada
drrajaashok@gmail.com

**Rajiv Aggarwal** Fellowship in Neonatology
Director and Senior Consultant
Department of Pediatrics and Neonatology
Narayana Health City, Bengaluru
drrajivaggarwal@hotmail.com

**Rajni Sharma** MD
Additional Professor
All India Institute of Medical Sciences
New Delhi
email:drrajnisharma@yahoo.com

**Rakesh Lodha** MD
Professor
Department of Pediatrics
All India Institute of Medical Sciences
New Delhi
rlodha1661@gmail.com

**Ranjith Kumar Manokaran** DM
Associate Professor
Sri Ramachandra Institute of Higher Education and Research
Porur, Chennai
doct.ranjith@gmail.com

**Ravneet Kaur** DM
Associate Consultant
Division of Medical Genetics
Fortis Hospital
Mohali, Punjab
docravneet@gmail.com

**Richie Dalai** DM
Assistant Professor
Department of Neonatology
All India Institute of Medical Sciences
Patna
richie.aiims@gmail.com

**Rinchen Zangmo** MD
Ex-Assistant Professor
Department of Obstetrics and Gynaecology
All India Institute of Medical Sciences
New Delhi
rinchhen.zn@gmail.com

**Rishika Potharaju** MBBS
Junior Resident
Department of Pediatrics
All India Institute of Medical Sciences
New Delhi

**Rohan Malik** DM
Additional Professor
All India Institute of Medical Sciences
New Delhi
dr.rohanmalik@gmail.com

**Sachit Anand** MCh
Assistant Professor
Department of Pediatric Surgery
All India Institute of Medical Sciences
New Delhi
kanu.sachit@gmail.com

**Sai Srinivas Gurram** MD
Senior Resident
Department of Neonatology
All India Institute of Medical Sciences
New Delhi
srinivassai982@gmail.com

**Satish Mishra** DM
Consultant Neonatologist and Pediatrician
NEO Center for Advanced Neonatology and Child Health
Sagar, Madhya Pradesh
drmishrasatish@gmail.com

**Satya Prakash** MD, DM
Senior Resident
Department of Neonatology
All India Institute of Medical Sciences
New Delhi
satyaprakash1994@gmail.com

**Saurabh Kumar Gupta**
MD (Pediatrics), DM (Cardiology)
Professor
Department of Cardiology
All India Institute of Medical Sciences
New Delhi
drsaurabhmd@gmail.com

**Seema Singhal** MD
Additional Professor
Department of Obstetrics and Gynaecology
All India Institute of Medical Sciences
New Delhi
drseemasinghal@gmail.com

**Shamnad Madathil** MD, DM
Consultant Neonatologist
Baby Memorial Hospital
Kozhikode
shamnadmadathil@gmail.com

**Shashank S Koundinya** MBBS
Junior Resident
Department of Pediatrics
All India Institute of Medical Sciences
New Delhi
shashankskoundinya007@gmail.com

**Shridhar Gopalakrishnan**
DM (Neonatology)
Professor
Department of Pediatrics
Armed Forces Medical College, Pune
shri27cat@gmail.com

**Sindhu Sivanandan** DM
Consultant Neonatologist and Clincal Lead
Kauvery Hospital, Chennai
drsindhusivanandan@gmail.com

**Soumya Devarapalli**
Senior Resident
Division of Neonatology
Department of Pediatrics
All India Institute of Medical Sciences
Ansari Nagar
soumya.devarapalli@gmail.com

**Srikanth Kulkarni** DM (Neonatology)
Consultant Neonatologist
Rainbow Children's Hospital
Marathahalli, Bengaluru
sskulkarni151@gmail.com

**Srinivasavaradan S Govindarajan** MD, DM
Senior Resident
Department of Pediatric Nephrology
All India Institute of Medical Sciences
New Delhi
kavisrini.1993@gmail.com

**Subhash Chandra Shaw** DM
Professor
Department of Pediatrics
Army Hospital Research and Referral
Delhi
drscshaw@rediffmail.com

**Subramanian Sreeram** DM
Consultant
Paramitha Children Hospital and
NEO BBC Children Hospital
Hyderabad
drsreeraman@yahoo.co.in

**Suman Chaurasia** MD, PhD
Assistant Professor
All India Institute of Medical Sciences
Rishikesh, Uttarakhand
sumanyss@gmail.com

**Suma S** DM
Consultant Neonatologist
Bai Jerbai Wadia Hospital for Children
Mumbai, suma.sund@gmail.com

**Sunil Kushwah** MD, DM
Senior Resident
Department of Pediatric Nephrology
Post Graduate Institute of
Medical Education and Research
(PGIMER), Chandigarh
drsunilkushwah04@gmail.com

**Sunil Saharan** MD
Assistant Professor
Division of Congenital Interventional
Cardiology, New York University
Langone Medical Center, New York
sunilsaharan@gmail.com

**Surjeet Kumar Bhardwaj** MD, DM
(Neonatology)
Assistant Professor
Department of Pediatrics
DrYSPGMC, Nahan, HP
drsurjeet99@gmail.com

**Suvasini Sharma** DM
Associate Professor
Lady Hardinge Medical College,
New Delhi
sharma.suvasini@gmail.com

**Tanushree Sahoo** MD, DM
Assistant Professor
Department of Neonatology
All India Institute of Medical Sciences
Bhubaneswar
tanushree_sony206@yahoo.co.in

**Tejo Pratap Oleti** DM
Senior Consultant and Head
Department of Neonatology
Fernandez Hospital, Hyderabad
tejopratap@gmail.com

**Umang Bhardwaj** MD
Senior Resident
Department of Neonatology
All India Institute of Medical Sciences
New Delhi
umangbhardwaj51@gmail.com

**Vandana Jain** MD
Professor
All India Institute of Medical Sciences
New Delhi
drvandanajain@aiims.edu

**Vasudha Kohli** MD
Senior Resident
Department of Pediatrics
All India Institute of Medical Sciences
New Delhi
kohli.vasudha@gmail.com

**Venkatesan Sampath Kumar** MS
Associate Professor
Department of Orthopaedics
All India Institute of Medical Sciences
New Delhi
venkatortho4@gmail.com

**Venkatnarayan Kannan** DM
Officer on Special Duty
NITI Aayog, Government of India
New Delhi
venkatnarayan_kannan@yahoo.co.in

**Vishesh Jain** MCh
Assistant Professor
Department of Pediatric Surgery
All India Institute of Medical Sciences
New Delhi
dr.vishesh79@gmail.com

**Vivek Kumar** MD
Consultant (Research)
Department of Pediatrics
All India Institute of Medical Sciences
New Delhi
vivekneoaiims@gmail.com

**Vivek Tiwari** MS
Senior Orthopaedic Consultant
Apollo Sage Hospital, Bhopal
vivek_tiwari50@yahoo.com

**V Prakash** MD
All India Institute of Medical Sciences
New Delhi

# Preface to the Third Edition

We take immense pleasure in presenting the third edition of *AIIMS Protocols in Neonatology*. In this updated edition, we have introduced 39 new protocols and deleted nine protocols from the second edition, expanding the compendium to encompass 106 protocols. Our primary aim is to provide valuable resources that enhance our readers' education and patient care.

These protocols are thoughtfully categorized into two distinct packages: Core Protocols, spanning two volumes, cater to the management of common neonatal conditions, while Additional Protocols are dedicated to practitioners handling critically ill neonates and to DM and DNB fellows. This categorization empowers readers to delve into all protocols or focus exclusively on the Core ones.

Our unwavering commitment throughout the development of this edition has been to ensure that these protocols are firmly rooted in evidence-based practices. Our team has diligently reviewed the extensive body of literature, including guidelines from reputed bodies such as the World Health Organization (WHO), American Academy of Pediatrics (AAP), American College of Obstetrics and Gynecology (ACOG), National Institute of Clinical Excellence (NICE), Government of India, and National Neonatology Forum (NNF), meticulously contextualized the information, and presented it in a user-friendly format.

We emphasize that the protocols primarily apply to our own or similar institutions and *may have to be adapted to the users' context*. We highly recommend appropriate diligence in this regard.

Creating this edition has demanded a monumental collaborative effort. Faculty members, fellows, residents from our division, colleagues from other divisions within our department and various departments across our institution, and colleagues from other institutions have invested their time and expertise into its development. We extend our heartfelt gratitude to all those who have contributed to this endeavor.

We are grateful to the readers of the second edition who provided us with their valuable feedback. Your insights have been instrumental in refining this edition. We have diligently incorporated relevant changes and rectified any errors to make this version more comprehensive and reliable.

We extend our heartfelt gratitude to Mr YN Arjuna and the dedicated team at CBS, our new publisher, for their exceptional commitment and hands-on involvement in supervising the entire publication process of this third edition.

We acknowledge the possibility of mistakes in this edition. We value your feedback, as it has been invaluable in the past. Please send any observations or suggestions to us via email at ra.aiims@gmail.com, jeevasankar@gmail.com, or dranuthukral@gmail.com.

**Ramesh Agarwal**
**Ashok Deorari**
**Vinod K Paul**
**M Jeeva Sankar**
**Anu Sachdeva**

# Preface to the First Edition

Protocols are instrumental for adoption of evidence-based practices and elimination of unnecessary or potentially harmful practices. Protocol based approach makes sure that there is a uniform clinical practice irrespective of disparate players and their views. Unit protocols also facilitate learning of the trainee doctors and nurses.

Protocols have been an integral part of NICU life at AIIMS right since its inception. As part of its philosophy of unrestricted sharing of the knowledge and resources, the neonatology faculty at AIIMS decided way back to publish the protocols in Indian Journal of Pediatrics. There was an overwhelming response from the neonatal fraternity to the extent that AIIMS protocols practically became part of majority of the neonatal units in India as well as other countries in South East Asia. For postgraduate students, it served as first hand resource for learning neonatology. The AIIMS protocols have been cited for over 400 times across the globe including in many major publications of recent times.

Initially, we published the protocols in Indian Journal of Pediatrics, which were periodically updated. Subsequently, the journal published them in form of a manual that enhanced their usability and outreach. The full texts of the protocols were made available on our website (wwwnewbornwhocc.org), which was one of the reasons of its popularity receiving nearly 200,000 hits over the last few years.

This publication is a manifestation of our desire to bring out a physician manual that contains relevant protocols based on context specific and updated evidence as well as other necessary resources and tools for day-to-day neonatology practice in level 2 and 3 neonatal units in South East Asia. The current manual has 33 protocols. These are focused on the operational aspects of a condition rather than discussing the theory. There are summaries of relevant evidence and management algorithms at appropriate places. There is a substantial amount of additional resource material such as resuscitation algorithm, hand hygiene poster, BP charts, drugs to be avoided in G6PD deficiency, online resources for self-learning and drugs use in pregnancy and lactation. There is a section that deals with main findings on chest X-ray of common conditions. A section on drug dosages has also been included.

India produces over 1200 postgraduate theses in pediatrics every year; however, the quality of research is too low to teach research methods to the students and generate a good piece of evidence. We have included a section that provides a number of research questions and optimum design to be used and relevant outcomes to be studied.

AIIMS protocols have been an outcome of intense efforts of the faculty, scientists and many past and present residents and fellows over a long time. All of them have shown an extraordinary commitment for this cause. We wish to acknowledge the immense contribution of Drs M Jeeva Sankar, Anu Thukral, Deepak Chawla, Kamal Arora and Aparna Chandrasekaran who not only contributed substantially in terms of contents but also in process of editing. We wish to thank Mr YN Arjuna of CBS Publishers who patiently accommodated our changing philosophy and style.

No book is flawless and we are unlikely to be exception. We would really appreciate your constructive criticism (ra.aiims@gmail.com).

**Ramesh Agarwal**
**Ashok Deorari**
**Vinod K Paul**

# Contents

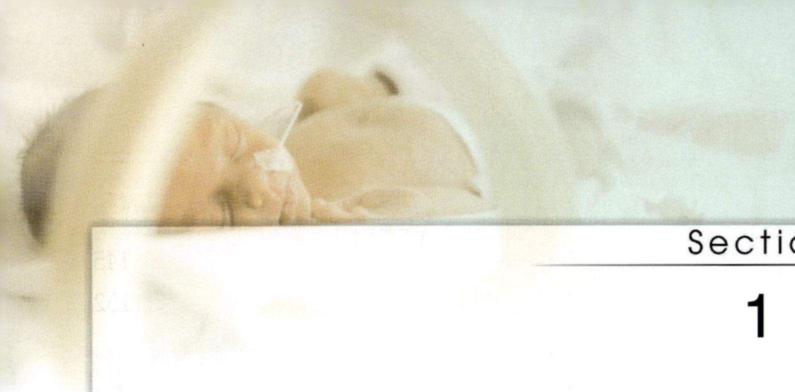

Section

1

# Fetal and Perinatal Care

CHAPTER

1

# Antenatal Fetal Monitoring

The antepartum fetal assessment aims to timely identify fetuses at risk of intrauterine death or other complications of intrauterine asphyxia and to prevent these adverse outcomes, if possible. An antepartum test needs to identify a compromised fetus such that the intervention is successful. The clinician must remember that no known assessment method can predict sudden events, such as a cord accident or placental abruption, which are frequent causes of fetal death.[1]

## PHYSIOLOGICAL BASIS OF ANTEPARTUM FETAL MONITORING

A compromised fetus undergoes a series of detectable physiological changes, such as the redistribution of blood flow or decreasing unnecessary movements (Fig. 1.1). Other factors may modify the progression of these changes such as gestational age, maternal medication, and smoking. In addition, there may be acute incidents like abruption leading to acute hypoxemia, which may not be detected on routine antepartum testing.

### Efficacy and Harms

Antepartum fetal assessment has been established in obstetrics since 1970s. However, its ability to improve pregnancy outcomes has not been evaluated by large, well-designed randomized trials. Various observational studies have reported lower fetal death rates in pregnancies that underwent fetal testing than among historical controls with the same indication for testing but no fetal testing or among the contemporary controls that were low-risk populations. The significant harm would be false-positive tests that lead to unnecessary additional fetal evaluation and intervention, particularly iatrogenic preterm birth. False-negative tests suggest a false sense of security and may again lead to potential harm.[2]

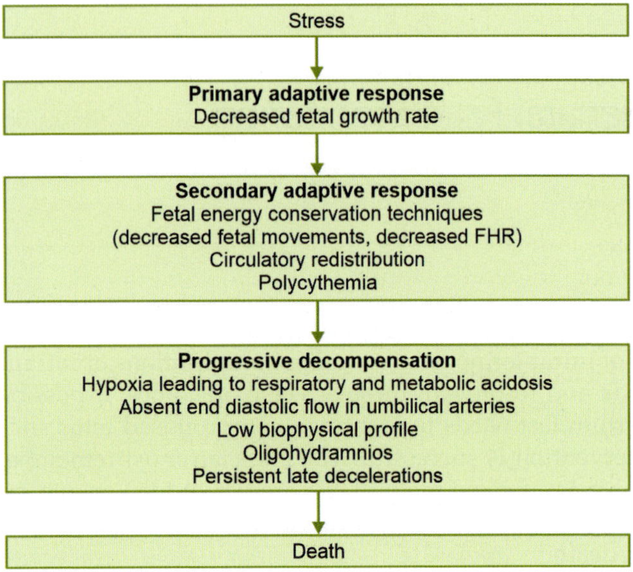


**Fig. 1.1:** Response of fetus to chronic hypoxia

## Indications[1]

### *Maternal Conditions*

- Pregestational diabetes mellitus
- Hypertension
- Systemic lupus erythematosus
- Chronic renal disease
- Antiphospholipid syndrome
- Hyperthyroidism (poorly controlled)
- Hemoglobinopathies (sickle cell, sickle cell–hemoglobin C, or sickle cell–thalassemia disease)
- Cyanotic heart disease

### *Pregnancy-related Conditions*

- Gestational hypertension
- Pre-eclampsia
- Decreased fetal movement
- Gestational diabetes mellitus (poorly controlled or medically treated)
- Oligohydramnios
- Fetal growth restriction

- Late-term or post-term pregnancy
- Isoimmunization
- Previous fetal demise (unexplained or recurrent risk)
- Monochorionic multiple gestations (with significant growth discrepancy)

## Techniques[3]

The main techniques for fetal assessment are the fetal movement count, nonstress test, biophysical profile, modified biophysical profile, and contraction stress test. Evaluation of amniotic fluid volume and Doppler velocimetry provide additional information about the fetal status.

### *Fetal Movement Counting*

It is a simple and inexpensive method of monitoring the fetus. There is a universal consensus that women with absent or reduced fetal movements should prompt the obstetrician for further fetal assessment, as decreased placental perfusion and fetal acidemia are associated with decreased fetal movements. However, available evidence does not support a clear fetal movement threshold or "alarm limit" indicating when the risk of fetal death or injury is increased. The fetal sleep cycle lasts about 20 to 40 minutes and practically never exceeds 90 minutes in a normal, healthy fetus. Hence, The American Congress of Obstetricians and Gynecologists (ACOG) recommends that less than ten movements within two hours are abnormal. There are two methods for fetal movement count:

a. The Cardiff method suggests a count to 10 movements in a fixed time frame (12 hours).
b. The Sadovsky method suggests counting movements in a specific time frame (usually 30 minutes to two hours).

### *Nonstress Test (NST)*

Fetal Heart Rate (FHR) accelerations, spontaneous or provoked (e.g. by vibroacoustic stimulation), indicate normal fetal autonomic function and absence of acidosis and neurologic depression. The non-stress test is performed during the antenatal period when the uterus is relaxed. The woman should empty her bladder and be positioned on either a bed or a reclining chair in the left lateral recumbent position. The recording should last at least 20 minutes. The baseline fetal heart rate should be within the normal range of 110 to 160 bpm. Moderate variability of 6 to 25 bpm is expected.

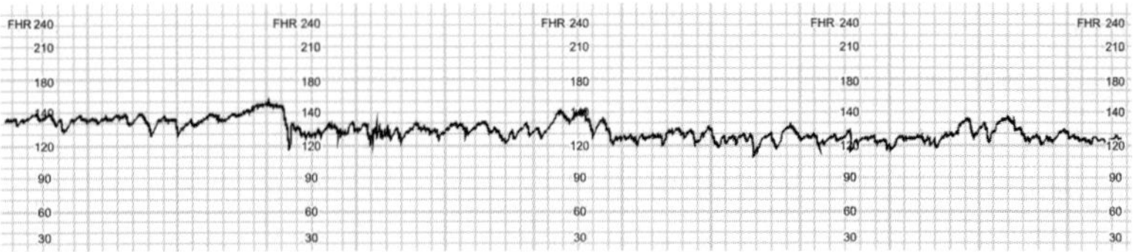

**Fig. 1.2:** Reactive non-stress test

A normal (reactive) non-stress test includes at least two accelerations from the baseline within the 20 minutes of testing that reach a peak of at least 15 bpm above the baseline and have a duration from onset to return to baseline of at least 15 seconds (Fig. 1.2).

A negative predictive value of the test for fetal and neonatal death is 99% within one week of testing. If the fetal heart acceleratory response does not meet the criteria after 20 minutes of testing, the recording should continue for another 20 minutes to account for the average period of non-rapid eye movement sleep when fetal movement and heart rate variability are reduced. If the criteria are still unmet, the test is reported as non-reactive NST, and a backup test, like a biophysical profile test, is performed.

### *Contraction Stress Test*

The contraction stress test (CST)/oxytocin challenge test is based on the fetal response to a transient reduction in fetal oxygen delivery during uterine contractions, which may manifest clinically as late decelerations.

Drawbacks of CST include the need to stimulate contractions with intravenous oxytocin with its contraindications (e.g. placenta previa), and the high false-positive rate (fetus goes on to tolerate labor without FHR changes necessitating intervention). The false-negative rate (rate of antepartum stillbirth within one week of a negative test) is meager, thus providing reassurance of adequate fetal oxygenation after a normal test result. The CST is seldom performed given the wide availability of other tests (e.g. nonstress test, biophysical profile) that do not have these drawbacks.

### *Biophysical Profile*[4]

The biophysical profile (BPP) combines the NST with fetal ultrasonographic assessment by assigning points to the following parameters: Amniotic fluid volume (AFV), fetal breathing movements, fetal body movements, and reflex/tone/flexion–extension movements (Tables 1.1 and 1.2). The modified biophysical

| Table 1.1: Scoring criteria for biophysical profile (Manning 1995) | | |
|---|---|---|
| *Biophysical variable* | *Normal (score=2)* | *Abnormal (score=0)* |
| Fetal breathing movements | 1 episode of at least 30 sec in 30 mins | Absent or no episode >30 sec in 30 mins |
| Fetal movements | 3 discrete body/limb movements in 30 mins | 2 or less in 30 mins |
| Fetal tone | 1 episode of active extension with return to flexion of limbs or trunk | Slow extension with return to partial flexion, or movement of limb in full extension, or no movement |
| Amniotic fluid | 1 pocket measuring at least 2 cm in 2 perpendicular | Either no pocket or a pocket < 2 cm in two perpendicular planes |
| Non-stress test | Reactive | Non-reactive |

| Table 1.2: Interpretation of biophysical profile scores | | |
|---|---|---|
| *Result* | *Interpretation* | *Action* |
| 10/10 OR 8/8 or 8/10 with normal amniotic fluid | Normal | No intervention |
| 6/10 with normal amniotic fluid (4 points for two of fetal movement, tone, and breathing, but +2 points for amniotic fluid) | Equivocal | The test is repeated within 24 hours to see if one of the absent acute variables returns to normal or, If the patient is at or near term, delivery is a reasonable option |
| 6/10 or 8/10 with oligohydramnios (6/10 or 8/10 with 0 points for amniotic fluid) | Abnormal | The risk of fetal asphyxia within one week is 89/1000 with expectant management Scores should be interpreted within the context of gestational age and maternal and obstetric factors |
| 0 to 4/10 | Abnormal | The risk of fetal asphyxia within one week is 91 to 600/1000 Delivery is usually indicated |

profile (mBPP) consists of the NST as a measure of acute oxygenation and the assessment of AFV as a measure of longer-term oxygenation.[5] Thus, this test assesses indicators of both acute hypoxia (NST, breathing, body movement, tone) and chronic hypoxia (AFV). The BPP score has a direct linear correlation with fetal pH. The false-negative rates for the BPP and mBPP are meager, but the false-positive rates are high (a false-negative BPP or mBPP is when an antepartum stillbirth occurs within one week of a high score; a false positive is a low score that is followed by a normal backup test and no fetal compromise).[6]

### *Amniotic Fluid Volume*

The rationale behind including AFI as a method of fetal assessment is that cardiac output is redirected to the brain, heart, and adrenals and away from less vital organs, such as the kidney, as a response to hypoxemia; the reduction in renal perfusion leads to decreased fetal urine production, which may result in reduced amniotic fluid volume (oligohydramnios) over time.

Various techniques can assess the amniotic fluid volume. One of them is the maximal vertical pocket depth. This approach identifies a pocket depth of 2 to 8 cm as normal, 1 to 2 cm as marginal, <1cm as decreased, and > 8 cm as increased. The second technique is the AFI. The AFI assesses amniotic fluid volume more broadly by summing the deepest vertical pocket of fluid in the four quadrants of the uterus. The AFI uses the 5th and 95th percentiles for gestational age to signify oligohydramnios and polyhydramnios, respectively. AFI, rather than pocket size, increases intervention frequency without improving outcomes.

### *Doppler Velocimetry*[7]

Measuring blood flow velocities in the maternal and fetal vessels provides information about uteroplacental blood flow and fetal responses to physiologic challenges. The important vessels studied are described in Table 1.3.

## Monitoring and Frequency

Antenatal fetal surveillance should start at $32^{0/7}$ *weeks* of gestation or later for most patients. However, for individuals with particularly worrisome high-risk conditions (e.g. chronic hypertension with suspected fetal growth restriction), antenatal fetal surveillance might begin at a gestational age when delivery would be considered for perinatal benefit.

### *Frequency of Tests*

The optimal frequency remains unknown; however, it is suggested that the frequency of antenatal fetal surveillance for each condition should be based on the approach of testing. It should be done at least

| Table 1.3: Doppler velocimetry and interpretation | | |
|---|---|---|
| *Vessel* | *Relevance* | *Remark* |
| Umbilical artery | Placental resistance, fetal cardiac afterload | Increased resistance correlates with the risk of hypoxia, and absent or reversed diastolic flow indicates a high risk of acidosis. |
| Middle cerebral artery | Cerebral hypoxia | Low pulsatility index indicates brain sparing effect and possible fetal hypoxia |
| Ductus venosus | The inflow of oxygenated blood to the fetus | Absent or reversed a wave associated with risk of fetal mortality and morbidity |
| Aortic Isthmus | The interface of oxygenated and deoxygenated blood—indicates oxygenation in the cranial supply | Abnormal flows indicate compromise of cerebral oxygenation—increased risk of neurological injury |
| Maternal uterine artery[8] | Placental resistance from the maternal side | High resistance indicates high placental resistance and suggests the etiology of poor uteroplacental perfusion |

weekly unless additional information is available that supports more frequent antenatal fetal surveillance (like abnormal Doppler results).

#### *The follow-up to an Abnormal Antepartum Surveillance Test Result*

These tests have high false-positive rates and low positive predictive values. Hence, abnormal antepartum fetal surveillance test results should be often followed by another test to evaluate fetal status. A holistic approach should be executed, including the antenatal fetal surveillance test results, overall maternal and fetal condition, and gestational age, if the decision for delivery has to be taken. Antenatal fetal surveillance must be interpreted with caution if performed before 32 weeks of gestation because the non-stress test of a normal preterm fetus is non-reactive in up to 50% of fetuses between 24 and 28 weeks and 15% of fetuses between 28 and 32 weeks gestation.

### Decision for Delivery Based on Doppler Monitoring in Growth Restricted Fetuses[9]

The monitoring in growth-restricted fetuses is depicted in Table 1.4, and the decision to deliver is based on Doppler velocimetry (Fig. 1.3). Delivery timing should consider short-term and long-term

**Table 1.4: Monitoring in growth-restricted fetuses**

| *Category* | *Risk of stillbirth* | *Monitoring* |
|---|---|---|
| SGA (EFW at 3rd–10th percentile, normal fluid, and Doppler studies) | Low | • Growth scan every two weeks<br>• Doppler (UA, MCA) every 1–2 weeks, BPP/NST once a week<br>• At ≥37 weeks, consider BPP/NST 1–2 times per week. |
| Uncomplicated FGR at <3rd Percentile or fall of AC/EFW by two quadrantile (normal liquor and normal Doppler studies) | Low | • Growth scan every two weeks<br>• Doppler (UA, MCA) 1–2 times per week, BPP/ NST 1–2 times per week |
| FGR with mild abnormalities:<br>1. Early Doppler changes: UA PI > 95th percentile, OR MCA PI <5th percentile OR CPR < 5th percentile OR UtA PI >95th percentile<br>2. Oligohydramnios<br>3. Suboptimal interval growth | Low | Consider inpatient monitoring, especially if other co-morbidities<br>• Consider steroids for fetal lung maturation if at risk of prematurity<br>• BPP/NST 2 times per week<br>• Doppler (UtA, UA, MCA, DV) 2 times per week<br>• Growth scan every two weeks |
| FGR with umbilical artery AEDF/REDF | Moderate with a median time of deterioration of 2–5 days | • Inpatient monitoring<br>• Steroids for fetal lung maturation<br>*Consider $MgSO_4$ if gestation is below 32 weeks.*<br>• BPP/NST once per day<br>• Doppler (UA, DV) every day.<br>*Consider delivery if a neonatal backup facility is available based on POG* |

(*Contd.*)

**Table 1.4: Monitoring in growth-restricted fetuses** (*Contd.*)

| *Category* | *Risk of stillbirth* | *Monitoring* |
| --- | --- | --- |
| FGR with abnormal ductus venosus Doppler | High | • Inpatient monitoring<br>• Consider delivery if a neonatal backup facility is available based on POG<br>• Steroids for fetal lung maturation<br>• Consider $MgSO_4$ if gestation is below 32 weeks.<br>• BPP/NST twice per day<br>• Daily Doppler |

*SGA:* Small for gestational age; *EFW:* Estimated fetal weight; *MCA:* Middle cerebral artery; *UA:* Umbilical artery; *Ut A:* Uterine artery; *BPP:* Biophysical profile; *NST:* Non-stress test

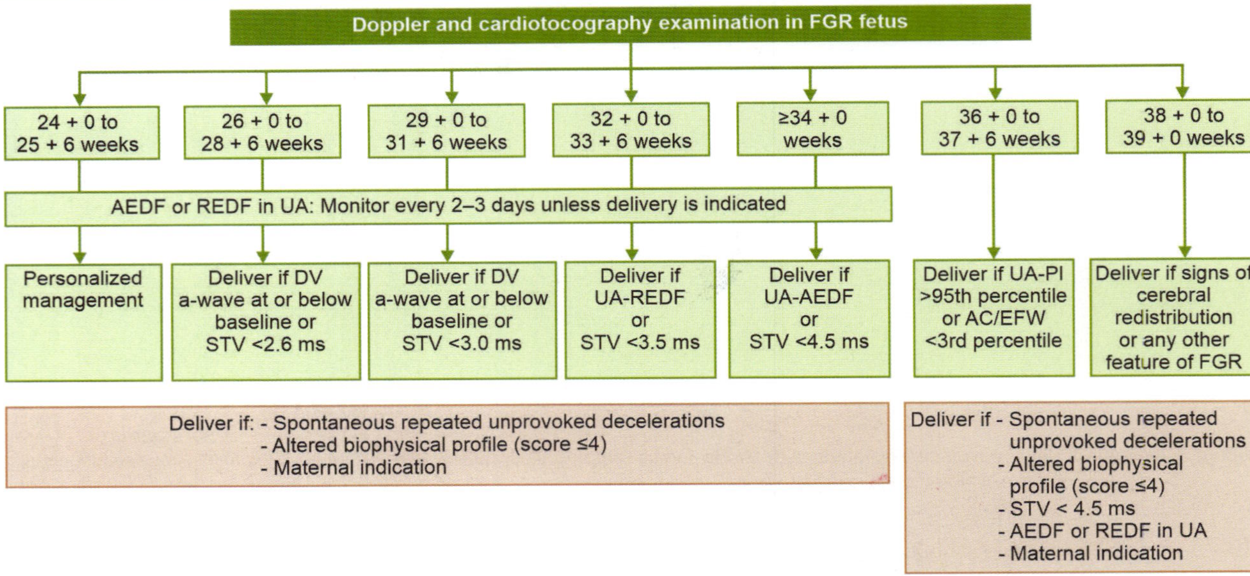


*FGR:* Fetal growth restriction; *AEDF:* Absent end diastolic flow; *REDF:* Reversed end diastolic flow; *UA:* Umbilical artery; *PI:* Pulsatility index; *STV:* Short-term variability (on computerized cardiotocography); *DV:* Ductus venosus; *EFW:* Estimated fetal weight; *AC:* Abdominal circumference

**Fig. 1.3:** Decision for delivery based on Doppler monitoring in growth-restricted fetuses

outcomes.[10] In most instances, all growth-restricted fetuses should be delivered by approximately 38 weeks.

## REFERENCES

1. Antepartum Fetal Surveillance: ACOG Practice Bulletin, Number 229. Obstetrics & Gynecology. 2021 Jun;137(6):e116–27.
2. Freeman RK, Anderson G, Dorchester W. A prospective multi-institutional study of antepartum fetal heart rate monitoring. American Journal of Obstetrics and Gynecology. 1982 Aug;143(7):771–7.
3. Devoe LD. Antenatal Fetal Assessment: Contraction Stress Test, Nonstress Test, Vibroacoustic Stimulation, Amniotic Fluid Volume, Biophysical Profile, and Modified Biophysical Profile—An Overview. Seminars in Perinatology. 2008 Aug;32(4):247–52.
4. Manning FA, Morrison I, Harman CR, Lange IR, Menticoglou S. Fetal assessment based on fetal biophysical profile scoring: In 19,221 referred high-risk pregnancies. American Journal of Obstetrics and Gynecology. 1987 Oct;157(4):880–4.
5. Miller DA, Rabello YA, Paul RH. The modified biophysical profile: Antepartum testing in the 1990s. American Journal of Obstetrics and Gynecology. 1996 Mar;174(3):812–7.
6. Clark SL, Sabey P, Jolley K. Nonstress testing with acoustic stimulation and amniotic fluid volume assessment: 5973 tests without unexpected fetal death. American Journal of Obstetrics and Gynecology. 1989 Mar;160(3):694–7.
7. Reddy UM, Abuhamad AZ, Levine D, Saade GR. Fetal Imaging: Executive Summary of a Joint Eunice Kennedy Shriver National Institute of Child Health and Human Development, Society for Maternal-Fetal Medicine, American Institute of Ultrasound in Medicine, American College of Obstetricians and Gynecologists, American College of Radiology, Society for Pediatric Radiology, and Society of Radiologists in Ultrasound Fetal Imaging Workshop. Obstetrics & Gynecology. 2014 May;123(5):1070–82.
8. Papageorghiou AT, Yu CKH, Cicero S, Bower S, Nicolaides KH. Second-trimester uterine artery Doppler screening in unselected populations: a review. The Journal of Maternal-Fetal & Neonatal Medicine. 2002 Jan;12(2):78–88.
9. Lees CC, Stampalija T, Baschat AA, Silva Costa F, Ferrazzi E, Figueras F, et al. ISUOG Practice Guidelines: diagnosis and management of small-for-gestational-age fetus and fetal growth restriction. Ultrasound Obstet Gynecol. 2020 Aug;56(2):298–312.
10. Ganzevoort W, Thornton JG, Marlow N, Thilaganathan B, Arabin B, Prefumo F, et al. Comparative analysis of 2-year outcomes in GRIT and TRUFFLE trials. Ultrasound Obstet Gynecol. 2020 Jan;55(1):68–74.

CHAPTER

# 2

# Intrapartum Fetal Monitoring

Some degree of hypoxemia occurs in almost all fetuses during labor. Still, it is the intensity, duration, and repetitive nature of the event, together with the individual variation in the capacity of each fetus to cope with the situation, that determines the severity of the resulting hypoxia.[1]

Fetal heart rate patterns are indirect markers of the fetal cardiac and medullary responses to blood volume changes, acidemia, and hypoxemia. Monitoring can help us provide timely intervention.[2] Fetal monitoring may be invasive or non-invasive.[3]

## NON-INVASIVE FETAL HEART RATE EVALUATION

It can be either with intermittent auscultation or by continuous electronic fetal monitoring which is performed using a cardiotocograph (CTG) with transducers attached for detecting fetal heart and uterine activity.

### Components of the CTG

1. Baseline FHR (normal 110–160 bpm).
2. Beat-to-beat variability (normal 6–25 bpm between contractions).
3. Accelerations.
4. Decelerations.

Interpretation of FHR tracings is subjective and not very reproducible. The comparison of cardiotocography (CTG) classification criteria in the FIGO, NICE, and ACOG guidelines is tabulated in Table 2.1.

| **Interobserver interpretation of CTG and accuracy of various guidelines in predicting fetal acidemia: What does the evidence say?** |
|---|
| In a study by Santo et al, a total of 27 clinicians performed the analysis of CTGs using the International Federation of Gynecology and Obstetrics (FIGO) 1987 guidelines, American College of Obstetricians and Gynecologists (ACOG) 2010 guidelines and the United Kingdom National Institute of Clinical Excellence |

(Contd.)

*(Contd.)*

(NICE) 2007 guidelines (Table 2.1). Reliability was significantly higher with FIGO (k=0.37, 95%CI 0.31-0.43), and NICE (k=0.33, 95%CI 0.28–0.39) than with ACOG (k=0.15, 95%CI 0.10–0.21), however, all represented only slight/fair reliability. FIGO and NICE showed a trend towards higher sensitivities in prediction of newborn acidemia (89% and 97% respectively) than ACOG (32%), but the latter achieved a significantly higher specificity (95%).[4]

## Initial Assessment

- An initial assessment of antenatal risk factors for fetal compromise would be needed at the onset of labor to determine whether intermittent auscultation or cardiotocography (CTG) is indicated.
- Risk assessment is continual, and the pregnant woman may become high risk even if low risk at the onset of labor.
- If continuous CTG is done in women with no identified risk factors, the risk–benefit ratio must be explained to the mother that the risks may outweigh the benefits.

## Deciding the Modality for Intrapartum Monitoring

The two commonly used modalities for intrapartum FHR monitoring are continuous electronic FHR monitoring and intermittent auscultation. Most obstetrics and gynecology societies agree that Continuous Electronic FHR monitoring (EFM) should be done for high-risk women. At the same time, intermittent auscultation (IA) is sufficient for low-risk women. Auscultation should be full of 60 seconds immediately after the contraction, every 15 to 30 mins in the first stage of labor and every 5 mins in the second stage of labor.[3]

**Continuous Versus Intermittent EFM : What Does the Evidence Say?**

A 2017 meta-analysis compared continuous electronic FHR monitoring with intermittent auscultation (13 randomized trials, >37,000 low- and high-risk pregnancies).Compared with intermittent auscultation, continuous cardiotocography showed no significant improvement in overall perinatal death rate (risk ratio (RR) 0.86, 95% confidence interval (CI) 0.59 to 1.23, N = 33,513, 11 trials, low quality evidence), but was associated with halving neonatal seizure rates (RR 0.50, 95% CI 0.31 to 0.80, N = 32,386, 9 trials, moderate quality evidence).[5] There was no difference in cerebral palsy. There was an increase in caesarean sections associated with continuous CTG and women were also more likely to have instrumental vaginal delivery. There was no difference in the incidence of cord blood acidosis or use of any pharmacological analgesia. Data for low risk, high risk, preterm pregnancy and high-quality trials subgroups were consistent with overall results. Access to fetal blood sampling did not appear to influence differences in neonatal seizures or other outcomes.

**Practice Point: Role of maternal oxygen administration in intrauterine resuscitation**

The theoretic rationale behind this practice is that maternal hyperoxia increases oxygen transfer to the fetus, thereby improving fetal hypoxia and preventing the transition to acidemia. However, routine and liberal use of maternal oxygen supplementation in the absence of maternal hypoxia must be carefully considered particularly because excess oxygen exposure is associated with increased free radical activity and subsequent cell damage.

### *Indications for Continuous Electronic Fetal Monitoring*

- Antenatal maternal risk factors
  - Previous cesarean birth or other total thickness uterine scar.
  - Any hypertensive disorder needing medication.
  - Prolonged ruptured membranes (but women who are already in established labor 24 hours after their membranes ruptured do not need CTG unless there are other concerns).
  - Any vaginal blood loss other than a show.
  - Suspected chorioamnionitis or maternal sepsis.
  - Pre-existing diabetes (type 1 or type 2) and gestational diabetes requiring medication.
- Antenatal fetal risk factors:
  - Non-cephalic presentation (including breech, transverse, oblique, and cord), including while a decision is made about the mode of birth.
  - Fetal growth restriction (estimated fetal weight below 3rd centile).
  - Small for gestational age (estimated fetal weight below 10th centile) with other high-risk features such as abnormal Doppler scan results, reduced liquor volume, or reduced growth velocity.
  - Advanced gestational age (more than 42 + 0 weeks at the onset of established labor).
  - Anhydramnios or polyhydramnios.
  - Reduced fetal movements before the start of contractions.
- Intrapartum risk factors
  - Contractions that last longer than 2 minutes, or five or more contractions in 10 minutes.
  - Presence of meconium.
  - Maternal pyrexia (a temperature of 38°C or above on a single reading or 37.5°C or above on two consecutive occasions 1 hour apart).

- Suspected chorioamnionitis or sepsis.
- Fresh vaginal bleeding that develops in labor.
- Blood-stained liquor not associated with the vaginal examination that is likely to be uterine in origin (and may indicate suspected antepartum hemorrhage).
- Maternal pulse over 120 beats a minute on two occasions 30 minutes apart.
- Hypertension (either systolic blood pressure of 140 mmHg or more or diastolic blood pressure of 90 mmHg or more on two consecutive readings taken 30 minutes apart, measured between contractions).
- A reading of 2+ of protein on urinalysis and a single reading of either raised systolic blood pressure (140 mmHg or more) or raised diastolic blood pressure (90 mmHg or more).
- Confirmed delay in the first or second stage of labor.
- Insertion of regional analgesia (for example, an epidural).
- Use of oxytocin.
- Other factors at the discretion of the healthcare providers.

## CTG Classification Criteria[6,7,8]

Various societies have recommended CTG classification criteria for identifying fetal hypoxia (Table 2.1).

## Representative CTG Traces

### *Taking Decisions Based on CTG Findings*[8]

CTG trace is normal:

- Continue CTG monitoring and usual care.
- Risk assessment is to be continued hourly, and findings documented.

CTG trace is suspicious:

- Perform risk assessment.
- Consider underlying reasons for change if CTG was previously normal.
- Undertake conservative measures.
  - Encourage the woman to mobilize or adopt an alternative position and avoid being supine.
  - If hypotensive secondary to epidural anesthesia, start IV fluids, shift to a left lateral position, and get an anesthetist review.

**Table 2.1: Comparison of cardiotocography (CTG) classification criteria**

| *FIGO* | *NICE* | *ACOG* |
|---|---|---|
| Normal pattern<br>• Baseline heart rate between 110 and 150 bpm<br>• The amplitude of heart rate variability between 5 and 25 bpm | Normal (a CTG where all of the following four reassuring features are present)<br>• Baseline rate: 110–160 bpm<br>• Variability: ≥5 bpm<br>• No decelerations<br>• Accelerations: Present | Category I (FHR tracings include all of the following)<br>• Baseline rate: 110–160 bpm<br>• Baseline variability: 6–25 bpm<br>• Late or variable decelerations: Absent<br>• Early decelerations: Present or absent<br>• Accelerations: Present or absent |
| Suspicious pattern<br>• Baseline heart rate between 150 and 170 bpm or between 100 and 110 bpm<br>• The amplitude of variability between 5 and 10 bpm for more than 40 min<br>• Increased variability above 25 bpm<br>• Variable decelerations | Suspicious (a CTG where one of the following features is present and all others fall into the reassuring category)<br>• Baseline rate<br>  – 100–109 bpm<br>  – 161–180 bpm<br>• Baseline variability<br>  – <5 bpm for 40–90 min<br>• Decelerations<br>  – Typical variable decelerations with >50% of contractions occurring for >90 min<br>  – Single prolonged deceleration for up to 3 min | Category II (Category II FHR tracings include all FHR tracings not categorized as Category I or Category III)<br>• Baseline rate<br>  – Bradycardia not accompanied by absent baseline variability<br>  – Tachycardia<br>• Baseline variability<br>  – Minimal variability<br>  – Absent variability with no recurrent decelerations<br>  – Marked variability<br>• Decelerations<br>  – Recurrent variable decelerations accompanied by minimal or moderate baseline variability<br>  – Prolonged deceleration 2–10 min |

(*Contd.*)

**Table 2.1: Comparison of cardiotocography (CTG) classification criteria** *(Contd.)*

| *FIGO* | *NICE* | *ACOG* |
|---|---|---|
| | • Accelerations<br>– The absence of accelerations with an otherwise typical trace is of uncertain significance | – Recurrent late decelerations with moderate baseline variability<br>– Variable decelerations with other characteristics, such as slow return to baseline, overshoots or shoulders<br>• Accelerations<br>– Absence of induced accelerations after fetal stimulation |
| Pathological pattern<br>• Baseline heart rate <100 or >170 bpm<br>• Persistence of heart rate variability of <5 bpm for >40 min<br>• Severe variable decelerations or severe repetitive early decelerations<br>• Prolonged decelerations<br>• Late decelerations: the most ominous trace is a steady baseline without baseline variability and with small decelerations after each contraction<br>• A sinusoidal pattern | Pathological (a CTG with one or more of the following features or two or more features in the previous category)<br>• Baseline rate<br>– <100 bpm<br>– >180 bpm<br>– Sinusoidal pattern ≥ 10 min<br>• Baseline variability<br>– <5 bpm for ≥ 90 min<br>• Decelerations<br>– Atypical variable decelerations with >50% contractions for >30 min<br>– Late decelerations for >30 min<br>– Prolonged deceleration >3 min | Category III (Category III FHR tracings include either)<br>• Absent baseline FHR variability and any of the following:<br>– Recurrent late decelerations<br>– Recurrent variable decelerations<br>– Bradycardia<br>• Sinusoidal pattern |

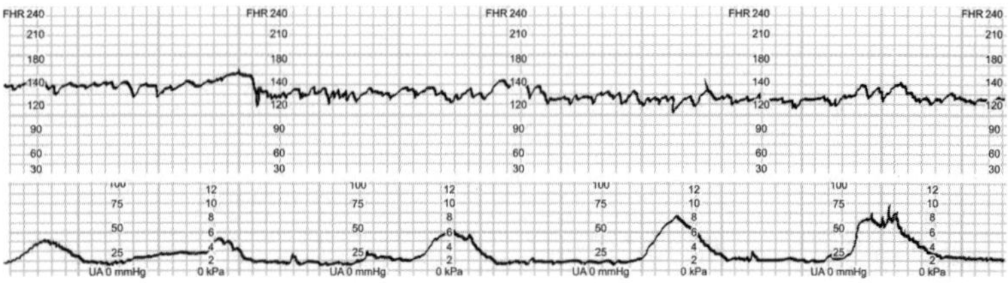


**Fig. 2.1:** Category I tracings: A baseline fetal heart rate of 110 to 160 bpm, absence of late or variable FHR decelerations, moderate FHR variability (6 to 25 bpm), Early decelerations, and accelerations may be present or absent

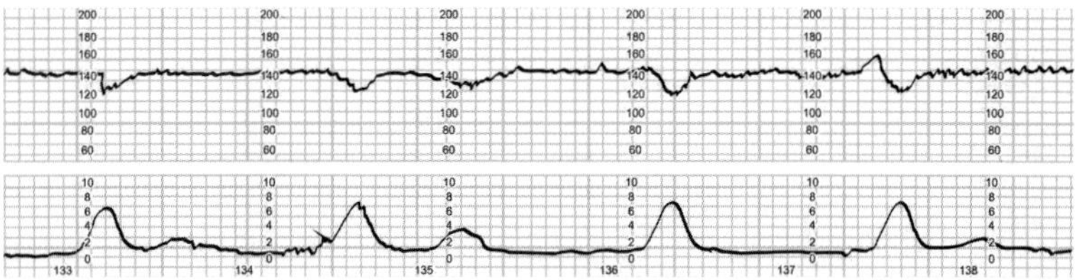


**Fig. 2.2:** Early decelerations: There is a gradual onset of deceleration in the early part of the contraction. The nadir of the deceleration usually coincides with the peak of the contraction, and the FHR usually returns to baseline at the end of the contraction

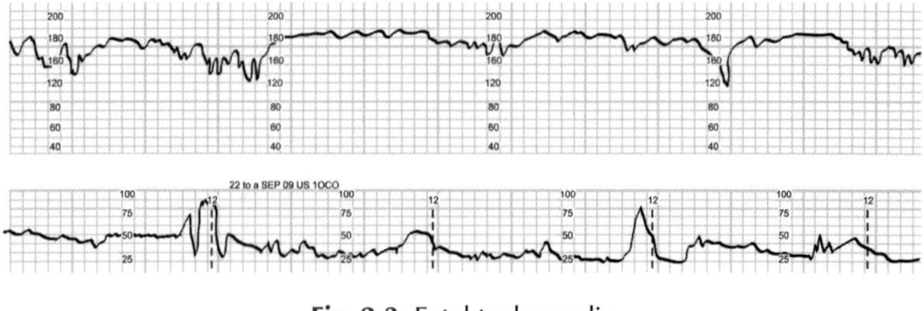


**Fig. 2.3:** Fetal tachycardia

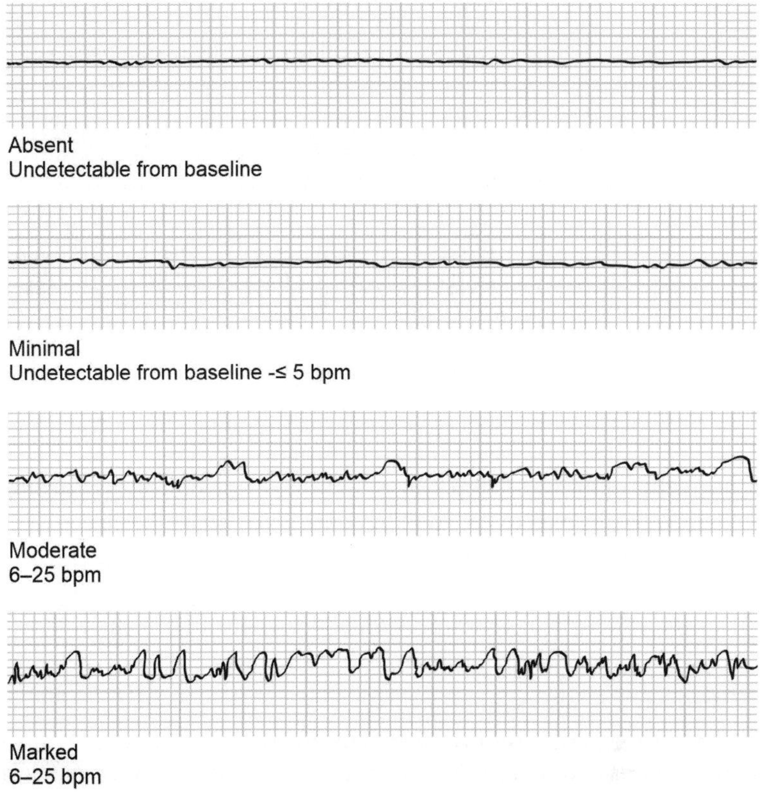


**Fig. 2.4:** Baseline variability

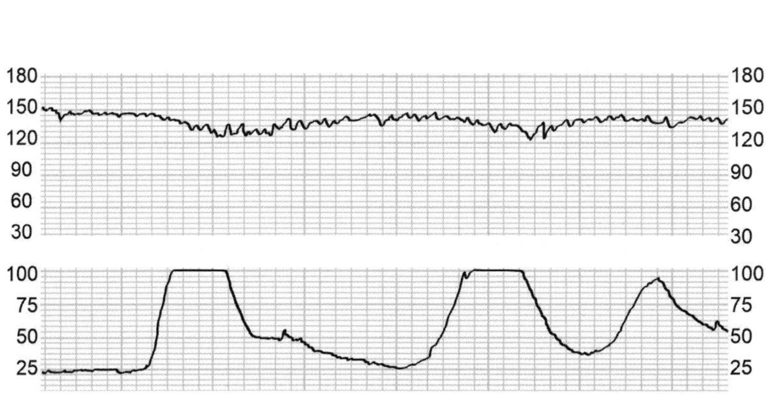


**Fig. 2.5:** Late decelerations. There is a gradual decrease in the FHR by at least 15 beats per minute below the baseline lasting for at least 15 seconds. It commences after the onset of the contraction, and it ends after the contraction has passed

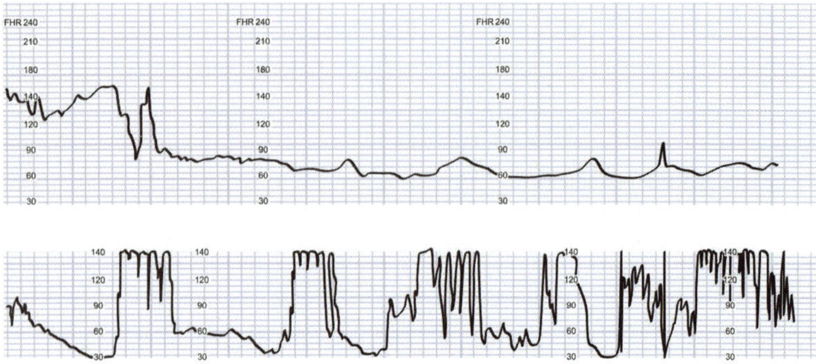


**Fig. 2.6:** Fetal bradycardia

- Stop or titrate oxytocin to reduce the frequency of contractions.
- Offer a tocolytic drug (i.e. s.cterbutaline 0.25 mg).

- Routine maternal facial oxygen should not be offered unless maternal hypoxia or as preoxygenation for anaesthesia.
- Amnioinfusion should not be offered.

If the CTG is suspicious with additional risk factors such as slow progress, sepsis, or meconium, consider expediting birth.

CTG trace is pathological:

- Perform risk assessment.
- Perform urgent senior obstetrician review.
- Exclude acute events (for example, cord prolapse, suspected placental abruption, or suspected uterine rupture) that need immediate intervention.
- Undertake conservative measures as above.

If CTG is still pathological after conventional methods, consider expediting delivery.

If there is acute bradycardia or a single prolonged deceleration for 3 minutes or more:

- Perform risk assessment.
- Perform urgent senior obstetrician review.
- Exclude critical events (for example, cord prolapse, suspected placental abruption, or suspected uterine rupture) that need immediate intervention.
- Undertake conservative measures as above.
- If there are significant antenatal or intrapartum risk factors for fetal compromise, expedite the birth if the acute bradycardia persists for 9 minutes or less.

## INVASIVE INTRAPARTUM FETAL MONITORING

A. **ST analysis (STAN) fetal heart monitor:** Internal measurement of FHR is invasive; thus, its use is restricted to the intrapartum period. The features are:

- A bipolar spiral electrode is inserted transcervical to penetrate the fetal scalp, and a second reference electrode is placed upon the maternal thigh to eliminate electrical interference.
- The internal electrode detects the fetal electrocardiogram (ECG) and calculates the FHR based on the interval between R waves.
- This signal is evident and provides an accurate measurement of beat-to-beat variability. Artifact is kept to a minimum, and there is a little need for autocorrelation.

A technical system, the STAN S31 fetal heart monitor, has been approved by the FDA for monitoring the fetal electrocardiogram (ECG) during labor. The use of this device is based on the principle that fetal hypoxemia can result in elevation or depression of the ST segment. The monitor's software automatically identifies and analyzes changes in the T wave and the ST segment of the fetal ECG obtained via a spiral electrode attached to the fetal scalp. The analysis is displayed in the lower section of the monitor's screen as a series of data points ('T/QRS crosses') and event markers.

STAN computerized interpretation of the FHR monitoring system has a sensitivity of 38 to 90 percent and a specificity of 83 to 100 percent for detecting fetal acidosis.

This technique is promising, but at this time, there are inadequate clinical and cost data from a variety of hospital settings to allow a recommendation for routine use.

B. **Fetal scalp blood sampling:** Fetal blood sampling is typically performed using a kit. The steps are:

- An amnioscope with a light source is used to expose the fetal scalp, which is cleansed of blood, mucous, and amniotic fluid.
- The scalp is smeared with silicone gel so that a droplet of blood forms when the scalp is punctured with a 2 mm blade.
- The blood is collected in long, heparinized capillary tubes.

| Table 2.2: Interpretation of fetal blood sampling results | | |
|---|---|---|
| *pH* | *Lactate (mmol/L)* | *Interpretation* |
| > 7.25 | < 4.2 | Normal |
| 7.20–7.25 | 4.2–4.8 | Intermediate |
| < 7.20 | > 4.8 | Abnormal |

- The test requires that the cervix be dilated at least 2 to 3 cm, which can be challenging to perform and uncomfortable for the parturient.

The degree of technical skill required, cost, need for the continuous availability of standardized equipment and trained personnel, and parturient discomfort has precluded using these tests in many labor and delivery units, despite their proven benefit in diagnosing fetal acidosis. Capillary blood collected from the fetal scalp usually has a pH lower than umbilical venous blood and correlates well with fetal arterial values.[9]

The test has poor sensitivity and positive predictive value (PPV) for predicting umbilical arterial pH <7.0 (sensitivity 35 percent, PPV 9 percent). The test also has poor sensitivity and PPV for identifying newborns with hypoxic-ischemic encephalopathy (sensitivity 50 percent, PPV 3 percent). In addition, logistics and skill in sampling, as well as laboratory capability, may affect results.

C. **Fetal pulse oximetry:** Data from human and animal studies suggest that fetal arterial oxygen saturation ($SaO_2$ by blood gas co-oximetry) >30 % is usually associated with pH >7.13. In humans, the mean fetal oxygen saturation ($SpO_2$ by fetal pulse oximetry) during the first and second stages of labor is 59±10 percent and 53±10 percent, respectively. In the setting of a nonreassuring FHR pattern, fetal $SpO_2$ <30 percent for greater than 10 minutes has been associated with an increased risk of fetal acidosis.

## REFERENCES

1. Pauliah SS, Shankaran S, Wade A, Cady EB, Thayyil S. Therapeutic hypothermia for neonatal encephalopathy in low- and middle-income countries: a systematic review and meta-analysis. PloS one. 2013 Mar 19;8(3):e58834.

2. Indian National Neonatal Perinatal Database. (National Neonatology Forum) (2002–2003). http://www.newbornwhocc.org/pdf/nnpd_report_2002-03.PDF. Accessed on September 4, 2013.
3. American Academy of Pediatrics, American College of Obstetricians and Gynecologists. Guidelines for Perinatal Care, 8th, 2017. p.240.
4. Santo S, Ayres-de-Campos D, Costa-Santos C, Schnettler W, Ugwumadu A, Da Graça LM, FM-Compare Collaboration. Agreement and accuracy using the FIGO, ACOG and NICE cardiotocography interpretation guidelines. Acta obstetricia et gynecologica Scandinavica. 2017 Feb;96(2):166–75.
5. Alfirevic Z, Devane D, Gyte G. ML, & Cuthbert, A.(2017). Continuous Cardiotocography (CTG) as a form of Electronic Fetal Monitoring (EFM) for fetal assessment during labor. Cochrane Database of Systematic Reviews.;2.
6. American College of Obstetricians and Gynecologists. ACOG Practice Bulletin No. 106: Intrapartum fetal heart rate monitoring: nomenclature, interpretation, and general management principles. ObstetGynecol 2009; 114:192.
7. Ayres-de-Campos D, Spong CY, Chandraharan E, FIGO Intrapartum Fetal Monitoring Expert Consensus Panel. FIGO consensus guidelines on intrapartum fetal monitoring: Cardiotocography. International Journal of Gynecology& Obstetrics. 2015 Oct;131(1):13–24.
8. Raghuraman N. Response to category II tracings: Does anything help?. In Seminars in Perinatology 2020 Mar 1 (Vol. 44, No. 2, p. 151217). WB Saunders.
9. Jørgensen JS, Weber T. Fetal scalp blood sampling in labor--a review. Acta ObstetGynecolScand 2014; 93:54.

CHAPTER

# 3

# Fetal Growth Restriction

Fetal growth restriction (FGR) is a common cause of adverse perinatal and neonatal outcomes. India accounts for the largest number of cases of FGR globally, with a prevalence of 47%.[1]

## DEFINITION

SGA and FGR should not be used interchangeably. FGR is defined as a fetus not reaching its biological growth potential due to environmental or genetic factors. Another important term is SGA (small for gestational age), which is defined as a birth weight below the 10th percentile on intrauterine growth charts. Taking this cutoff of weight below the 10th percentile does not differentiate between a constitutionally small fetus likely to achieve normal growth potential, from a similarly small fetus whose growth is restricted.

### Symmetric Versus Asymmetric FGR

Around 80% of FGR infants are asymmetric, i.e. caused by an intrauterine insult that occurs later in gestational age. These cases are characterized by a reduction in cell size rather than number, a relative sparing of the head, and a ponderal index of less than 2.

A small proportion of FGR infants are symmetric. These can be small but normally nourished fetuses with no evidence of placental disease ("constitutionally small") or those with congenital malformations, infections, or genetic causes. The ponderal index in these cases is more significant than two and uniformly affects weight, length, and head circumference.

## PATHOPHYSIOLOGY

The mechanisms leading to FGR depend upon the onset of growth restriction: Early start (<32 weeks) and late-onset (≥32 weeks) (Table 3.1).

| Table 3.1: Doppler changes in fetal growth restriction | | |
|---|---|---|
| *Site* | *Changes* | |
| Uterine artery | PI > 95th centile* | 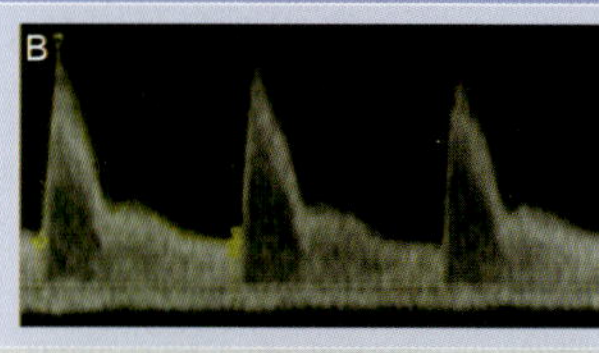  |
| Umbilical artery | Absent end-diastolic flow (AEDF)<br>Reversed end-diastolic flow (REDF) | 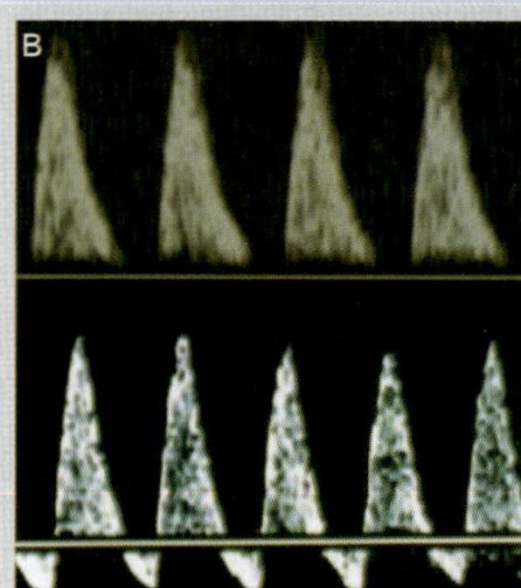  |
| Middle cerebral artery | PI <5th centile* | 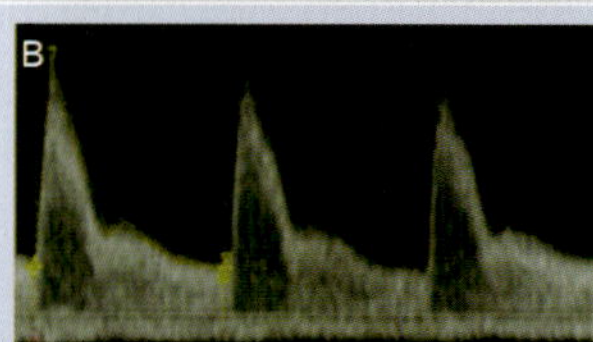  |
| Ductus venosus | Absent a wave<br>Reversed a wave | 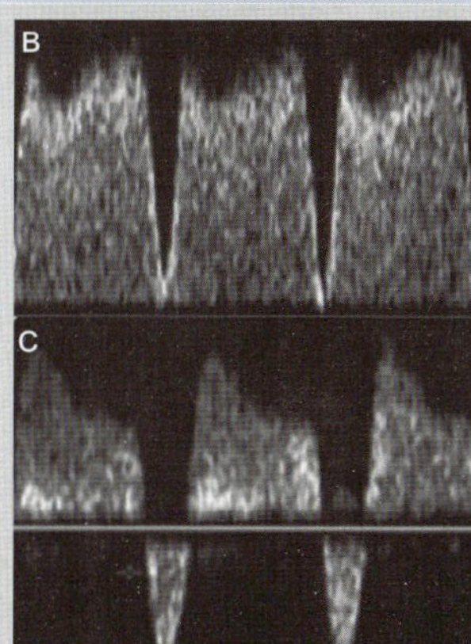  |
| Cerebro-placental ratio | The ratio of MCA PI to UtA PI—a surrogate marker of the brain-sparing effect <5th centile | |

**PI (Pulsatility Index): Ratio of difference between systolic (S) and diastolic (D) velocity to the mean velocity (S-D/Mean), PI: Pulsatility index*

## Pathogenesis and Doppler Abnormalities

A reduction in umbilical venous flow initiates hemodynamic changes in early FGR. Redistribution of blood flow from the liver causes a reduction in abdominal circumference (the *first biometric sign of FGR*). An elevated placental resistance decreases umbilical artery end-diastolic flow, increasing the pulsatility index (PI). A progressive increase in placental resistance initially leads to diastolic absence and later flow reversal in the umbilical artery.

Due to systemic cardiovascular adaptation, the blood is channeled to perfuse the vital organs (e.g. the brain). As a result, end-diastolic flow increases in the cerebral arteries. Worsening hypoxia leads to loss of brain-sparing effect, and PI in the middle and cerebral arteries normalizes or is falsely elevated.

Chronic hypoxia, nutritional deprivation, and acidosis decrease the diastolic flow in umbilical veins (particularly ductus venosus), culminating in absent, and in severe cases, reversal of a wave. With impending acidosis and death, aortic arch flow reversal and tricuspid regurgitation ensue pre-terminally. The hemodynamic changes are not as profound in late-onset FGR owing to mild placental disease. The umbilical artery Doppler changes are characteristically absent in the late-onset type.

Systemic cardiovascular (early onset) or isolated cerebrovascular (late onset) adaptation due to growth restriction forms the basis of performing Doppler studies to ensure timely detection of FGR and delivery. The Doppler changes in different vessels are depicted in Table 3.1.

## Early and Late-onset FGR

Although early and late fetal growth restriction has been suggested to be distinct entities, the optimal gestational age cut-off that differentiates them is unclear. Table 3.2 lists the differences in pathophysiology and Doppler abnormalities in early-onset and late-onset FGR. Table 3.3 lists the consensus definition.

## Etiology

FGR usually results from a complex interplay between maternal, placental, fetal, or endocrine causes (Table 3.4). While maternal and placental conditions cause 2/3rd cases, 1/3rd are genetic, and the etiology remains unknown in nearly 40% of cases.

| Table 3.2: Differences in early-onset and late-onset FGR | | |
|---|---|---|
| | *Early onset FGR* | *Late-onset FGR* |
| Prevalence | Low (1–3%) | High (3–5%) |
| Pathogenesis | Impaired trophoblastic invasion<br>Reduced villous surface area | Defective villous maturation |
| Placental disease | Severe | Mild |
| Hypoxia | Marked<br>*'Systemic cardiovascular adaptation'* | Mild or absent<br>*'Central cardiovascular adaptation'* |
| Doppler changes | UtA PI → CPR → UA PI → MCA PI → UA-AEDF → UA-REDF → DV absent 'a' → DV reversal → CTG decelerations → Poor manning → Death | UtA PI → CPR → MCA PI → CTG decelerations → Poor manning → Death |
| Outcome | High mortality<br>High morbidity | Low mortality<br>Late stillbirth<br>High morbidity |

*UtA:* Uterine artery; *UA:* Umbilical artery; *MCA:* Middle cerebral artery; *AEDF:* Absent end diastolic flow; *REDF:* Reversed end diastolic flow; *DV:* Ductus venosus; *CTG:* Cardiotocograph

*CPR (Cerebro-placental ratio):* Ratio of MCA PI to UtA PI; Surrogate marker of brain sparing effect (<5th centile)

| Table 3.3: Consensus definition of fetal growth restriction[2] | |
|---|---|
| *Early FGR: GA <32 weeks, in absence of congenital anomalies* | *Late FGR: GA ≥32 weeks, in absence of congenital anomalies* |
| AC/EFW <3rd centile or UA-AEDF<br>**OR**<br>AC/EFW <10th centile combined with<br>1. UtA-PI >95th centile and/or<br>2. UA-PI >95th centile | AC/EFW <3rd centile<br>**OR**<br>*At least two out of three of the following:*<br>1. AC/EFW <10th centile<br>2. AC/EFW crossing centiles >2 quartiles<br>3. CPR <5th centile or UA-PI 95th centile |

*FGR:* Fetal growth restriction; *GA:* Gestational age; *AC:* Abdominal circumference; *EFW:* Estimated fetal weight; *UtA:* Uterine artery; *UA:* Umbilical artery; *PI:* Pulsatility index; *CPR:* Cerebro-placental ratio

| Table 3.4: Causes of fetal growth restriction | |
|---|---|
| Maternal causes | Maternal age < 16 and > 36 years<br>Lower socio-economic status<br>Lower pre-pregnancy BMI < 20 kg/m$^2$<br>Smoking<br>Drug abuse/alcohol abuse<br>Chronic hypertension/pre-eclampsia<br>Diabetes mellitus<br>Chronic renal/pulmonary/cardiac/gastrointestinal disease<br>Maternal SLE<br>Use of assisted reproductive technologies<br>Previous history of SGA or mother being SGA at birth |
| Fetal | Chromosomal abnormalities (trisomy 13, 18)<br>Congenital malformations (1–2%): CDH, TEF, abdominal wall defects, neural tube defects, anorectal malformations<br>Congenital infections (5%)<br>Multiple gestations (more common in monochorionic) |
| Placental | Low placental weight<br>Vascular anomalies (true knots, velamentous cord insertion)<br>Placental infections<br>Placental mosaicism |
| Endocrine | Insulin deficiency<br>Decreased IGF-I, IGF-II, and IGFBP-2 expression<br>Reduced levels of thyroid hormone<br>Endothelin deficiency |

*CDH:* Congenital diaphragmatic hernia; *TEF:* Tracheoesophageal fistula; *IGF:* Insulin-like growth factor; *IGFBP:* Insulin-like growth factor binding protein

## Antenatal Diagnosis

A. **Clinical examination**

1. **Abdominal palpation** of limited value due to the advent of ultrasound. The sensitivity is poor (30–50%).
2. **Symphysio-fundal height (SFH):** The distance from the symphysis pubis to the highest level of the fundus in the supine position is a sensitive marker to detect FGR at 32–34 weeks. A difference of more than three weeks between SFH and the gestation period has a variable

sensitivity (30–70%) but reasonable specificity (80–92%). However, it has limited value at very early onset and late onset FGR.[3]

B. **Fetal biometry:** The growth of a fetus is assessed using various parameters like abdominal circumference (AC), biparietal diameter, head circumference (HC), femur length, HC/AC ratio, and femur length to AC ratio. These parameters estimate the fetal weight (EFW) using computerized software incorporating fetal growth charts. An AC < 10th centile or an EFW <10th centile are highly specific markers (90%) to detect FGR.

C. **Doppler studies:** The use of Doppler has now become the cornerstone of managing and diagnosing FGR.[4] The rate of detection of SGA is significantly increased when EFW < 10th centile is combined with either an abnormal CPR or UtA velocities, especially in late FGR cases. CPR is affected in 25% of the cases and is a better predictor of adverse perinatal outcomes. The diagnosis of early onset can be made by abnormal UA velocities.

| Evidence |
|---|
| A Cochrane review on 19 trials (~10667 women) revealed a significant reduction in perinatal mortality (29%) in high-risk pregnancies with use of routine Doppler versus no Doppler. Also, the rate of indicated cesarean section was lowered by 10%.[4] |

## Management

A. **Timing of delivery:** DV changes are the most vital single parameter to predict the short-term risk of fetal death in early-onset FGR. This sign is considered sufficient to recommend delivery at any gestational age after the completion of steroids. A stage-based management protocol has been proposed to adequately time the delivery weighing the risks of fetal compromise and prematurity[5] (Table 3.5).

B. **Neonatal management:** Neonates born with intrauterine growth restriction are at a higher risk of short- and long-term complications.
   - Short-term complications include hypoglycemia, polycythemia, and hypocalcemia. Those associated with Doppler abnormalities, especially A/REDF, have a 3–4 times higher incidence of feed intolerance and a 2.5 times higher risk of necrotizing enterocolitis.

**Table 3.5: Stage-based management protocol[5]**

| *Stage* | *USG/Doppler criteria* | *Monitoring* | *Timing of delivery* | *Mode of delivery* |
|---|---|---|---|---|
| SGA | EFW < 10th centile | Fortnightly | 40 weeks | Labor induction |
| Stage I FGR (Mild placental insufficiency) | CPR <5th centile<br>UA PI > 95th centile<br>MCA PI < 5th centile<br>UtA PI > 95th centile | Weekly | 37 weeks | Labor induction |
| Stage II FGR (Severe placental insufficiency) | UA-AEDF | Biweekly | 34 weeks | Cesarean section |
| Stage III FGR (Low-suspicion signs of fetal acidosis) | UA-REDF | 1–2 days | 30 weeks | Cesarean section |
| Stage IV FGR (High-suspicion of fetal acidosis) | DV reversal<br>Decelerations | 12 hourly | 26 weeks | Cesarean section |

*FGR:* Fetal growth restriction; *EFW:* Estimated fetal weight; *UtA:* Uterine artery; *UA:* Umbilical artery; *MCA:* Middle cerebral artery; *DV:* Ductus venosus; *PI:* Pulsatility index; *CPR:* Cerebro-placental ratio; *AEDF:* Absent end diastolic flow; *REDF:* Reversed end diastolic flow

**Evidence**

A large multicenter study done in 20 European centres (TRUFFLE), randomized cases of FGR with abnormal Doppler to deliver at different times based on short term variations on CTG, early changes on DV Doppler or late changes on DV Doppler. The study resulted in significantly higher proportion of neonates with survival free of neurodevelopmental impairment at 2 years in the group delivered on the basis of late DV changes.[6]

- Preterm babies with growth restriction are at 45% higher risk of bronchopulmonary dysplasia and respiratory complications.
- SGA babies have a significant neurodevelopmental disadvantage, with approximately twice the risk of cerebral palsy.
- In cases of A/REDF, feeding needs special consideration and should be initiated with a high index of suspicion and monitored stringently (*see* protocol on 'feeding in A/REDF babies').

- Further, SGA babies have an increased risk of metabolic complications later in life with adequate catch-up growth. These complications include hypertension, insulin resistance, coronary artery disease, and cerebrovascular stroke. The proposed mechanism is a series of epigenetic changes in response to fetal malnutrition followed by postnatal overnutrition (Barker's hypothesis).[7]

C. **Risk of recurrence:** Women with a growth-restricted fetus have a 20–30% chance of recurrence in future pregnancies.[8]

### Prevention

Since no definitive treatment for FGR exists, the search for preventive strategies remains crucial. Many strategies have been tried, and many more are still experimental. The most important strategies include decreasing the risk factors for FGR, including optimal maternal age at delivery, maternal nutrition and micronutrient supplementation, calcium supplementation, timely diagnosis and treatment of maternal diseases (diabetes, hypertension, renal, etc.) and cessation of smoking, alcohol and drug abuse.

## ROLE OF ASPIRIN IN PREGNANCY

Aspirin inhibits platelet aggregation and enhances nitric oxide levels, causing a reduction in uteroplacental resistance by vasodilatory effect. A meta-analysis studying the impact of aspirin suggested significant benefits in severe pre-eclampsia and FGR, with a dose-response effect. It is, therefore, recommended to all women with risk factors for placental insufficiency or pre-eclampsia at a dose of 81 mg started at 12–28 weeks (preferably before 16 weeks) till 36 weeks of gestation.[9]

## EMERGING ANTENATAL THERAPIES

Interventions under investigation for the prevention of FGR include those targeting an increase in nitric oxide (NO donors, nitrates), increase in VEGF (gene therapy, statins, proton pump inhibitors), decrease in thrombotic mediators (heparin, thromboxane) and an increase in cGMP (sildenafil, tadalafil). Other therapies include lactoferrin, melatonin, and insulin growth factor-I and II.

## REFERENCES

1. Lee AC, Katz J, Blencowe H, Cousens S, Kozuki N, Vogel JP et al. CHERG SGA-Preterm Birth Working Group. National and regional estimates of term

and preterm babies born small for gestational age in 138 low-income and middle-income countries in 2010. Lancet Glob Health. 2013 Jul;1(1):e26-36. doi: 10.1016/S2214-109X(13)70006-8. Epub 2013 Jun 25. Erratum in: Lancet Glob Health. 2013 Aug;1(2):e76. PMID: 25103583; PMCID: PMC4221634.

2. Beune IM, Damhuis SE, Ganzevoort W, Hutchinson JC, Khong TY, Mooney EE, Sebire NJ, Gordijn SJ. Consensus Definition of Fetal Growth Restriction in Intrauterine Fetal Death: A Delphi Procedure. Arch Pathol Lab Med. 2021 Apr 1;145(4):428-436. doi: 10.5858/arpa.2020-0027-OA. PMID: 32882006.
3. Pay ASD, Wiik J, Backe B, Jacobsson B, Strandell A, Klovning A. Symphysis-fundus height measurement to predict small-for-gestational-age status at birth: A systematic review. BMC Pregnancy Childbirth. 2015 Dec 1;15.
4. Alfirevic Z, Stampalija T, Dowswell T. Fetal and umbilical Doppler ultrasound in high-risk pregnancies. Cochrane Database of Systematic Reviews 2017, Issue 6. Art. No.: CD007529. DOI: 10.1002/14651858.CD007529.pub4.
5. Figueras F, Gratacós E. Update on the diagnosis and classification of fetal growth restriction and proposal of a stage-based management protocol. Fetal Diagn Ther. 2014;36(2):86-98. doi: 10.1159/000357592. Epub 2014 Jan 23. PMID: 24457811.
6. Lees C, Marlow N, Arabin B, Bilardo CM, Brezinka C, Derks JB, et al. Perinatal morbidity and mortality in early-onset fetal growth restriction: cohort outcomes of the trial of randomized umbilical and fetal flow in Europe (TRUFFLE). Ultrasound Obstet Gynecol Off J Int Soc Ultrasound Obstet Gynecol. 2013 Oct;42(4):400–8.
7. Malhotra A, Allison BJ, Castillo-Melendez M, Jenkin G, Polglase GR, Miller SL. Neonatal Morbidities of Fetal Growth Restriction: Pathophysiology and Impact. Front Endocrinol (Lausanne). 2019 Feb 7;10:55. doi: 10.3389/fendo.2019.00055. PMID: 30792696; PMCID: PMC6374308.
8. Blue NR, Page JM, Silver RM. Recurrence Risk of Fetal Growth Restriction: Management of Subsequent Pregnancies. Obstet Gynecol Clin North Am. 2021 Jun;48(2):419–36.
9. ACOG Committee Opinion No. 743: Low-Dose Aspirin Use During Pregnancy. Obstet Gynecol. 2018 Jul;132(1):e44-e52. doi: 10.1097/AOG.0000000000002708. PMID: 29939940.

CHAPTER

4

# Preterm Labor and Triple I

## Preterm Labour

Preterm labor is the onset of regular uterine contractions before 37 weeks of gestation with cervical changes such as dilatation or effacement. Maternal risk factors include history of previous preterm birth, infection (genital tract infections, sexually transmitted diseases etc), short interpregnancy interval (< 18 months), undernutrition (BMI < 18.5), chronic medical disorders and short cervical length. Fetal factors, including multiple pregnancy, polyhydramnios, congenital anomalies, along with environmental and genetic risk factors, are other causes of preterm labor.[1]

### *Diagnosis*

A diagnosis of preterm labor should be made in a woman if she has regular uterine contractions with one of the following: Premature rupture of membranes, cervical dilatation > 2 cm, and cervical effacement > 50%. Threatened preterm labor is documented uterine contractions with no evidence of cervical changes. All women should undergo ultrasound for fetal presentation, liquor assessment, fetal weight and cervical length estimation. To look for cervical length, a transvaginal ultrasound is useful in women with suspected preterm labor but without cervical changes on per speculum examination.

### *Management*

The management includes prompt and accurate diagnosis, proper referral to a center with NICU facility, and appropriate treatment including antenatal corticosteroids for fetal lung maturity, short-term tocolytic therapy till steroid cover, magnesium sulphate for neuroprotection and transfer to the appropriate facility.

Non-pharmacological treatment (bed rest in left lateral position, hydration, abstention from intercourse) to prevent preterm birth in women with preterm labor has been recommended historically; however, effectiveness of these interventions is lacking.

*Tocolysis*

The American College of Obstetricians and Gynaecologists (ACOG) and the Society of Maternal-Fetal-Medicine (SMFM) recommend tocolysis between 24 and 34 weeks of gestation.[1] The contraindications of tocolytic therapy include chorioamnionitis, maternal sepsis, significant antepartum hemorrhage with hemodynamic instability, cervical dilatation more than 4 cm, abnormal cardiotocography (CTG) status, any specific allergy to certain tocolytic drugs, intrauterine demise, lethal congenital anomaly/chromosomal malformations, eclampsia and contraindications to drugs with specific co-morbidities (beta-agonists should not be given in case of cardiac disease, hyperthyroidism, and uncontrolled diabetes, magnesium sulphate is contraindicated in myasthenia gravis, nifedipine is contraindicated in heart disease).[2]

*Antenatal Corticosteroids (ACS)*

Antenatal corticosteroids are administered when there is a high probability of imminent delivery such as spontaneous preterm labor with cervical dilatation ≥3 cm, spontaneous preterm prelabor rupture of membranes or a pregnancy complication (e.g. pre-eclampsia with severe features, bleeding placenta previa) warranting planned delivery (e.g. induction, cesarean) within 48 hours to improve maternal and/or neonatal outcomes. The timing, doses, schedule, and efficacy have been covered in the relevant chapter.

*Magnesium Sulfate*[3,4,5]

- It is administered to women at risk of preterm delivery between 24 and 32 weeks period of gestation within 24 hours of delivery.
- Contraindications include myasthenia gravis (which can precipitate crisis), myocardial compromise or cardiac conduction defects (anti-ionotropic effects), and impaired renal function (loading dose can be given).
- Dose: Intravenous 4 grams loading dose followed by 1 gram/hour infusion continued for up to 24 hours or delivery, whichever is earlier. Monitoring includes hourly urine output, deep tendon reflexes and respiratory rate.
- Caution:
  - Avoid treatment in threatened preterm labor or preterm premature rupture of membranes without preterm labor.
  - Aim for 6–12 hours of maintenance therapy prior to elective caesarean section.

- Do not delay emergency delivery if life-threatening maternal or fetal indication.

| **Practice tip** |
|---|
| Antibiotics should not be routinely prescribed for women in spontaneous preterm labour with intact membranes without evidence of clinical infection.[6] |

### *Mode of Delivery[7]*

It depends on fetal and maternal indications. Counseling the couple regarding the mode of delivery and documenting the plan of management is essential. There is no evidence that caesarean delivery improves the survival or decreases the morbidity. However, it is the safest mode of delivery in preterm labor with a singleton extremely preterm breech fetus. Delayed cord clamping should be performed where feasible.[8]

### *Preterm Labour in Twin: Special Situation*

Routine prophylactic use of tocolytics, pessary, cerclage, or supplemental progesterone in twin pregnancies with normal cervical length in 2nd trimester does not reduce the chances of preterm birth.

A short course of tocolytics may be indicated for patients with acute preterm labour. The use of magnesium sulphate and antenatal corticosteroids is similar to singleton pregnancy.

## Preterm Premature Rupture of Membranes

Preterm premature rupture of membranes (PPROM) is defined as the spontaneous rupture of fetal membranes before 37 weeks of gestation and before labor. Apart from preterm labor, it can lead to pulmonary hypoplasia, skeletal or joint deformities due to oligohydramnios and result in chorioamnionitis. Intra-uterine infection can be both a cause and a consequence of PPROM. Antenatal management aims to reduce adverse consequences of intra-uterine infection and prematurity.

### *Diagnosis*

Initial evaluation includes history taking, confirming dates, evaluation of risk factors, detailed physical and obstetric examination along with a single sterile per speculum examination. A direct observation of a gush of clear fluid from the vagina on per speculum examination is a definitive diagnosis of PPROM. In cases where it is not seen, cough or valsalva can provoke leaking and make it demonstrable.

### *Management*

- **Gestation less than 24 weeks**
  - Administer antibiotics (Table 4.1).
  - Expectant management with careful monitoring for signs of maternal and/or fetal infection.
  - Administration of antenatal steroids is reasonable if delivery is anticipated in the next seven days and the family desires aggressive neonatal intervention.
  - Magnesium sulphate for neuroprotection is offered.
  - Termination of pregnancy is an option in these previable pregnancies.
  - Shared decision making is vital.
- **Gestation between 24 and $33^{+6}$ weeks:** The management strategy includes in patient management with appropriate antibiotics, antenatal corticosteroids for fetal lung maturity, magnesium sulfate for fetal neuroprotection, strict maternal and fetal surveillance. Expectant management is recommended if there are no maternal or fetal contraindications. Observe for clinical signs of chorioamnionitis including maternal pulse, temperature, uterine tenderness, foul smelling discharge, and fetal tachycardia.

**Table 4.1: Suggested regimens for antibiotics for prophylaxis in PPROM**

| *Guidelines* | *Suggested regimen for antibiotics** |
|---|---|
| RCOG[9] | Erythromycin 250 mg 6 hourly PO for 10 days |
| ACOG[10] | Inj. ampicillin 2 g IV every 6 hours + Inj. erythromycin 250 mg every 6 hours × 48 hours followed by Oral amoxycillin 250 mg every 8 hours + Oral erythromycin base 333 mg every 8 hours for 5 days. |
| SOGC[11] | Inj. ampicillin 2 g IV every 6 hours + Inj. erythromycin 250 mg IV every 6 hours × 48 hours followed by oral amoxicillin 250 mg orally every 8 hours + oral erythromycin 333 mg orally every 8 hours × 5 days or oral erythromycin 250 mg orally every 6 hours for 10 days. |

**Azithromycin 1g orally can replace erythromycin due to ease of administration, better gastrointestinal tolerance and cost effectiveness and similar efficacy and coverage of organisms. Women with penicillin allergy can be offered cephalosporin and clindamycin.*
*ACOG:* American College of Obstetricians and Gynecologists; *RCOG:* Royal College of Obstetricians and Gynaecologists; *SOGC:* Society of Obstetricians and Gynaecologists of Canada

The indication of tocolysis is only for the administration of antenatal corticosteroids for fetal lung maturity.

- Fetal monitoring should be done by non-stress test and biophysical profile.
- Ultrasound evaluation of fetal growth every two weeks.
- Women with history of prior preterm birth due to PPROM may benefit from progesterone in the next pregnancy.
- Indications of delivery include fetal distress, placental abruption, chorioamnionitis, cord prolapse, preterm labour.
- Expectant management till $34^{+0}$ weeks is suggested.
- Spontaneous or induced vaginal delivery is preferred in absence of contraindications. Caesarean delivery is performed for standard indications.

• **Period of gestation between 34 and $36^{+6}$ weeks:**
  - Consider delivery at 34 weeks and beyond.
  - Administer appropriate antibiotics.
  - Spontaneous or induced vaginal delivery is preferred in absence of contraindications. Caesarean delivery is performed for standard indications.
  - Fetal monitoring is practiced with daily NST and/or BPP.

## Intrauterine Inflammation, Infection, or Both (Triple I)

It is defined as acute inflammation of the fetal membranes and chorion due to infection in women with PPROM. It also involves the amniotic fluid, fetus, placenta, and cord. This term replaces the original term chorioamnionitis.[12] There are clinical criteria to define triple I and isolated maternal fever does not classify as triple I.[13]

### *Isolated Maternal Fever (Not Triple I)*

- Maternal oral temperature 39.0°C or greater (102.2°F) on any one occasion.
- If oral temperature is between 38.0°C (100.4°F) and 39.0°C (102.0°F), repeat the measurement in 30 min; if the repeat value remains at least 38.0°C (100.4°F), it is documented fever.

### *Classification of Triple I*

- **Suspected triple I:** Fever either 39.0°C [102.2°F] once or 38.0°C [100.4°F] to 38.9°C [102.02°F] on two or more measurements (ideally taken orally) 30 minutes apart without a clear source of infection plus any of the following:

- Baseline fetal tachycardia (>160 beats per min for 10 min or longer, excluding accelerations, decelerations, and periods of marked variability).
- Maternal white blood cell (WBC) count greater than 15,000/$mm^3$ in the absence of corticosteroids.
- Definite purulent fluid from the cervical os.

• **Confirmed triple I:** Suspected triple I plus objective laboratory findings of infection, such as:
  - Positive amniotic fluid Gram stain for bacteria, low amniotic fluid glucose (e.g. ≤14 mg/dl), high amniotic fluid white cell count in the absence of a bloody tap (e.g. >30 cells/$mm^3$), or positive amniotic fluid culture results, or
  - Histopathologic evidence of infection or inflammation or both in the placenta, fetal membranes, or the umbilical cord vessels (funisitis).

### *Management*

• *In utero* Management:
  - Admission or transfer to tertiary facility.
  - Administer appropriate broad spectrum antibiotics.
  - Antipyretics for symptomatic treatment.
  - Caesarean delivery for standard obstetric indications.
  - Placenta should be sent for histopathological examination.

## REFERENCES


1. American College of Obstetricians and Gynecologists' Committee on Practice Bulletins—Obstetrics. Practice Bulletin No. 171: Management of Preterm Labor. Obstet Gynecol. 2016 Oct;128(4):e155–64.
2. Anotayanonth S, Subedar NV, Neilson JP et al. Betamimetics for inhibiting preterm labor. Cochrane Database Syst Rev.2004;(4):CD004352.
3. Crowther CA, Hiller JE, Doyle LW, et al. Effect of magnesium sulphate given for neuroprotection before preterm birth: a randomized controlled trial. JAMA.2003;290(20):2669–76.
4. Rouse DJ, Hirtz DG, Thom E, et al. A randomized, controlled trial of magnesium sulphate for the prevention of cerebral palsy. N Engl J Med. 2008;359(9):895–905.
5. Marret S, Marpeau L, Zupan-Simunek V, et al. Magnesium sulphate given before very-preterm birth to protect infant brain: the randomized controlled PREMAG trial. BJOG. 2007;114(3):310–8.
6. Kenyon SL, Taylor DJ, Tarnow-Mordi W, et al. Broad spectrum antibiotics for spontaneous preterm labor: the ORACLE II randomized trial. Lancet 2001 Mar 31;357 (9261):989–94.

7. Skupsi DW, Greenough A, Don SM, et al. Delivery mode for the extremely premature fetus: a statement of the prematurity working group of the World Association of Perinatal Medicine. J Perinatal Med. 2009;37(6):583–6.
8. Committee on Obstetric Practice, American College of Obstetrician and Gynecologists. Committee Opinion No. 543: Timing of umbilical cord clamping after birth. ObstetGynecol 2012;120:1522–6.
9. Royal College of Obstetricians and Gynaecologists. Preterm Prelabor Rupture of Membranes. Green -Top guideline No.44, November 2006.
10. The American College of Obstetricians and Gynecologists. Premature Rupture of Membranes. Practice Bulletin No. 172, October 2016.
11. Yudin MH, van Schalkwyk J, Eyk NV, et al. Antibiotic therapy in preterm premature rupture of the membranes. J ObstetGynaecol Can.2009; 31(9):863–7.
12. Committee Opinion No. 712: Intrapartum Management of Intraamniotic Infection. ObstetGynecol 2017; 130:e95.
13. Higgins RD, Saade G, Polin RA, et al. Evaluation and Management of Women and Newborns With a Maternal Diagnosis of Chorioamnionitis: Summary of a Workshop. ObstetGynecol 2016; 127:426.

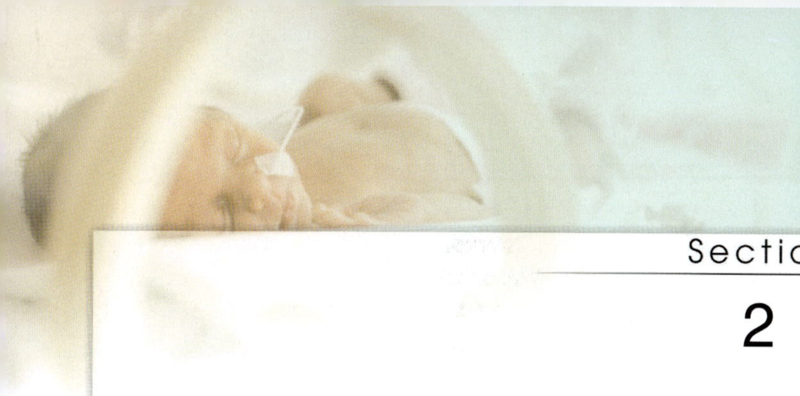

Section

2

# Central Nervous System

5. Neural Tube Defects

CHAPTER

5

# Neural Tube Defects

Spinal dysraphism is the most common congenital disorder of the central nervous system with an incidence of 0.3–5 per 1000 live births worldwide and 4–5 per 1000 live births in India.[1,3] The level of defect is lumbosacral in 90% cases, thoracic in 6–8%, and cervical in 2–4%. Meningomyelocele (MMC) is the most common neural tube defect compatible with life.[2] It is often associated with hydrocephalus (85% cases) and Arnold-Chiari malformation type 2.

## CLASSIFICATION

The neural tube defects (NTDs) are classified into open or closed defects depending on the embryological basis of the failure of primary neurulation or secondary neurulation.[2]

a. **Open NTDs:** Anencephaly, iniencephaly, encephalocele, rachischisis and spina bifida aperta/cystica (myeloschisis, meningomyelocele, meningocele)
b. **Closed NTDs:** Spina bifida occulta, lipomatous malformations (lipoma, lipomeningomyelocele), split cord malformations (diastematomyelia, diplomyelia), neurenteric cysts, dermal sinuses, tethered spinal cord and sacral agenesis and caudal regression.

## ETIOLOGY

Genetic and environmental factors play a central role in the etiology of NTDs. However, many other contributing factors like obesity, diabetes, immune dysregulation, folic acid antagonists, dihydrofolate reductase inhibitors, antiepileptic drugs, socioeconomic status, geography, and ethnicity are also implicated.

The most important genetic risk factor for NTDs described is a single nucleotide polymorphism (C677T) in the MTHFR gene, which leads to a mildly dysfunctional enzyme, increased levels of homocysteine in plasma, and an increased risk of NTDs in those affected.[4]

Periconceptional folic acid supplementation (4 mg/day in mothers with a previous history of NTD) is associated with a 72% risk reduction in recurrence.[5]

## CLINICAL PRESENTATION

The presentation can be antenatal or postnatal. Postnatally, the child usually presents with a swelling in the midline of the back. History should include: Any rupture or discharge, fever, vomiting or abnormal increase in head size, abnormal body or eye movements, irritability or lethargy, posturing of the body, constant fecal soiling, urinary retention, or continuous dribbling, weakness or reduced movements in any limb or foot deformity.

## ASSESSMENT OF NEONATES WITH NEURAL TUBE DEFECTS[6,7]

### General

1. Infant's general state and vitals examination.
2. Around one-third of the cases are associated with other congenital anomalies, e.g. cleft palate, undescended testis, omphalocele, talipes equinovarus, etc.[9]

### Spinal Lesion

1. The type of NTD and the vertebral level must be noted. The size of the swelling must be measured. The width of the bony defect and the availability of skin for surgical repair are of obvious concern.
2. The membrane overlying the swelling must be carefully inspected for any breaks/tears which occur in 10% of the cases and predisposes the baby to meningitis.
3. Positive transillumination of the lesion is suggestive of a meningocele or meningomyelocele.
4. Cutaneous stigmata of spina bifida occulta: Lumbosacral hypertrichosis (i.e. hairy patch), dermal sinus tract, sacral dimple, capillary hemangioma, caudal appendage, subcutaneous lipoma, and skin tags should be noted.

### Cerebral Function

1. Infant's state of alertness and the ability to fixate objects.
2. Signs of hydrocephalus: The occipitofrontal circumference above the 90th centile is indicative of severe hydrocephalus. One must also appreciate the separation of the sutures (especially the

lambdoidal and petrosquamous suture), a tense bulging anterior fontanelle, distended scalp veins, and papilloedema.

3. The asymmetrical tonic neck reflex is very strong if ventricular pressure is high and may return after the age of 6 months in a child with a blocked cerebrospinal fluid shunt.
4. Signs of associated Chiari II malformation—central or obstructive apnea, stridor, opisthotonus, etc.

Sensory and motor neurologic examination is carried out with the baby lying prone on the bed or held prone by the examiner's hand supporting the abdomen and the lower limb movements are noted after stimulation. The power should be charted according to MRC grading. It is always important to determine the spinal level of the defect, which does not always correspond to the anatomical level of the lesion.

## Spinal Cord Function

### *1. Motor Examination*

a. The active movements of muscle groups according to their segmental innervations are recorded.
b. Motor testing for the neurological level evaluates each possible level of involvement from L1-2 to S2-3 by assessing the action of joints of the lower limb: Hip flexion (T12-L3), hip extension (S1), hip adduction (L2-4), hip abduction (L5), knee extension (L2-4), knee flexion (L5, S1), ankle dorsiflexion (L4, 5), ankle plantar flexion (S1, 2), ankle inversion (L4), and ankle eversion (S1).
c. Initially 'voluntary' or rather spontaneous movement is assessed, and for this purpose it is permissible to activate the child by stimulation of the upper limbs. By appropriate positioning, each muscle can be made to operate with gravity eliminated or against gravity and, by palpation, the strength of contraction can be graded, on the MRC scale.[8]
d. With involvement of the lower sacral segments, inactivity of pelvic floor muscles (S3-S4) results in a flat-bottomed appearance with absence of the natal cleft and a patulous anus.
e. If L3 segment and above are affected—the lower limbs are completely paralysed.
f. If L4-L5 are affected with a normal L3—the baby has a characteristic posture with flexion of the hip and extension of the knee, but essentially no other limb movement.

g. When the L4-L5 spinal segments are preserved, there is movement of the hip and knee, and the foot can dorsiflex but cannot plantar flex.
h. When S1 and S2 are preserved, leg movements are essentially normal but bowel and bladder incontinence is likely to persist: This is usually the case in low sacral lesions.

*2. Sensory Testing*

Sensory testing is best carried out with the infant quiet. The first aim is to determine the lowest level of normal sensation. Starting in the lowest sacral territory, i.e. the perianal region, the skin is stimulated over the posterior aspect of the buttocks, thighs, and legs, and then upwards over successive dermatomes of the anterior surface and on to the abdomen. Observe the baby closely for a facial grimace, a cry, or a Moro response.

*3. Bladder and Bowel Assessment*

a. Look for a palpable or expressible bladder in the suprapubic region.
b. Frequent small volume dribbling of urine that increases by crying, movement, or suprapubic pressure is a warning of future incontinence.
c. Constant leakage of meconium from a patulous anus.
d. Infants who have neither voluntary nor reflex function in muscles innervated from S2-4 (lateral hamstrings, calf, and anal sphincter) tend to have complete bladder paralysis. Those with either partial voluntary function or purely reflex activity in S2-4 usually have an active detrusor but an efficient automatic reflex bladder is rare and outlet obstruction common.
e. Examine reflexes—anocutaneous reflex, bulbospongiosus (females) or cremasteric reflex (males). Eliciting these reflexes is an essential component of the neurological examination.

## Management

### *Perinatal Care*

1. The best route of delivery is controversial. The majority of the published evidence suggests that vaginal delivery does not adversely affect neonatal outcome with meningomyelocele.[11] Delivery at term by cesarean section is also preferred by some obstetricians.

2. Late pre-term to early term delivery is preferred in cases of fetal surgery.[11]
3. For infants and newborns with neural tube defects, immediate precautions should be taken after delivery to minimize the risk of meningitis.
   a. A sterile, saline moistened gauze dressing should be used to cover the neural placode. If possible, latex precautions should be used uniformly.
   b. Prophylactic antibiotics are recommended.
   c. Infant should be positioned prone or on his/her side in order to avoid pressure on the neural placode.
   d. Doughnut ring is used to prevent rupture of sac.
   e. Regular monitoring for head circumference, anterior fontanelle, brain stem compression symptoms.

## Investigations

### *A. Antenatal Diagnosis*

- **Maternal serum alpha fetoprotein:** Specificity 97–98%
- Second trimester (16–18 weeks): 60–70% accuracy for open NTD when MSAFP is elevated to 2.5 multiples of median or greater, with false positive rates of 1–3%.[10]
- **Antenatal ultrasonography (18–20 weeks):** Sensitivity: > 90%[12]
  i. Assessment of cranial features
  ii. Assessment of spine
  iii. Assessment of lower extremities
- **Fetal MRI:** Most sensitive as it is not dependent on maternal obesity, fetal position and oligohydramnios. However, it is not recommended by ACOG for screening or routine evaluation.[11,13]

### *B. Postnatal Evaluation*[12]

- Associated cardiac/renal anomalies: 2D echocardiography and ultrasound KUB must be done.
- X-ray spine: To screen whole spine and locate the spinal defect.
- USG cranium: To evaluate ventriculomegaly and hydrocephalus, resistive index of middle cerebral arteries, associated anomalies in the brain including Arnold-Chiari malformation.
- USG spine: For the level of spinal defect and the contents of sac, level of conus, tethering, syrinx, split cord malformations, lipomatous component.

- MRI: In complicated anomaly for better delineation of the anomaly and the craniospinal axis.

## Surgical Repair

Fetal surgery prevents chemical and physical damage to the exposed cord. Surgery is done before the end of the 24th week of gestation by open/minimally invasive approach. The MOM trial (Management of Myelomeningocele Study) showed a lower incidence of hind brain herniation and lesser need for VP shunt at one year of age. Walking without support was improved in prenatal surgery group.[14,15]

Complications of fetal surgery include increased risks of prematurity, oligohydramnios, premature pre-labor rupture of membranes (PPROM), placental abruption and fetal death.

## Postnatal Repair

For best neurological outcomes, the repair should be done within 48–72 hours: 37% risk of ventriculitis beyond 72 hours compared to 7% before 72 hours. If surgery is delayed, the CSF cultures should be obtained prior to repair. In case of positive cultures, the defect closure must be postponed.

### *Ventriculoperitoneal Shunting*

Hydrocephalus occurs in 85–90% cases with open NTDs.[16] Early shunting before spinal surgery is done in case of severe hydrocephalus. If no hydrocephalus, close follow-up is done postoperatively as 60–80% will need shunting later.

Postoperatively, the baby is nursed prone or lateral position. Head end to be kept low to prevent elevation of CSF pressures in already operated site. Monitor for limb movements/apnea/brain stem compression symptoms. Monitor head circumference charting, anterior fontanelle shape, and pulsation for hydrocephalus. Prevent fecal soiling of the wound by barrier dressing. Assess motor and sensory function regularly. USG cranium on post-operative day 7 for RI (<0.7). The elevated intracranial pressure may need drugs like mannitol, acetazolamide and glycerol. Clean intermittent catheterization (CIC) is needed for a few months after repair. Early initiation of CIC (proactive approach) is crucial to prevent renal damage.[17]

## Outcomes

- Untreated cases: 20% of the cases don't survive the first year if left untreated. 40% of the cases die before puberty[19]

- 70–80% require pressure relieving shunt[16]
- 40–70% have neurological deficit needing orthotics[20]
- 30–50% have neurogenic bowel and bladder (incidence reported up to 90%)[20]

  Bladder management and continence outcomes from National Spina Bifida registry 2009–2015[18] (Wiener et al.)

  a. 76.8% performed CIC for continence.
  b. Bowel dysfunction was present in 80% requiring daily enema.

### Poor Prognosis (Lorber's Criteria)[21]

1. Severe paraplegia
2. Gross enlargement of the head
3. Severe kyphosis or scoliosis
4. Associated gross congenital anomalies (such as complex heart diseases or major birth injuries)

### Good Prognosis

1. Distal lesions: Lesions beyond T11-L1
2. Skin covered lesions
3. No hydrocephalus or Arnold-Chiari malformation
4. Normal leg movement without any deformity
5. No associated abnormalities

### Follow-up Evaluation

a. Hydrocephalus—with fundoscopy or CT scan.
b. Patency of VP shunt (if present).
c. Ambulatory status—physiotherapy and rehabilitation.
d. Bowel and bladder dysfunction: Evaluation and management of neurogenic bladder and bowel.
e. Growth and intelligence.
f. Sensory loss and prevention of pressure sores.
g. Sexual status.

## REFERENCES

1. Allagh KP, Shamanna BR, Murthy GV, Ness AR, Doyle P, Neogi SB, Pant HB, Wellcome Trust-PHFI Folic Acid project team. Birth prevalence of neural tube defects and orofacial clefts in India: a systematic review and meta-analysis. PloS one. 2015 Mar 13;10(3):e0118961.
2. Reghunath A, Ghasi RG, Aggarwal A. Unveiling the tale of the tail: an illustration of spinal dysraphisms. Neurosurg Rev. 2021 Feb;44(1):97-114. doi: 10.1007/s10143-019-01215-z. Epub 2019 Dec 7. PMID: 31811517.

3. Frey L, Hauser WA (2003) Epidemiology of neural tube defects. Epilepsia 44:4–13.
4. van der Put NM, Steegers-Theunissen RP, Frosst P et al (1995) Mutated methylenetetrahydrofolate reductase as a risk factor for spina bifida. Lancet 346:1070–1071.
5. Prevention of neural tube defects: results of the Medical Research Council Vitamin Study (1991) MRC Vitamin Study Research Group. Lancet 338:131–1.
6. Hutson JM, Beasley SW. The surgical examination of children. Springer Berlin Heidelberg; 2013.
7. Stark GD. Neonatal assessment of the child with a myelomeningocele. Archives of disease in childhood. 1971 Aug;46(248):539.
8. No MM. Aids to the examination of the peripheral nervous system. HMSO, London; 1976.
9. Dai L, Zhu J, Zhou GX, Wu YQ, Wang YP, Miao L, Liang J. [Clinical features of 3798 perinatals suffering from syndromic neural tube defects]. Zhonghua Fu Chan Ke Za Zhi. 2003 Jan;38(1):17–9.
10. Vintzileos AM, Ananth CV, Fisher AJ, Smulian JC, Day- Salvatore D, Beazoglou T, Knuppel RA. Cost-benefit analysis of targeted ultrasonography for prenatal detection of spina bifida in patients with an elevated concentration of second-trimester maternal serum alpha-fetoprotein. Am J Obstet Gynecol 1999;180: 1227–1233.
11. American College of Obstetricians and Gynecologists. ACOG practice bulletin no. 187: neural tube defects. Obstet Gynecol. 2017;130(6):e279–90.
12. Cameron M, Moran P (2009). Prenatal screening and diagnosis of neural tube defects. Prenat Diagn 29:402–411.
13. Hüsler MR, Danzer E, Johnson MP, Bebbington M, Sutton L, Adzick NS, Wilson RD. Prenatal diagnosis and postnatal outcome of fetal spinal defects without Arnold-Chiari II malformation. Prenat Diagn. 2009 Nov;29(11):1050–7.
14. Adzick, N. S., Thom, E. A., Spong, C. Y., Brock, J. W., Burrows, P. K., Johnson, M. P., Howell, L. J., Farrell, J. A., Dabrowiak, M. E., Sutton, L. N., Gupta, N., Tulipan, N. B., D'alton, M. E., & Farmer, D. L. (2011). A Randomized Trial of Prenatal versus Postnatal Repair of Myelomeningocele. N Engl j Med, 364, 993–1004.
15. Houtrow AJ, Thom EA, Fletcher JM, Burrows PK, Adzick NS, Thomas NH, Brock JW, Cooper T, Lee H, Bilaniuk L, Glenn OA. Prenatal repair of myelomeningocele and school-age functional outcomes. Pediatrics. 2020 Feb 1;145(2).
16. Myelomeningocele-associated hydrocephalus: nationwide analysis and systematic review David J. McCarthy, MSc, Dallas L. Sheinberg, MSc, Evan Luther, MD, and Heather J. McCrea, MD, PhD.
17. Elzeneini W, Waly R, Marshall D, Bailie A. Early start of clean intermittent catheterization versus expectant management in children with spina bifida. Journal of pediatric surgery. 2019 Feb 1;54(2):322–5.

18. Wiener JS, Suson KD, Castillo J, Routh JC, Tanaka ST, Liu T, Ward EA, Thibadeau JK, Joseph DB, National Spina Bifida Patient Registry. Bladder management and continence outcomes in adults with spina bifida: results from the National Spina Bifida Patient Registry, 2009 to 2015. The Journal of urology. 2018 Jul;200(1):187–94.
19. Hunt GM. 'The median survival time in open spina bifida'. Developmental medicine and child neurology. 1997 Aug 1;39(8):568.
20. Masini L, De Luca C, Noia G, Caruso A, Lanzone A, Rendeli C, Ausili E, Massimi L, Tamburrini G, Apicella M, De Santis M. Prenatal diagnosis, natural history, postnatal treatment and outcome of 222 cases of spina bifida: experience of a tertiary center. Ultrasound in Obstetrics & Gynecology. 2019 Mar;53(3):302–8.
21. Lorber J. Neurologic Assessment of Neonates with Spina Bifida: Notes on Some Diagnostic and Therapeutic Considerations. Clinical Pediatrics. 1968 Nov;7(11):676–9.

Section

3

# Cardiovascular System

6. Neonatal Hypertension

CHAPTER

6

# Neonatal Hypertension

Advances in neonatology and improved survival of premature infants have led to increased recognition of neonatal hypertension (HTN). Hypertension has been reported in 0.2% of healthy-term neonates compared to 0.8 to 3% in NICU-admitted neonates.[1–3] In a large multicentric study, hypertension in NICU-admitted neonates was documented in 1.8% and an additional 3.7% were identified as undiagnosed hypertension.[4] Incidence is increased in high-risk conditions like indwelling umbilical arterial catheters, bronchopulmonary dysplasia (BPD), patent ductus arteriosus, intraventricular hemorrhage, acute kidney injury, and congenital anomalies of the kidneys and urinary tract (CAKUT).[5] HTN may be detected during NICU stay or may present after discharge.

## DEFINITION

It is difficult to define normal blood pressure (BP) in neonates because of considerable variation in the first weeks of life and lack of robust normative data. In preterm neonates, BP on the first day varies with birthweight and gestational age.[6] In healthy term neonates, however, such pattern is not seen.[7] BP also varies with post-conceptional age. After initial decrease in BP in 1st three hours, it increases rapidly during 1st two weeks. The systolic blood pressure (SBP) increases by 2.2 to 2.7 mm Hg per day and diastolic blood pressure (DBP) increases by 1.6 to 2.0 mm Hg per day during initial five days, and thereafter increase by 0.2 to 0.3 and 0 to 0.2 mm Hg per day respectively.[8] Rate of rise of BP in preterm neonates is higher than term neonates.

Hypertension in children and adolescents (1–13 years) has been defined by AAA[9] in 2017 as:

- **Normal BP:** SBP and/or DBP <90th percentile for age, sex and height.
- **Elevated BP:** 90th percentile to <95th percentile or 120/80 mm Hg to <95th percentile (whichever is lower).

- **Stage 1 HTN:** 95th percentile to <95th percentile + 12 mmHg, or 130/80 to 139/89 mm Hg (whichever is lower).
- **Stage 2 HTN:** 95th percentile + 12 mm Hg, or 140/90 mm Hg (whichever is lower).

In neonates, the definition of HTN is derived from that of children and adolescents as follows[10]:

- **Hypertension:** SBP or DBP 95th percentile as per PCA (GA at birth + postnatal age in weeks) on 3 separate occasions.
- **Severe hypertension:** SBP or DBP >99th percentile.

## MEASUREMENT OF BP

BP can be measured invasively by intra-arterial catheter or non-invasively by oscillometric method, ultrasonic Doppler, and a sphygmomanometer.

Intra-arterial BP monitoring is the gold standard method and is recommended in sick babies. Oscillometric method has been shown to overestimate BP in sick neonates but underestimate systolic BP in small for gestational age infants. However, in relatively stable babies oscillometric method is commonly used. Oscillometric method measures the mean arterial pressure (maximum arterial pulsation amplitude), and then uses an algorithm to project the systolic and diastolic BP. This method has a good correlation (correlation coefficient of 0.8 to 0.85) with intra-arterial BP. Ultrasonic Doppler used in some older studies tends to underestimate systolic BP and is no longer used. Sphygmomanometry is not recommended as Korotkoff sounds are not heard reliably in neonates.[6,8,9,11,12]

The 4th task force on HTN recommended a BP cuff size of $4 \times 8$ cm$^2$ size for neonates.[12] Neonatal BP cuffs come in different sizes (# cuff size number 1: 3 to 6 cm; #2: 4 to 8 cm; #3: 6 to 11 cm; #4: 7 to 13 cm; #5: 8 to 14 cm) but an appropriate BP cuff with a bladder length that covers 80% to 100% of arm circumference and a cuff width to arm circumference ratio of 0.5 (0.44 to 0.55) should be used.[9]

A recent systematic review found upper arm to be least variable and the most accurate location for oscillometric BP measurement. Thigh BP did not correlate with arm BP and is not recommended. Calf BP is similar to arm BP in the first few days of life but more variable at a later age.[11]

The standardized method of non-invasive BP measurement is described as follows[13]:

- Measure BP one and half hour after feeding or any medical intervention/procedure.

- Tie appropriate size BP cuff on right upper arm. Wait for 15 minutes.
- Baby should be asleep or quietly awake.
- Take mean of three readings taken at two-minute intervals.
- If first reading is discrepant, discard it and take average of next two readings.

## Who are at Risk?

**Antenatal risk factors:** Prematurity (most common risk factor), small for gestational age, LBW, babies born to mothers with pre-eclampsia and cocaine intake.

**Postnatal risk factors:** History of umbilical arterial or venous catheterization, intake of drugs, e.g. steroids, caffeine, theophylline, and phenylephrine. Bronchopulmonary dysplasia (BPD) is the most significant non-renal cause of hypertension in VLBW infants (incidence: 12% to 40%). In high-risk babies with BPD, HTN can appear from 15 days to 15 months of postnatal age.[14]

In the study from AWAKEN group, AKI, hyperbilirubinemia, Caucasian race, outborn, vaginal delivery, and congenital heart disease were identified as risk factors. Protective factors identified were multiple gestations, small for gestational age, and antenatal steroid coverage.

The causes of HTN are enlisted in Table 6.1.

## Which Reference Charts to Use?

Defining HTN is a cumbersome task as there is lack of comprehensive normative data in neonates. Zubrow et al. developed reference curves in 608 neonates using oscillometric method defining mean BP (± 95% confidence limits) for different gestational ages (22 to 42 weeks), post-menstrual ages (24 to 46 weeks) and birth weights (750 to 4000 gm) during the first 99 days of life and found significant correlation of BP with post menstrual age (PMA).[8] Similarly, Pejovic et al. had given reference values for BP in neonates, i.e. mean (±95% confidence limits) for neonates with GA from 24 to 44 weeks and birth weight from 500 to 5000 gm.[6]

With existing scarcity of data for defining and staging persistent hypertension, Dionne et al. pooled data from 7 studies and generated BP values (50th, 95th and 99th) after two weeks of age in neonates of 26 to 44 weeks of PMA.[9] Out of 7 studies, four used oscillometry and the remaining used Doppler methods for

| Table 6.1: Causes of neonatal HTN[2,3,5,6,14–16] | |
|---|---|
| Renal | **Reno-vascular:** Thromboembolism, renal venous thrombosis, fibromuscular dysplasia, renal artery stenosis, renal artery compression.<br>**Renal parenchymal:** Acute kidney injury, acute tubular necrosis, interstitial nephritis, hemolytic-uremic syndrome, nephrolithiasis, congenital nephritic syndrome, CAKUT (polycystic kidney diseases, ureteropelvic junction obstruction, renal hypoplasia). |
| Pulmonary | Bronchopulmonary dysplasia. |
| Cardiovascular | Coarctation of aorta, interrupted aortic arch, patent ductus arteriosus (PDA), fibromuscular dysplasia, post-PDA ligation. |
| Endocrine | Congenital adrenal hyperplasia, hyperaldosteronism, hyperthyroidism. |
| CNS | Intraventricular hemorrhage, subdural hematoma, raised intracranial pressure, neonatal seizures. |
| Tumors | Wilms tumor, neuroblastoma. |
| Iatrogenic | Pain, umbilical artery and vein catheterization, total parenteral nutrition. |
| Drugs | Dexamethasone, phenylephrine, caffeine/theophylline, vasopressors, indomethacin, hypervitaminosis D.<br>Maternal drugs: Antenatal steroids, substance abuse -cocaine and heroin. |
| Miscellaneous | Hypercalcemia, closure of anterior abdominal wall defects, ECMO, birth asphyxia, adrenal hemorrhage. |
| Idiopathic | |

BP measurement. For studies reporting mean and SD, mean was assumed as the 50th percentile, 2 SD as the 95th percentile, and 3 SD as the 99th percentile.[15]

AAP recommends using the normative data from Dionne et al till 44 weeks and BP curves from the 1987 second task force report for infants aged 1–12 months.[9]

*We use Zubrow charts for the first two weeks of age and Dionne's BP percentiles thereafter for management of HTN.*

## CLINICAL FEATURES

In most neonates, HTN is an incidental finding detected during routine BP measurement. The signs and symptoms of HTN overlap with other neonatal illnesses. Clinical features include feeding difficulties, unexplained tachypnea, apnea, lethargy, irritability and seizures. Features of severe hypertension include hypertensive retinopathy, left ventricular hypertrophy, congestive cardiac failure, seizures, stroke, and renal dysfunction. At-risk neonates need meticulous BP monitoring. In case of persistent hypertension, pediatric nephrology and cardiology consultation must be taken.[2,3,5,6,10]

## DIAGNOSTIC WORK UP

It involves detailed history taking, examination and laboratory investigations (Table 6.2).

## TREATMENT

Management of HTN includes correction of iatrogenic causes, control of BP with antihypertensive drugs (Table 6.3) and treatment of underlying aetiology (Fig. 6.1).

### Treatment is Indicated if

1. Severe HTN with BP >99th percentile or
2. BP ≥95th percentile with symptoms or
3. Persistence of BP ≥95th percentile (asymptomatic) more than 4 to 6 weeks.

### Goals of Treatment

1. To reduce BP to <95th percentile for age
2. To reduce BP <90th percentile, if evidence of end organ damage or if comorbid conditions (e.g. renal cystic disease) are present.

**Table 6.2: Evaluation of neonate with HTN[2,3,5,6,10]**

| | |
|---|---|
| History | Antenatal risk factors, perinatal insult, NICU procedures and neonatal morbidities |
| Examination | Peripheral pulses, radio-radial and radio-femoral delay, 4 limb BP, heart murmur (cardiac causes), any lump in abdomen (palpable kidney), bruit in lumbar area (renal causes).<br>Genital hyperpigmentation (congenital adrenal hyperplasia), facial dysmorphism. |
| Laboratory investigations | Serum sodium, potassium, calcium, urine RBC, urine routine (albumin/RBC), protein/creatinine, renal function test, fundus, ECG, CXR, USG kidney, renal and aortic Doppler study, echocardiography. |
| Investigations depending on the cause | |

**Table 6.3: Commonly used anti-hypertensive drugs[5,10,12,15,16]**

| *Class* | *Drug* | *Route* | *Dose* | *Interval* | *Comment* |
|---|---|---|---|---|---|
| Vasodilators | Hydralazine | IV | 0.1–0.6 mg/kg/dose | 4 hourly | Occasional tachycardia |
| | | Oral | 0.25 to 7 mg/kg/day | QID | |
| | Sodium nitroprusside | IV | 0.3–8 μg/kg/min (in 5% dextrose) | Infusion | Renal failure, monitor for cyanide toxicity |
| Calcium channel blocker | Amlodipine | Oral | 0.05–0.3 mg/kg/dose (max 0.6 mg/kg/day) | OD | May cause tachycardia |
| | Nicardipine | IV | 1–4 μg/kg/min Infusion | Infusion | |
| Diuretic | Chlorothiazide | Oral | 10–30 mg/kg/day | BID | Monitor electrolytes |
| | Hydrochlorthiazide | Oral | 1–3 mg/kg/day | BID | |
| | Spironolactone | Oral | 1–3 mg/kg /day | OD | |
| α and β antagonist | Labetalol | Oral | 0.5–1.0 mg/kg/dose max 10 mg/kg/day | BD-TDS | Monitor heart rate. Avoid in BPD |
| | | IV | infusion 0.25–3.0 mg/kg/hr | Infusion | |
| | Propranolol | Oral | 0.5–1.0 mg/kg/dose max 6 mg/kg/day | BD-TDS | |
| Central α agonist | Clonidine | IV | 3–10 μg/kg/day | BD-TDS | CNS depression and bradycardia |
| ACE inhibitors | Enalapril | Oral | 0.08–0.6 mg/kg/day | BD | May cause rapid drop in BP, especially if receiving diuretics. Monitor serum creatinine and Na, K. Avoid use in preterm infants, aortic arch anomalies, renal artery stenosis. Do not use in neonates with GFR<30 mg/min/1.73 $m^2$ |

Hypertension with severe symptoms, i.e. hypertensive emergency should be treated with IV drugs like sodium nitroprusside, labetalol, or hydralazine. The goal of treatment is to reduce mean arterial pressure (MAP) to 95th percentile gradually over 36 to 48 hours, i.e. 25% reduction in MAP (difference between observed MAP and 95th percentile) over first 8 hours and rest 75% reduction over the next 36 to 48 hours. After initial control of hypertensive crisis, an oral antihypertensive drug is instituted within 12 hours of parenteral therapy and later is gradually withdrawn over next 12–48 hours.

Daily monitoring of BP is warranted in admitted neonates until BP is controlled. On outpatient basis, BP should be monitored every 1–2 weeks until it is controlled, and every 4 to 8 weeks thereafter. Monitoring for side effects of antihypertensive drugs during treatment is crucial. After treatment of secondary causes and achieving adequate BP control, antihypertensive drugs may be de-escalated. During de-escalation strict BP monitoring is required as HTN may recur after discontinuation of antihypertensive therapy. Parents should be taught regarding BP measurement and monitoring at home.[5,10,12,15]

## FOLLOW-UP

Around 2.6% of babies with history of NICU stay develop HTN within 3 years of discharge.[2] In neonates with risk factors, BP should be checked at discharge from NICU and at 1st follow-up visit. If infant is normotensive or prehypertensive, monitor BP six monthly.

Steroid-induced hypertension tends to resolve as early as 2 weeks after stopping therapy. However, patients with renovascular hypertension need to be followed up to 5 years of age. Most of the cases of neonatal hypertension get resolved by six months of age. Small for gestational age and IUGR babies are at risk of developing hypertension in adolescence and adult life, hence six monthly follow-up monitoring is required.[2,3,5,6,15]

AAP recommends routine BP monitoring only after 3 years of age.[9] However, BP monitoring prior to 3 years should be done in the following conditions:

1. History of prematurity <32 weeks gestation or small for gestational age, very low birth weight, other neonatal complications requiring intensive care, history of umbilical artery catheter.
2. Congenital heart disease (repaired or unrepaired).
3. Recurrent urinary tract infections, hematuria, or proteinuria.

4. Known renal disease or urologic malformations.
5. Family history of congenital renal disease.
6. Treatment with drugs known to raise BP.
7. Other systemic illnesses associated with HTN.

## Approach to Management of Neonatal Hypertension

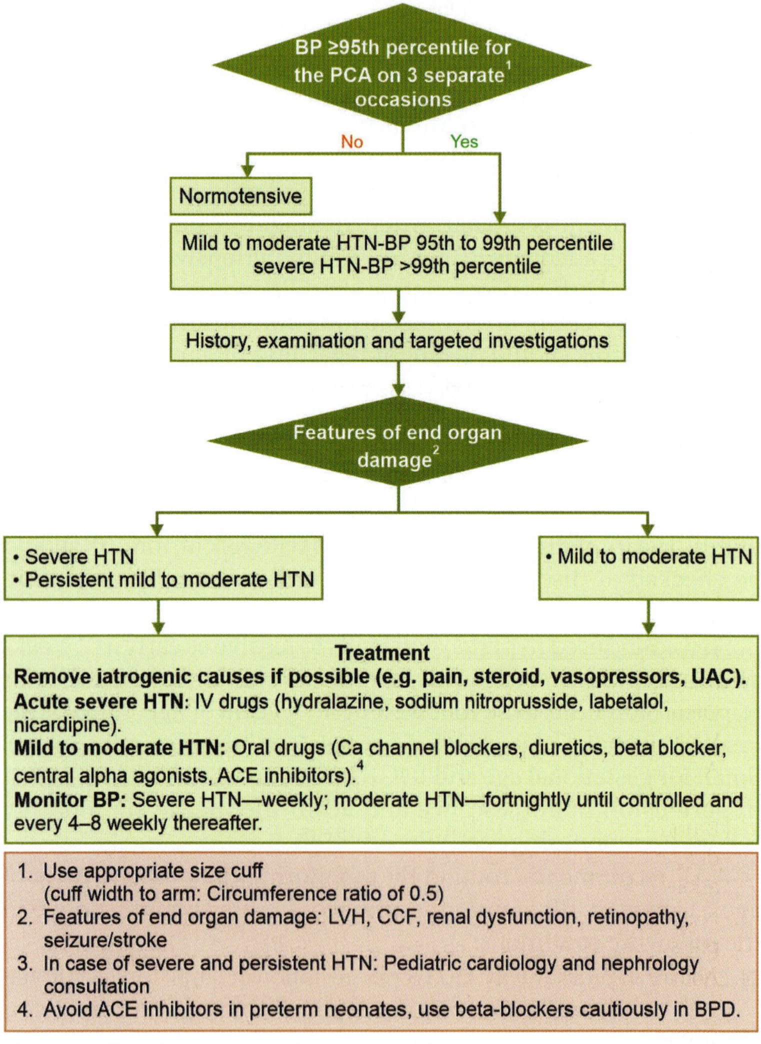


**Fig. 6.1:** Algorithmic approach to neonatal hypertension (HTN). *PCA:* Post-conceptional age; *LVH:* Left ventricular hypertension; *CCF:* Congestive cardiac failure; *UAC:* Umbilical artery catheter

## REFERENCES


1. American Academy of Pediatrics Committee on Fetus and Newborn: Routine evaluation of blood pressure, hematocrit, and glucose in newborns. Pediatrics. 1993 Sep;92(3):474–6.
2. Friedman AL, Hustead VA. Hypertension in babies following discharge from a neonatal intensive care unit. A 3-year follow-up. Pediatr Nephrol Berl Ger. 1987 Jan;1(1):30–4.
3. Seliem WA, Falk MC, Shadbolt B, Kent AL. Antenatal and postnatal risk factors for neonatal hypertension and infant follow-up. Pediatr Nephrol Berl Ger. 2007 Dec;22(12):2081–7.
4. Kraut EJ, Boohaker LJ, Askenazi DJ, Fletcher J, Kent AL, Neonatal Kidney Collaborative (NKC). Incidence of neonatal hypertension from a large multicenter study [Assessment of Worldwide Acute Kidney Injury Epidemiology in Neonates-AWAKEN]. Pediatr Res. 2018 Aug;84(2):279–89.
5. Mistry K, Gupta C. Neonatal Hypertension. NeoReviews. 2017 Jun 1;18(6):e357–71.
6. Pejovic B, Peco-Antic A, Marinkovic-Eric J. Blood pressure in non-critically ill preterm and full-term neonates. Pediatr Nephrol Berl Ger. 2007 Feb;22(2):249–57.
7. Kent AL, Kecskes Z, Shadbolt B, Falk MC. Normative blood pressure data in the early neonatal period. Pediatr Nephrol Berl Ger. 2007 Sep;22(9):1335–41.
8. Zubrow AB, Hulman S, Kushner H, Falkner B. Determinants of blood pressure in infants admitted to neonatal intensive care units: a prospective multicenter study. Philadelphia Neonatal Blood Pressure Study Group. J Perinatol Off J Calif Perinat Assoc. 1995;15(6):470–9.
9. Flynn JT, Kaelber DC, Baker-Smith CM, Blowey D, Carroll AE, Daniels SR, et al. Clinical Practice Guideline for Screening and Management of High Blood Pressure in Children and Adolescents. Pediatrics. 2017 Sep;140(3):e20171904.
10. Hjorten R, Flynn JT. Neonatal Hypertension. Clin Perinatol. 2022 Mar;49(1):27–42.
11. Dionne JM, Bremner SA, Baygani SK, Batton B, Ergenekon E, Bhatt-Mehta V, et al. Method of Blood Pressure Measurement in Neonates and Infants: A Systematic Review and Analysis. J Pediatr. 2020 Jun;221:23-31.e5.
12. National High Blood Pressure Education Program Working Group on High Blood Pressure in Children and Adolescents. The fourth report on the diagnosis, evaluation, and treatment of high blood pressure in children and adolescents. Pediatrics. 2004 Aug;114(2 Suppl 4th Report):555–76.
13. Nwankwo MU, Lorenz JM, Gardiner JC. A standard protocol for blood pressure measurement in the newborn. Pediatrics. 1997 Jun;99(6):E10.
14. Abman SH, Warady BA, Lum GM, Koops BL. Systemic hypertension in infants with bronchopulmonary dysplasia. J Pediatr. 1984 Jun;104(6):928–31.
15. Dionne JM, Abitbol CL, Flynn JT. Hypertension in infancy: Diagnosis, management and outcome. Pediatr Nephrol Berl Ger. 2012 Jan;27(1):17–32.
16. Giri P, Roth P. Neonatal Hypertension. Pediatr Rev. 2020 Jun 1;41(6):307–11.

Section

# 4

# Respiratory System

CHAPTER

7

# Bronchopulmonary Dysplasia

Bronchopulmonary dysplasia (BPD) occurs in preterm infants who require mechanical ventilation or oxygen therapy for a primary lung disorder. Though the incidence of BPD has largely remained unchanged over the years, improved survival of more immature infants has led to an increased absolute number of infants with BPD. These infants are more likely to have persistent respiratory symptoms requiring frequent hospital admissions in the first two years after birth and neurodevelopmental impairment.

## DEFINITION

Since its first description by Northway et al. fifty years ago, the definition of BPD has undergone a significant transformation. In 2001, the National Institute of Child Health and Human Development (NICHD) definition of BPD suggested the need for oxygen for >28 days and at 36 weeks' PMA to identify the severity of BPD. Given that the criteria for supplemental oxygen might vary across the units, Walsh proposed a physiological definition based on "room air challenge" to define BPD. However, the previous definitions could not classify infants dying from severe respiratory failure before 36 weeks' PMA and did not consider the newer modes of noninvasive ventilation. To overcome these pitfalls, the NICHD proposed a revised definition of BPD in 2018 (Table 7.1).[1]

## INCIDENCE

A recent systematic review reported the global incidence of BPD to be 10–89% in extremely preterm infants (varies from 18–82% in the Asian population).[2] A few reports are available from the centers in India; a recent study from South India showed an incidence of 31% in neonates <32 weeks' gestation according to the 2001 NICHD criteria (76% mild; 20% moderate; 4% severe). In a prospective cohort study conducted at AIIMS (2013–2014), the incidence of BPD

**Table 7.1: Definition of BPD[1]**

*A preterm infant (<32 weeks gestational age) with BPD has persistent parenchymal lung disease, radiographic confirmation of parenchymal lung disease, and at 36 weeks PMA requires one of the following $FiO_2$ ranges/oxygen levels/$O_2$ concentrations for ≥3 consecutive days to maintain arterial oxygen saturation in the 90–95% range.*

| *Grades* | *Invasive IPPV** | *N-CPAP, NIPPV, or nasal cannula ≥3 L/min* | *Nasal cannula flow of 1 to <3 L/min or hood $O_2$* | *Nasal cannula flow of <1 L/min* |
|---|---|---|---|---|
| I | – | 21 | 22–29 | 22–70 |
| II | 21 | 22–29 | >30 | >70 |
| III | >21 | >30 | | |
| III(A) | Early death (between 14 days of postnatal age and 36 weeks) owing to persistent parenchymal lung disease and respiratory failure that cannot be attributable to other neonatal morbidities (e.g. necrotizing enterocolitis, intraventricular hemorrhage, redirection of care, episodes of sepsis, etc.). | | | |

**Excluding infants ventilated for primary airway disease or central respiratory control conditions.*

*CPAP:* Continuous positive airway pressure; *IPPV:* Intermittent positive pressure ventilation; *N-CPAP:* Nasal continuous positive airway pressure; *NIPPV:* Noninvasive positive pressure ventilation

(2001 NICHD criteria) in infants <32 weeks' gestation was 33% (mild 32.4%; moderate 27.3%; severe 40.3%).

## PATHOGENESIS

BPD has a multi-factorial etiology. The most crucial factor in the pathogenesis of BPD is prematurity. The other major risk factors include oxygen therapy, mechanical ventilation, infection, patent ductus arteriosus (PDA), and genetic predisposition. Recently, genetic polymorphisms and antenatal factors, especially placental dysfunction, are also thought to play a role.

## PATHOLOGY: *'OLD' VS.'NEW' BPD*

'Old' BPD (rarely seen nowadays) refers to a severe form of BPD in infants who received aggressive ventilation and is characterized by extreme morphological changes, including emphysema, atelectasis, fibrosis, and smooth muscle hypertrophy in the airways and pulmonary vasculature. In contrast, the milder form or 'new BPD' arises mainly from incomplete lung development coupled with various postnatal insults. It is characterized by a striking decrease in alveolar septations and impaired vascular development. An increasing role of growth factors (such as thyroid transcription factor 1 and VEGF in the sacculation, alveolarization, and vasculogenesis of peripheral lung) and epigenetics (such as SP-B i4 deletion, polymorphism in genes coding pro and anti-inflammatory cytokines) is being recognized in the pathogenesis of new BPD.[3]

## CLINICAL AND RADIOLOGICAL FEATURES

Respiratory signs in infants with BPD include fast but shallow breathing, retractions, and paradoxical breathing. Rales and coarse rhonchi are usually heard on auscultation.

**Radiographic features of 'old' and 'new' BPD are different. 'Old' BPD has four distinct stages:** Stage 1, consistent with hyaline membrane disease; stage 2, opaque lung fields with air bronchograms due to areas of atelectasis alternating with emphysema; stage 3, small radiolucent fields; and stage 4, hyperinflated lungs with generalized cystic areas and dense fibrotic strands. In contrast, infants with new BPD show only haziness reflecting diffuse loss of lung volume or increased lung fluid. Occasionally they have dense areas of segmental or lobar atelectasis, or pneumonic infiltrates, but they do not show severe hyperinflation.

## MANAGEMENT

### Prevention

#### *Before Birth*

The use of antenatal steroids (ANS) in mothers at risk for delivering a premature infant reduces the incidence of neonatal deaths and RDS but not BPD, probably due to increased survival of very immature infants at high risk of BPD.

#### *After Birth*

**In the delivery room:** The management principles in the 'golden hour after delivery include establishing functional residual capacity (FRC), improving pulmonary blood flow, and ensuring adequate tissue oxygenation. The crux is to achieve these with minimal lung injury.

i. **Delivery room CPAP:** The establishment of FRC at birth can be ensured by providing adequate CPAP/PEEP to infants with respiratory distress. This results in better recruitment of collapsed alveoli. Provision of early CPAP followed by selective use of surfactant is associated with lower rates of BPD and death than prophylactic surfactant therapy.[4]

ii. **Gentle ventilation in the delivery room:** The Cochrane review comparing prophylactic CPAP with intubation and mechanical ventilation shows a slight reduction in the incidence of BPD at 36 weeks. In cases where PPV in the delivery room is unavoidable, gentle ventilation with a T-piece resuscitator may help decrease lung injury. Recent studies have shown that tidal volume measurement (respiratory function monitor) in preterm infants requiring PPV in the delivery room is feasible, but its effect on BPD is still unknown.

iii. **Restricted use of oxygen:** Current recommendations for preterm infants below 35 weeks'gestation suggest initiating resuscitation at 21–30% $FiO_2$. However, the exact time-specific oxygen targets for preterm infants are still lacking.[5]

*In the NICU*

A. **Fluids and nutrition**

i. **Fluid restriction:** Anecdotal data indicate that fluid restriction in preterm infants reduces the incidence of BPD; however, the Cochrane review did not find any significant reduction. Using plastic barriers (e.g. cling wrap), humidification and caps and socks would help minimize the insensible water loss and fluid requirement.

ii. **Nutrition:** Early aggressive parenteral nutrition with an early transition to enteral feeding may help decrease the incidence of BPD. When expressed breast milk is used, fortification with human milk fortifier (HMF) or preterm formula powder often makes up for deficiencies of micronutrients and protein. The role of specific nutrients such as inositol, vitamin E, selenium, glutamine, lactoferrin, probiotics, and docosahexaenoic acid in preventing BPD is still speculative.

B. **Ventilator strategies**

i. **CPAP:** Use of nasal CPAP as the initial mode of respiratory management in preterm infants, compared to IMV, has been associated with a lower incidence of BPD, the need for surfactant, and subsequent mechanical ventilation.[6]

ii. **Nasal intermittent positive pressure ventilation (NIPPV):** The Cochrane review found a decreased risk of respiratory failure and intubation rate but no reduction in rates of BPD in preterm infants treated with early NIPPV compared to early CPAP.

iii. **Patient triggered modes of ventilation:** Patient-triggered modes of ventilation (e.g. SIMV, assist-control, and pressure support ventilation) improve infant ventilator synchrony, thereby reducing the risk of ventilator-induced lung injury (VILI). Though the Cochrane review on PTV did not find any reduction in the incidence of BPD following these modes, it is still a good practice to use PTV whenever possible.

iv. **High-frequency ventilation (HFV):** A recent meta-analysis of the individual patient data of RCTs revealed that HFV was equally effective in preventing BPD as conventional ventilation. However, earlier initiation of HFV (between 1 and 4h) when indicated would probably be more beneficial than starting it as a primary mode (<1 h) or later (after 4 h).

v. **Volume-targeted (VT) ventilation:** The Cochrane review on volume ventilation showed a significant reduction of BPD or death (NNT=8) and borderline reduction of BPD with VT ventilation modes.[7] If available and the health care providers are experienced, VT modes should preferably be used in preterm infants.

vi. **Permissive hypercapnia:** 'Minimal' ventilation to achieve mild hypercapnia ($PaCO_2$ 45–55 mm Hg) using low tidal volumes/less peak inflation pressures, though safe, has not been proven to decrease the incidence of BPD.

vii. **Permissive hypoxemia:** Recent meta-analysis shows that restricted oxygen (target $SpO_2$ 85–89%) in preterm infants born before 28 weeks' gestation results in higher mortality rates and NEC with no consistent benefits in reduction of BPD (though rates of ROP of prematurity decreased). The current recommendation is to target $SpO_2$ of 91–95% until 36 weeks PMA.[8]

C. **Pharmacological strategies**

i. **Exogenous surfactant:** Surfactant should be used selectively after the establishment of adequate FRC by using CPAP; routine use of prophylactic surfactant may cause potential harm. The early rescue strategy is more beneficial than delayed surfactant therapy in reducing the incidence of BPD.[9] Several approaches are being evaluated to administer the surfactant without intubation, including less invasive surfactant administration (LISA), minimally invasive surfactant therapy (MIST), and aerosolized surfactant. LISA/MIST has been shown to reduce the risk of death or BPD.[10]

In our unit, we practice the MIST technique using poractant (200 mg/kg) in preterm neonates who do not require intubation at birth and fulfil the criteria for surfactant therapy.

ii. **Vitamin A:** Studies indicate a decreased risk of BPD in VLBW infants who received either enteral or parenteral vitamin A supplementation, but this effect was limited to infants with a baseline vitamin A intake of <1500 U/kg/day.[11]

We do not use either enteral or parenteral vitamin A in our unit to prevent BPD.

iii. **Methylxanthines:** A multi-centric RCT on caffeine in infants with birth weights of 500–1250 g showed a significant reduction in the incidence of BPD. The probable reason was the reduced duration of mechanical ventilation and reduction in apneic episodes following caffeine.[12]

We use prophylactic caffeine in <28 weeks GA and therapeutic caffeine to treat apnea of prematurity and after extubation in preterm infants <32 weeks GA.

iv. **Postnatal systemic steroids:** Steroid therapy for BPD is conventionally categorized into two groups based on the timing of initiation: Early (up to the first seven days of life) or late (after seven days of life). Meta-analyses of RCTs of both groups have reported short-term (hypertension, gastrointestinal perforation, poor somatic growth) and long-term (cerebral palsy) side effects of the therapy. The reviews concluded that the benefits of postnatal steroids might not outweigh these potential harms.[13] Thus, it is prudent to use steroids only as a late strategy in ELBW infants on invasive mechanical ventilation in the second week of life. A recent network meta-analysis found that moderately early (8–14 days) dexamethasone at a cumulative dose of 2–4 mg/kg might be the best strategy for decreasing death or BPD at 36 weeks' PMA.[14]

We use early low dose hydrocortisone (PREMILOC regime) in <28 weeks GA and late low dose dexamethasone (DART regime) in ELBW infants who continue to be on mechanical ventilation even after 10–14 days of life.

v. **Inhaled steroids:** The meta-analysis that included 16 trials with substantial heterogeneity in the inclusion criteria found a significant reduction in the incidence of BPD, with no effect on mortality rates. The long-term effects of such therapy on growth, respiratory and developmental outcomes are still unclear.[15]

We do not routinely use inhaled steroids in our unit to prevent BPD.

vi. **Inhaled nitric oxide (iNO):** A recently conducted large trial has shown that iNO has no substantial role in preventing BPD. Sub-group analysis suggested that a potential effect probably still exists in 'black' infants when given between 7 and 14 days. But the optimal dose, the timing of therapy, and the sub-group of infants who may benefit from iNO remain unclear.

vii. **Diuretic therapy:** With the inherent long-term complications associated with chronic use, diuretics cannot be recommended to prevent BPD. They can, however, be used sparingly if there are clinical/radiographic features of pulmonary edema in an infant with evolving or established BPD.

We use 0.5–1 mg/kg/day of furosemide in infants with features suggestive of excess lung fluid; we stop after 24–48 hours if no improvement is noted.

viii. **PDA management:** Prophylactic closure of PDA has not reduced the risk of BPD. In contrast, medical treatment of hemodynamically significant PDA using indomethacin, ibuprofen, or paracetamol could reduce the incidence of BPD. Recently reported RCTs have found that drugs used routinely to close moderate to large PDA at the end of the first week did not affect the risk of BPD.[16] However, the secondary analysis revealed that the persistence of a PDA shunt beyond ten days in extreme preterm infants requiring mechanical ventilation for >10 days was associated with an increased risk of BPD.

ix. **Emerging therapies:** Several novel therapies are being evaluated and are currently in phase 2/3 trials. They include antioxidants (superoxide dismutase), macrolide antibiotics, inositol, leukotriene receptor antagonists, intratracheal corticosteroids, late surfactant, DHA, and stem cell therapy. A few trials on intratracheal administration of budesonide with surfactant have shown encouraging results, but further studies are needed. Intratracheal administration of mesenchymal stem cells has been shown to reduce the incidence of BPD in phase-2 trials.

D. **Non-pharmacological strategies:** A comprehensive focus on improving protocols incorporating multiple standards of care, such as increasing the use of CPAP, reducing the time to surfactant administration, and reducing mechanical ventilation, has resulted in a substantial reduction in BPD rates amongst 19 participating NICUs in Vermont Oxford Network. The use of developmentally supportive care, such as NIDCAP (Neonatal Individualized Developmental Care and Assessment Program), when conducted in an appropriate environment with a focus on the quality of intervention, has also been shown to reduce BPD in a few settings.

## Treatment of Established BPD

The primary goal in the treatment of established BPD is to maintain adequate gas exchange with as minimal support as possible. CPAP and NIPPV should be attempted whenever possible. The settings should be titrated for infants on ventilators, keeping in mind the rapidly changing pulmonary mechanics (increasing airway resistance and improving lung compliance). Often, slow rates with long Ti are needed as the disease progresses. Volume-targeted ventilation is preferred, especially in neonates with marked variability in compliance and resistance. Accepting a relatively high $PaCO_2$ (45–55 mm Hg, provided that pH >7.25) would help minimize the ventilator settings and early extubation.

The role of drugs in established BPD is minimal. Infants with 'BPD spells'(sudden episodes of deterioration due to marked expiratory airflow limitation) may require sedation and muscle relaxation to reduce agitation. Infants developing BPD require 20% to 40% more calories than their age-matched healthy controls. Their caloric requirement varies from 120 to 150 kcal/kg/day. This can be achieved by fortifying breast milk with HMF or infant formula. For infants who require more calories, fat supplementation (e.g. MCT oil) is preferable to adding carbohydrates because of the less pronounced effects on $CO_2$ levels.

## Complications of BPD

**Pulmonary hypertension:** Recent studies have highlighted that pulmonary hypertension (PH) increases the morbidity, duration of hospitalization, and mortality associated with BPD. Prospective studies have shown that PH affects 16–25% of infants with BPD. The pathogenesis is multifactorial and results from a complex interplay between maternal, genetic, epigenetic, and environmental factors.[17] The pediatric pulmonary hypertension network recommends that an echocardiogram be performed to screen for PH at the time of formal BPD diagnosis, i.e. at 36 weeks PMA.[18] Management of PH includes maintaining $SpO_2$ between 92–95%. Some case series have demonstrated a reduction in mortality by adding sildenafil in infants with PH associated with BPD. However, long-term safety and mode of administration are yet to be established.

**Other long-term outcomes:** With more BPD infants surviving, the long-term consequences of BPD are becoming more apparent. Follow-up studies in adult survivors of classic BPD have demonstrated compromised pulmonary functions, asthma-like symptoms, pulmonary hypertension, and exercise intolerance with altered responses to hypoxia.[19] Up to 49% of infants require rehospitalization in the initial two years of life. Increased susceptibility to respiratory infections, particularly RSV ALRI, has been observed in infants with BPD. Central airway diseases like acquired tracheomalacia, glottis, and subglottic damage are not uncommon. These infants also have a significantly higher risk of mortality and neurodevelopmental impairment. Therefore, weight gain, linear growth, and neurodevelopment are important considerations at each follow-up visit. Higher rates of healthcare use and impairments in quality of life that extend into adulthood have been noted in BPD.[20]

Figure 7.1 summarizes the steps of preventing and treating BPD in preterm VLBW infants.

**Antenatal period**

Antenatal corticosteroids

**At birth**

If resuscitation required, avoid excessive pressure and volume (i.e. avoid excessive chest rise); delay cord clamping & ensure optimal FRC

**Birth to 24 hours**

- Early CPAP, try to avoid intubation
- If surfactant is to be used, use early surfactant
- **Fluids:** 60–80 ml/kg/d
- **Nutrition:** Oral feeds—breast milk (MEN/full feeds) to be initiated in stable infants
- If on ventilator:
    - Early rescue surfactant and early extubation
    - **Settings:** Rapid rates (50–60/min), moderate PEEP (4–6 cm $H_2O$), short Ti (0.25–0.4 s). Consider volume targeted ventilation (4–5 ml/kg)
    - Target values—$SpO_2$: 91–95%; $PaCO_2$ 45–55 mmHg; pH: 7.25–7.35
    - Use methylxanthines to facilitate extubation

*(Contd.)*

(*Contd.*)

| | |
|---|---|
| **24 hours to 1 week** | • **Fluids:** Daily increment of 15–20 ml/kg/d to reach a maximum of 140–150 ml/kg/d by day 7<br>• **Nutrition:**<br>- Parenteral: TPN for ELBW infants till full enteral feeds are achieved<br>- Enteral: Gradually increase feed volume by 20–30 ml/kg/d if accepting well; give only breast milk; fortify with HMF after reaching 100 ml/kg/d<br>• If on ventilator:<br>- **Settings** and **target values** as above<br>- Extubate to CPAP/ NIPPV as early as possible<br>- Methylxanthines to facilitate extubation<br>• Initiate developmentally supportive care |
| **2–4 weeks** | • **Fluids:** 150–160 ml/kg/d<br>• **Nutrition:** Fortify breast milk with HMF; Increase calorie intake to 120–150 kcal/kg/d<br>• If on ventilator:<br>- **Settings:** PTV mode; slow rates (25–40/min), moderate PEEP (4–5 cm $H_2O$), moderate Ti (0.35–0.45 s), low tidal volume (4–6 ml/kg)<br>- **Target values:** $SpO_2$: 91–95%; $PaCO_2$ 45–55 mm Hg; pH: 7.25–7.35<br>• **Steroids:** Consider in ELBW infants on ventilator support even after 10–14 days of age<br>• Diuretics for features of pulmonary edema<br>• Bronchodilators for bronchospasm<br>• Diagnose and treat pulmonary hypertension, gastroesophageal reflux |
| **>4 weeks** | • **Fluids:** 150–160 ml/kg/d<br>• **Nutrition:** Fortify breast milk with HMF; add more calories if needed<br>• **If on ventilator:** Mild/moderate BPD<br>- **Settings:** PTV mode; slow rates (20–40/min), moderate PEEP (6–8 cm $H_2O$), Ti (0.35–0.45 s), tidal volume (5–8 ml/kg);<br>- **Target values:** $SpO_2$: 92–98%; $PaCO_2$ 45–60 mm Hg; pH>7.25<br>**Severe-chronic BPD**<br>- **Settings:** PTV mode; slow rates (15–30/min), high PEEP (up to 8–10 cm $H_2O$), longer Ti (0.5–1.0 s), large tidal volume (6–12 ml/kg);<br>- **Target values:** $SpO_2$: 92–98%; $PaCO_2$ 50–60 mm Hg; pH>7.25<br>• Bronchodilators for bronchospasm<br>• Sedation and muscle relaxation for 'BPD spells'<br>• Consider sildenafil for established pulmonary arterial hypertension. |

*FRC:* Functional residual capacity; *CPAP:* Continuous positive airway pressure; *NIPPV:* Noninvasive positive pressure ventilation; *PEEP:* Positive end-expiratory pressure; *MEN:* Minimal enteral nutrition; *ELBW:* Extremely low birth weight infants; *TPN:* Total parenteral nutrition; *HMF:* Human milk fortifier; *PTV:* Patient triggered ventilation; *Ti:* Inspiratory time

**Fig. 7.1:** Flowchart for management of BPD

## REFERENCES

1. Higgins RD, Jobe AH, Koso-Thomas M, Bancalari E, Viscardi RM, Hartert TV, et al. Bronchopulmonary Dysplasia: Executive Summary of a Workshop. The Journal of Pediatrics. 2018 Jun;197:300–8.
2. Siffel C, Kistler KD, Lewis JFM, Sarda SP. Global incidence of bronchopulmonary dysplasia among extremely preterm infants: a systematic

literature review. J Matern Fetal Neonatal Med. 2021;34(11):1721-1731. doi:10.1080/14767058.2019.1646240.
3. Merritt TA, Deming DD, Boynton BR. The 'new' bronchopulmonary dysplasia: challenges and commentary. Semin Fetal Neonatal Med. 2009 Dec;14(6):345-57.
4. Rojas-Reyes MX, Morley CJ, Soll R. Prophylactic versus selective use of surfactant in preventing morbidity and mortality in preterm infants. Cochrane Database Syst Rev. 2012;3(3):CD000510.
5. Escobedo MB, Aziz K, Kapadia VS, et al. 2019 American Heart Association Focused Update on Neonatal Resuscitation: An Update to the American Heart Association Guidelines for Cardiopulmonary Resuscitation and Emergency Cardiovascular Care. Pediatrics. 2020;145(1):e20191362.
6. Schmölzer GM, Kumar M, Pichler G, Aziz K, O'Reilly M, Cheung P-Y. Noninvasive versus invasive respiratory support in preterm infants at birth: systematic review and meta-analysis. BMJ. 2013;347:f5980.
7. Wheeler KI, Klingenberg C, McCallion N, Morley CJ, Davis PG. Volume-targeted versus pressure limited ventilation in the neonate. Cochrane Database Syst Rev 2010;(11):CD003666.
8. Askie LM, Darlow BA, Finer N, et al. Association Between Oxygen Saturation Targeting and Death or Disability in Extremely Preterm Infants in the Neonatal Oxygenation Prospective Meta-analysis Collaboration. JAMA. 2018;319(21):2190–2201.
9. Bahadue FL, Soll R. Early versus delayed selective surfactant treatment for neonatal respiratory distress syndrome. Cochrane Database Syst Rev. 2012;11(11):CD001456.
10. Abdel-Latif ME, Davis PG, Wheeler KI, De Paoli AG, Dargaville PA. Surfactant therapy via thin catheter in preterm infants with or at risk of respiratory distress syndrome. Cochrane Database Syst Rev. 2021;5(5):CD011672.
11. Rakshasbhuvankar AA, Pillow JJ, Simmer KN, Patole SK. Vitamin A supplementation in very-preterm or very-low-birth-weight infants to prevent morbidity and mortality: a systematic review and meta-analysis of randomized trials. Am J Clin Nutr. 2021;nqab294.
12. Schmidt B, Roberts RS, Davis P, Doyle LW, Barrington KJ, Ohlsson A, et al. Caffeine for Apnea of Prematurity Trial Group. Caffeine therapy for apnea of prematurity. N Engl J Med 2006;354:2112–2121.
13. Barrington KJ. The adverse neuro-developmental effects of postnatal steroids in the preterm infant: a systematic review of RCTs. BMC Pediatrics 2001; 1: 1–14.
14. Ramaswamy VV, Bandyopadhyay T, Nanda D, et al. Assessment of Postnatal Corticosteroids for the Prevention of Bronchopulmonary Dysplasia in Preterm Neonates: A Systematic Review and Network Meta-analysis. JAMA Pediatr. 2021;175(6):e206826.
15. Shinwell ES, Portnov I, Meerpohl JJ, Karen T, Bassler D. Inhaled Corticosteroids for bronchopulmonary dysplasia: A Meta-analysis. Pediatrics. 2016 Dec;138(6). pii: e20162511.
16. Clyman RI, Liebowitz M, Kaempf J, Erdeve O, Bulbul A, Håkansson S, et al. PDA-TOLERATE Trial: An Exploratory Randomized Controlled Trial of

Treatment of Moderate-to-Large Patent Ductus Arteriosus at 1 Week of Age. The Journal of Pediatrics. 2019 Feb;205:41–48.e6.

17. Mourani PM, Abman SH. Pulmonary Hypertension and Vascular Abnormalities in Bronchopulmonary Dysplasia. Clinics in Perinatology. 2015 Dec;42(4):839–55.
18. Krishnan U, Feinstein JA, Adatia I, Austin ED, Mullen MP, Hopper RK, et al. Evaluation and Management of Pulmonary Hypertension in Children with Bronchopulmonary Dysplasia. The Journal of Pediatrics. 2017 Sep;188:24–34.e1.
19. Bhandari A, McGrath-Morrow S. Long-term pulmonary outcomes of patients with bronchopulmonary dysplasia. Seminars in Perinatology. 2013 Apr;37(2):132–7.
20. Homan TD, Nayak RP. Short- and Long-Term Complications of Bronchopulmonary Dysplasia. Respir Care. 2021 Oct;66(10):1618-1629. doi: 10.4187/respcare.08401. PMID: 34552015.

CHAPTER

8

# Airway and Lung Malformations (Other than CDH and TEF)

Malformations of the airway and lung, often arising from defects in bronchopulmonary development, constitute a broad spectrum of abnormalities. Earlier clubbed under a blanket umbrella term of congenital cystic lung diseases, these abnormalities are now categorized based on their pathology.

## TYPES AND PATHOLOGY

1. **Congenital pulmonary airway malformations (CPAM)**, earlier known as congenital cystic adenomatoid malformations (CCAM),[1] are hamartomatous lesions that comprise cystic and adenomatous elements arising from tracheal, bronchial, bronchiolar, or alveolar tissue.
   - CPAMs are more common in the lower lobes. Although the lesions are usually limited to one lobe, they rarely involve multiple lobes. Bilateral involvement is rare.
   - The incidence ranges from 1 per 8300 to 35000 live births.[2] There is no particular etiological factor or causal genetic predisposition.
   - CPAM was classified by Adzick et al. into macrocystic lesions (single or multiple cysts 5.0 mm or larger on ultrasonography) and microcystic lesions (appearing as a solid echogenic mass on sonography)[3].
   - The currently used Stocker classification: (1) Classifies the cysts into five subtypes depending on the tissue from where the cysts[4] originate. The characteristic features are described in Table 8.1.
2. **Bronchopulmonary sequestration** is a rare abnormality arising from the lower airway, occurring in approximately 1 in 10000 to 35000 live births.[5] It consists of a mass of non-functioning lung tissue that lacks a bronchial connection to the native tracheobronchial tree and is supplied by an anomalous systemic

| Table 8.1: Stocker's classification of CPAM and their salient features | | | |
|---|---|---|---|
| *Type* | *Prevalence* | *Origin* | *Salient Features* |
| 0 | 1–3% | Tracheal or bronchial tissue | Rarest form; small cysts (0.5 cm diameter); diffuse—involving the entire lung resulting in impaired gas exchange; most die at birth |
| 1 | 60–70% | Distal bronchi or proximal bronchioles | Most common; well-differentiated tissue within the lesion; thin-walled cyst (2–10 cm diameter); single but rarely multiloculated. The large cyst can cause mass effect and respiratory distress, or fetal hydrops; may have malignant potential. Adjacent lung normal. |
| 2 | 15–20% | Terminal bronchioles | Multiple cysts (0.5–2 cm diameter) with solid areas; resemble extralobar pulmonary sequestration; 60% have associated congenital abnormalities. |
| 3 | 5–10% | Distal airways and acinar | Mixture of solid and cystic areas involving the entire lung with numerous cysts (0.5 cm in diameter). May present with severe cyanosis and respiratory distress resulting in death in the neonatal period. |
| 4 | 5–10% | Alveolar | Large cysts (maximum diameter of 7 cm); variable presentation—asymptomatic, infection, or tension pneumothorax; strongly associated with pleuropulmonary blastoma. |

artery. The vascular supply generally arises from the lower thoracic or upper abdominal aorta. The venous drainage is usually normal (to the left atrium), but abnormal drainage to the right atrium, vena cava, and azygous vein has also been documented. Various subtypes described are:

- **Intralobar sequestration (ILS) (75%):** It is incorporated into the surrounding normal lung and lacks visceral pleura. Approximately 60% of ILS involve the left lower lobe, the majority in the posterior basal segment. It may rarely have an abnormal connection to the bronchial tree, leading to repeated infections.
- **Extralobar sequestration (ELS) (25%):** It is located outside the normal lung and has its visceral pleura. Occasionally, it is located below the diaphragm (13–15%). ELS is more likely to occur in males and is associated with other congenital anomalies. Most ELS involves the left hemithorax.

- **Hybrid BPS/CPAM lesions:** Hybrid lesions have histologic CPAM features and blood supply from a systemic artery and have been reported in a substantial proportion (28–50%) of cases of BPS.[5,6]
- **Bronchopulmonary foregut malformation:** This term is usually used to refer to a rare variant of sequestration in which the sequestered lung tissue is connected to the gastrointestinal tract, which may occur in either ILS or ELS.

3. **Congenital lobar emphysema** is characterized by hyperinflation of one or more pulmonary lobes. With a prevalence of 1 in 20000 to 30000 live births, it is found more commonly in males. It occurs due to a disruption in the bronchopulmonary development, which leads to an abnormal bronchus creating a "ball-valve" mechanism, in which a greater volume of air enters the affected lobe during inspiration than leaves during expiration, producing air trapping. The bronchus may be affected by intrinsic, extrinsic, or intraluminal causes. The left upper lobe is commonly affected (40–50%), followed by the right middle (25–35%), right upper (20%), and lower lobes (2–10%).[7] Pathologically they range from simple, uniformly enlarged distal airways and airspaces to a polyalveolar form, lacking proper emphysematous changes.
4. **Bronchogenic cysts** arise from anomalous budding of the foregut during development and represent part of the spectrum of bronchopulmonary foregut malformations. They can occur at any location in the tracheobronchial tree.
5. **Other airway and lung malformations** include tracheomalacia, bronchomalacia, and rare abnormalities such as tracheal atresia, tracheal bronchus, congenital tracheal stenosis, bronchial atresia, and stenosis.

## CLINICAL PRESENTATION

1. **Antenatal**
   - CPAM may be detected antenatally as a cystic lesion. It is evaluated using MRI, and CPAM Volume Ratio (CVR) can be calculated to predict the outcome. CVR is estimated by the formula for the volume of a prolate ellipse and normalizing it for gestational age by dividing by the head circumference.[8] Severe forms with CVR > 1.6 may progress to fetal hydrops. Fetuses with values >1 have been shown to require respiratory support and early resection.[9] Spontaneous resolution has been noted to occur in CPAM.

- BPS generally presents as a solid appearing lesion in the lower hemithorax. It may be difficult or impossible to distinguish from microcystic CPAM unless a systemic arterial feeder can be identified. The outcome can range from spontaneous resolution to hydrops.

2. **Postnatal**
   - CPAM may either be asymptomatic (75%) or present with respiratory distress in the neonatal period. Those with higher CVR and antenatally detected mediastinal shift, polyhydramnios, or ascites are at increased risk of developing respiratory distress after birth. The severity of postnatal presentation also depends on the type of lesion, as described in Table 9.1. Those detected outside the neonatal period (1/3rd of all cases) generally present with recurrent pulmonary infections.
   - Neonates with large BPS may be symptomatic at birth. Rarely, it results in high-output cardiac failure if the lesion causes an excess flow through it, creating a left-to-right shunt. Other BPS may either remain asymptomatic or present with infection or hemoptysis after the neonatal period.
   - Neonates affected with CLE usually are symptomatic in the neonatal period, with 25–33% of cases presenting at birth, 50% by one month, and remaining by six months of age. Like in other cystic lesions, severity depends on the size of the affected lobe and the extent of the mediastinal shift. Milder forms may present with poor feeding, failure to thrive, and recurrent LRTI.
   - Bronchogenic cyst generally presents during childhood with cough, pneumonia, and wheezing; however, neonates with a rapidly enlarging cyst located centrally may present with respiratory distress, cyanosis, and poor feeding.
3. Other congenital anomalies are often associated and should be looked for during evaluation. Detailed family history of any cancers or cystic lesions should be obtained.

## MANAGEMENT

1. **When to Suspect?**
   A high index of suspicion at birth must be kept in those without an antenatal diagnosis in the presence of any of the following:
   - Sudden onset respiratory distress with cyanosis.

- Respiratory distress presenting after birth and gradually worsening.
- Respiratory distress in a child with other congenital anomalies.

2. **How to Investigate?**
   - Antenatal diagnosis is usually made with USG and further confirmed with MRI.
   - All neonates with an antenatal diagnosis need to be evaluated postnatally with radiological imaging, even if the lesion was noted to be prenatally resolved.
   - Chest X-ray is the first investigation to be performed in these neonates.
   - Advanced imaging with computed tomography or MRI may be required in some neonates; however, this can be deferred to the post-neonatal period in asymptomatic neonates. The investigations for each lesion and specific findings are mentioned in Table 8.2.
   - It has been recommended to perform imaging immediately in symptomatic neonates. If antenatally detected CPAM is asymptomatic and without any risk factors,[10] such as large cysts, bilateral or multifocal lesions, or family history of cancer,[6] definite imaging like CT scan can be delayed till 3–6 months of age.
3. **Management Strategies**
   - Resection and surgical excision of the lung lesion is the treatment of choice in symptomatic cases. It may be needed to be performed on an emergency basis in some neonates.
   - Lobectomy is the surgery of choice for CPAM, CLE, and ILS; ELS can be treated with simple excision. Bronchogenic cysts are managed by excision of cysts or partial/total lobectomy.[11]
   - An intercostal drainage tube is often placed post-operatively in most neonates.
   - Minimally invasive surgery has low complications and may be preferred, if possible.
   - In asymptomatic neonates, immediate surgery vs. observation is decided based on the following considerations:
     - Early surgical resection is advocated if the neonate has high-risk features: Large lesion, bilateral or multifocal involvement, family history of cancer, or development of pneumothorax.

**Table 8.2: Radiological investigations and the appearance of cystic lesions of the airway**

| *Lesion type* | *Chest X-ray* | *Computed tomography* | *Other additional imaging/ investigations* |
|---|---|---|---|
| CPAM | • Type 1 and 4 CCAMs show evidence of large air and fluid-filled cysts.<br>• Type 2 cysts are smaller giving a "bubbly" appearance.<br>• Type 3 CCAMs may appear as a more solid space-occupying lesion.<br>• Mediastinal shift, ipsilateral lung hypoplasia seen in all. | • Often correlates well with pathological findings<br>• Confirms complete regression of an antenatally detected but resolved lesion<br>• Identify additional microcystic surrounding area | MRI |
| CLE | • Distension of the affected lobe.<br>• Asymmetry in parenchymal translucency with hyperlucent zone.<br>• Mediastinal shift.<br>• Compression and atelectasis of the contralateral lung.<br>• Diaphragm appears flattened.<br>• Opacified lobe (immediately after birth). | • Helps confirm diagnosis and identify the source of airway obstruction | • MRI<br>• Angiography: To demonstrate any vascular causes<br>• Echocardiography |

(*Contd.*)

**Table 8.2: Radiological investigations and the appearance of cystic lesions of the airway (*Contd.*)**

| *Lesion type* | *Chest X-ray* | *Computed tomography* | *Other additional imaging/ investigations* |
|---|---|---|---|
| BPS | • Uniformly dense mass within the thoracic cavity.<br>• Cystic areas within the mass (recurrent infection) +/– air-fluid levels.<br>• Usually lower lobes. | • Variable appearance, homogenous/ heterogenous solid mass with cystic changes<br>• Cystic mass with air-fluid levels<br>• Emphysematous changes at the margin<br>• Aberrant systemic artery | • MRI<br>• MR/CT angiography: for aberrant systemic supply<br>• USG Doppler |
| Bronchogenic cyst | • Round cystic +/– air-fluid levels (associated with previous or current infection). | • Well marginated cystic mediastinal mass<br>• Soft tissue or water attenuation | |

   - In a low-risk neonate, imaging is often performed after 3 months with a plan of delayed elective surgical excision, usually by 6–12 months of age. Practices vary among centres, and there is no consensus on the optimal timing of resection.[12] Early resection has the advantage of allowing more time for the remaining lung to undergo compensatory hypertrophy. On the other hand, some advocate delayed resection because a few lesions undergo spontaneous resolution, and older children tolerate general anaesthesia better than young infants.
   - A small extra lobar sequestration can be considered for observation alone.
   - Conservative management may be considered in infants with CLE with no or minimal symptoms but is usually not recommended.
- The risk of malignant degeneration in almost all forms of congenital cystic abnormalities should be explained to parents before initiating observational management.

### Complications if Untreated

1. Risk of infection.
2. Association with malignancy.
   a. Pleuropulmonary blastoma
   b. Bronchoalveolar carcinoma
3. Sudden hemorrhage/rupture of a tense bronchogenic cyst.
4. Cardiac failure due to shunting from the aberrant systemic vessel in BPS.
5. Sudden respiratory decompensation during intubation and positive pressure ventilation in CLE (often requiring urgent thoracotomy to decompress).

## FOLLOW-UP AND OUTCOMES

Operated infants are called once during the early postoperative period—usually after two weeks—to examine the wound and check for any other complaints; subsequent follow-up is less frequent to watch for any complications or recurrence. Those waiting for surgery are followed up on an elective basis and started on hematinics pre-operatively.

Generally, favorable outcomes are expected with excellent survival in most neonates; however, the prognosis depends on several factors:

- Antenatally detected cases that develop hydrops could have a fatal outcome.
- Compared to other histopathological variants, a better prognosis is noted for type 1 CPAM lesions. The other types may have a fatal outcome during the neonatal period and may develop pulmonary hypertension due to hypoplasia of the contralateral lung.
- The absence of other congenital abnormalities is another factor that portends a good outcome.
- The extent of lung resection also has a role in determining long-term pulmonary outcomes.

There is a compensatory hypertrophy of the remaining lung parenchyma, which leads to near-normal pulmonary function in many neonates. Almost 50–80% have a normal pulmonary function test; some patients may have mildly impaired exercise tolerance.[13] Thoracotomy may be associated long-term complications such as the development of winging of the scapula, abnormality of the breast bud, and development of scoliosis and other thoracic deformities.

## REFERENCES

1. Stocker JT. Congenital pulmonary airway malformation - a new name for and an expanded classification of congenital cystic adenomatoid malformation of the lung. Histopathology 2002;41(Suppl2):424–30.
2. Gornall AS, Budd JLS, Draper ES, Konje JC, Kurinczuk JJ. Congenital cystic adenomatoid malformation: accuracy of prenatal diagnosis, prevalence and outcome in a general population. Prenat Diagn 2003;23:997–1002. https://doi.org/10.1002/PD.739.
3. Adzick NS, Harrison MR, Crombleholme TM, Flake AW, Howell LJ. Fetal lung lesions: management and outcome. Am J Obstet Gynecol 1998;179:884–9. https://doi.org/10.1016/S0002–9378(98)70183–8.
4. Priest JR, Williams GM, Hill DA, Dehner LP, Jaffé A. Pulmonary cysts in early childhood and the risk of malignancy. Pediatr Pulmonol 2009;44:14–30. https://doi.org/10.1002/PPUL.20917.
5. Durell J, Thakkar H, Gould S, Fowler D, Lakhoo K. Pathology of asymptomatic, prenatally diagnosed cystic lung malformations. J Pediatr Surg 2016;51:231–5. https://doi.org/10.1016/J.JPEDSURG.2015.10.061.
6. Conran RM, Stocker JT. Extralobar sequestration with frequently associated congenital cystic adenomatoid malformation, type 2: report of 50 cases. Pediatr Dev Pathol 1999;2:454–63. https://doi.org/10.1007/S100249900149.
7. Shanti CM, Klein MD. Cystic lung disease. Semin Pediatr Surg 2008;17:2–8. https://doi.org/10.1053/J.SEMPEDSURG.2007.10.002.
8. Crombleholme TM, Coleman B, Hedrick H, Liechty K, Howell L, Flake AW, et al. Cystic adenomatoid malformation volume ratio predicts outcome in

prenatally diagnosed cystic adenomatoid malformation of the lung. J Pediatr Surg 2002;37:331–8. https://doi.org/10.1053/jpsu.2002.30832.
9. Ehrenberg-Buchner S, Stapf AM, Berman DR, Drongowski RA, Mychaliska GB, Treadwell MC, et al. Fetal lung lesions: can we start to breathe easier? Am J Obstet Gynecol 2013;208:151.e1-151.e7. https://doi.org/10.1016/J.AJOG.2012.11.012.
10. Priest JR, Williams GM, Hill DA, Dehner LP, Jaffé A. Pulmonary cysts in early childhood and the risk of malignancy. Pediatr Pulmonol 2009;44:14–30. https://doi.org/10.1002/PPUL.20917.
11. Choudhury SR, Chadha R, Mishra A, Kumar V, Singh V, Dubey NK. Lung resections in children for congenital and acquired lesions. Pediatr Surg Int 2007;23:851–9. https://doi.org/10.1007/S00383–007–1940–8.
12. Jelin EB, O'Hare EM, Jancelewicz T, Nasr I, Boss E, Rhee DS. Optimal timing for elective resection of asymptomatic congenital pulmonary airway malformations. J Pediatr Surg 2018;53:1001–5. https://doi.org/10.1016/J.JPEDSURG.2018.02.032.
13. Hijkoop A, van Schoonhoven MM, van Rosmalen J, Tibboel D, van der Cammen-van Zijp MHM, Pijnenburg MW, et al. Lung function, exercise tolerance, and physical growth of children with congenital lung malformations at 8 years of age. Pediatr Pulmonol 2019;54:1326–34. https://doi.org/10.1002/PPUL.24345.

CHAPTER

9

# Persistent Pulmonary Hypertension of the Newborn

Successful adaptation to extra-uterine life involves a rapid fall in pulmonary vascular resistance at birth and a simultaneous increase in pulmonary blood flow. Failure of this normal circulatory transition leads to elevated pulmonary vascular resistance resulting in right-to-left shunting of blood and hypoxemia. Persistent pulmonary hypertension of the newborn (PPHN) is a cardiopulmonary disorder characterized by high pulmonary vascular resistance and systemic arterial hypoxemia. The incidence of PPHN is around 2 per 1000 live *births*[1] and is associated with mortality ranging from 5–30%.

## ETIOLOGY

- **Primary or idiopathic PPHN:** Remodeled or mal-developed pulmonary vasculature due to in-utero fetal stress, hypoxia, premature closure of ductus due to maternal nonsteroidal anti-inflammatory drug (NSAID) exposure. The pulmonary parenchyma is normal and appears black in X-ray—"black lung" PPHN.
- **Secondary PPHN:** It is secondary to parenchymal lung diseases such as meconium aspiration syndrome, respiratory distress syndrome (RDS), pneumonia, or sepsis. It can also be due to lung hypoplasia due to prolonged oligohydramnios or congenital diaphragmatic hernia (hypoplastic pulmonary vasculature). It is more common than primary PPHN.

## ASSESSMENT

PPHN should be suspected in any neonate with respiratory distress complicated by labile oxygen saturations, severe hypoxia, and differential cyanosis. One should differentiate PPHN from congenital cyanotic heart disease in all such cases. Evaluation should include history, physical examination, simultaneous pre- and post-ductal oxygen saturation measurements, chest radiography, and arterial blood gas analyses. Echocardiography is used to confirm the diagnosis (Table 9.1).

| Table 9.1: History and clinical examination findings in PPHN |
|---|
| **History**<br>1. Severe or prolonged oligo-hydramnios or premature rupture of membranes in early gestation: Pulmonary hypoplasia.<br>2. Absent or decreased fetal movements or non-reactive fetal heart rate: Fetal hypoxia or acidosis.<br>3. Prolonged fetal bradycardia and marked anemia: Twin-twin transfusion syndrome, hemolysis, feto-maternal or fetoplacental hemorrhage.<br>4. History of maternal drug intake like aspirin, nonsteroidal anti-inflammatory drugs (NSAIDs), selective serotonin reuptake inhibitors (SSRIs), and lithium<br>5. Premature or prolonged rupture of membranes, maternal chorioamnionitis: Neonatal sepsis/pneumonia.<br>6. Findings of antenatal ultrasound: Congenital diaphragmatic hernia, congenital pulmonary airway malformations (CPAM), congenital heart disease. |
| **Events at delivery**<br>1. Need for positive pressure ventilation: Pneumothorax.<br>2. Need for resuscitation, including chest compression: Perinatal asphyxia.<br>3. Meconium-stained liquor: Meconium aspiration syndrome. |
| **Physical examination**<br>1. *Clinical findings:* Labile oxygen saturations (fluctuating saturations with handling or agitation) and oxygen requirement out of proportion to lung disease and differential cyanosis ($SpO_2$ that is 5–10% higher in the right arm than in post-ductal limbs).<br>2. *Respiratory system:* Tachypnea with cyanosis without retractions (or respiratory distress) points to congenital cyanotic heart disease or idiopathic PPHN, whereas presence of retractions, grunting or nasal flaring suggest pulmonary parenchymal disease.<br>3. *Cardiovascular system:* Single S2, which can be loud; systolic murmur of tricuspid regurgitation (tricuspid regurgitation associated with PPHN or because of asphyxial myocardial dysfunction). BP of four limbs should be taken to determine aortic obstruction (coarctation, interrupted aortic arch). |

(*Contd.*)

**Table 9.1: History and clinical examination findings in PPHN** *(Contd.)*

**Pulse-oximeter**

- Pre-ductal $SpO_2$ greater than post-ductal $SpO_2$ by 10% or more indicates increased shunting of blood from the pulmonary artery to descending aorta through PDA due to higher pulmonary vascular resistance (compared to systemic circulation).
- Absence of pre-post ductal $SpO_2$ difference does not rule out PPHN. It may be due to R->L shunting occurring at the atrial level (patent foramen ovale) or intra-pulmonary shunting alone or because the ductus is closed.

**Chest X-ray**

- Findings depend on the underlying condition. Patchy infiltrates in pneumonia, heterogenous opacity with localized hyperinflation in MAS, diffuse homogenous ground glass appearance in RDS.
- If the severity of the hypoxemia is out of proportion to the CXR findings, one might be dealing with idiopathic or "black lung PPHN" (lung fields appear oligemic due to poor pulmonary blood flow) or it can be cyanotic heart disease.
- Abnormal cardiac silhouette in cyanotic heart disease.

**Other investigations**

a. Arterial blood gas analysis for pH, $PCO_2$, $HCO_3$, BE and lactate levels. Pre-post ductal $PaO_2$ difference > 20 mmHg can be noted in PPHN.

b. Hyperoxia test: This test helps to determine whether heart disease is a likely etiology in the infant with cyanosis and can be useful in centers where echocardiography is not available. A rise in $PaO_2$ >80 to 120 mm Hg above baseline or an absolute $PaO_2$ >150 mmHg after 100% oxygen administration suggests that cyanotic CHD is unlikely. $PaO_2$ <50 mmHg in 100% oxygen is highly suggestive of cyanotic CHD, whereas $PaO_2$ between 50 and 150 mmHg with 100% oxygen administration necessitates further evaluation.

c. Oxygenation index $(MAP \times FiO_2)/(PaO_2 \times 100)$: Oxygenation index > 15 despite adequate lung recruitment suggests a severe failure of oxygenation; $AaDO_2$ > 200 is also considered abnormal.

d. Complete blood count, sepsis screen, and blood culture to rule out infection.

*(Contd.)*

**Table 9.1: History and clinical examination findings in PPHN** *(Contd.)*

**Echocardiography**

Echocardiography is the gold standard investigation. Initial echo should be done in a stepwise approach which should include.

- Step 1: Ruling out congenital heart disease by confirming the situs, origin of great arteries and venous return.
- Step 2: Confirming the presence and severity of PPHN by documenting increased pulmonary artery pressure (30–60 mm Hg). It can be calculated from the tricuspid regurgitation (TR) jet. In cases where a TR jet may not be seen due to poor right ventricular contractility, interventricular septum configuration and LV systolic eccentricity index can be informative. Along with these the direction of shunt through PDA and PFO provide useful information.
- Step 3: To look for right or left or biventricular dysfunction which seen by tricuspid annular plane systolic excursion (TAPSE) and fractional area change (FAC) for RV and fractional shortening (FS) or ejection fraction (EF) for LV.

Echocardiography also helps to serially evaluate the pulmonary vascular pressures once pulmonary vasodilatory therapies are instituted. If the response to inhaled nitric oxide is sub-optimal, echocardiography helps to rule out CHD and to evaluate LV dysfunction.

## MANAGEMENT

Early recognition of PPHN and initiation of therapy are vital to prevent worsening, and management starts in the delivery room itself. In neonates with significant antenatal risk factors, delivery room resuscitation should focus on optimal lung recruitment and ventilation. Supplemental oxygen should be administered guided by a preductal pulse oximeter in the range recommended by the neonatal resuscitation program. Hypothermia, hypoxia, and hyperoxia should be avoided. Postnatal management of PPHN involves supportive care—eliminating factors exacerbating pulmonary vasoconstriction, improving oxygenation with oxygen therapy, and ensuring adequate lung recruitment—and using specific pulmonary vasodilator therapy.

**Supportive care** is as crucial as other therapies in a neonate with PPHN. It involves.

- Maintenance of normothermia.
- Avoidance of stress—minimal and gentle handling and nursing in quiet surroundings with low noise and direct lighting. Some neonates may require sedation as agitation can aggravate hypoxia.
- Optimal nutrition—intravenous nutrition and correction of hypoglycemia, hypocalcemia, and acidosis
- Maintenance of adequate intravascular volume and systemic blood pressure using fluids and inotropes. Blood pressures should be maintained in the normal range because the right to left shunt size depends partly on systemic BP. An invasive arterial line should be in place for continuous blood pressure monitoring and blood gas analysis.

Muscle paralysis is associated with increased mortality, while alkali infusion is associated with an increased need for extracorporeal membrane oxygenation and should be avoided.

**Improving oxygenation:** The underlying lung condition should be managed appropriately. The spectrum of PPHN varies from mild hypoxia to severe labile hypoxia with cardiovascular collapse. Some neonates may need only oxygen and non-invasive ventilation, while others require invasive mechanical ventilation with adequate MAP. The optimal saturation target in the management of PPHN is unclear. Both hypoxia and hyperoxia are deleterious. A preductal saturation target of 91–95% is recommended during acute PPHN management, and $FiO_2$ is best adjusted based on preductal $SpO_2$.[2]

Similarly, arterial oxygen tension from the preductal site (preductal $PaO_2$) has better utility as it dictates oxygen delivery to the cerebral and coronary circulation. The target preductal $PaO_2$ is between 50–80 mmHg. Blood gases from umbilical arterial lines provide post-ductal $PaO_2$ and could be at least 10–20 mm Hg lower than preductal values in severe PPHN with labile hypoxemia with ductal shunts.

**Ventilatory strategies** should provide adequate lung recruitment and maintenance of FRC because both atelectasis and over-distension result in hypoxemia and acidosis. Gentle ventilation strategies with optimal PEEP, relatively low PIP, and some permissive hypercapnia are recommended with a target pH of 7.25–7.35 and $PCO_2$ of 40–50 mm Hg. Hyperventilation (risk of sensorineural hearing loss and impaired cerebral perfusion) and alkalosis (higher risk of mortality and ECMO use) are harmful and should be avoided.[3] In PPHN associated with pulmonary parenchymal involvement like RDS and MAS, lung recruitment is better achieved with high-frequency ventilation (HFV), and the combination of HFV with inhaled nitric oxide (NO) works better than either therapy alone.[4] Early surfactant therapy for late preterm or term infants with parenchymal lung disease (meconium aspiration syndrome and RDS) and PPHN is associated with a 3-fold reduction in the risk of ECMO and death.[5] Benzodiazepines (except in extremely preterm neonates) such as midazolam and opioid analgesics like morphine or fentanyl can be judiciously used in neonates on mechanical ventilation.

## Cardiovascular Support

PPHN can be associated with systemic hypotension. If the cardiac function is good, fluid bolus (10 ml/kg normal saline) followed by vasopressors like dopamine, nor-epinephrine, or vasopressin can be considered. If the blood pressure is normal with evidence of LV dysfunction, an inodilator such as milrinone is considered (Table 9.2). Hypotension with cardiac dysfunction is associated with high mortality.

**Pulmonary vasodilator therapy:** PPHN is associated with an impaired balance between vasodilators (NO and prostacyclin) and constrictors (endothelin-1) of the pulmonary vasculature. Selective pulmonary vasodilation without affecting systemic circulation improves pulmonary blood flow and oxygenation. Such therapies should be initiated only after adequate lung recruitment. Examples of pulmonary vasodilators include inhaled nitric oxide and sildenafil, which act via the cGMP pathway; prostacyclin and milrinone, which act via the cAMP pathway; bosentan, an endothelial receptor antagonist; and arginine vasopressin[6] (Table 9.1).

## Inhaled Nitric Oxide (NO)

Inhaled NO causes selective pulmonary vasodilation without effects on systemic circulation (it gets inactivated after combining with hemoglobin to form methemoglobin). It also has a micro-selective effect because it preferentially enters well-ventilated alveoli, thereby improving V/Q matching.

**Evidence for the use of inhaled nitric oxide in PPHN**

In term and near-term infants with hypoxemic respiratory failure with evidence of pulmonary hypertension, inhaled nitric oxide improves oxygenation and reduces the combined outcome of death and the need for ECMO. The improved outcome is mainly because of the reduction in ECMO (RR 0.63, 95% CI 0.54, 0.75) rather than a reduction in mortality. The OI drops by an average of 15 points within 30 and 60 minutes of administration, and $PaO_2$ increases by about 50 mmHg.[7]

**Indications for use:** NO should be initiated in term and near-term infants with severe hypoxemic respiratory failure, i.e. OI of 25 or more when the risk of requiring ECMO or mortality is 50%. Both idiopathic and secondary PPHN show improvement with NO.

### *Role of NO in Preterm Infants and CDH*

Use of NO in preterm neonates early in life for BPD prevention or later for those at higher risk of BPD is not recommended.[8] In preterm infants with severe hypoxemia secondary to PPHN physiology or pulmonary hypoplasia, using NO resulted in better oxygenation as measured by $PaO_2$ and oxygenation index. A therapeutic trial can be considered in selected preterm infants with severe hypoxemia without alternative therapeutic options. Clinical decision-making should be guided by echocardiography, prior experience and physiologic rationale. Although NO therapy has not been shown to reduce mortality or ECMO requirement in infants with CDH, it may still have a role in stabilizing some infants by improving oxygenation temporarily. It thus may act as a bridge before ECMO or surgery.

**Contraindications:** NO is contraindicated in congenital heart disease with duct-dependent systemic circulation like hypoplastic left heart syndrome or interrupted aortic arch where pulmonary vasodilatation further compromises systemic blood flow. Other contraindications include severe left ventricular dysfunction (NO therapy can increase the risk of pulmonary edema), severe congenital methemoglobinemia, intracranial hemorrhage, and life-threatening congenital malformations.

**Timing of therapy:** Starting NO early when the OI is between 15 and 25 has been shown to improve oxygenation without reducing the need for ECMO or mortality. Some recommend NO therapy when OI is ≥20 on at least two occasions. While we generally initiate therapy when OI is 25, it is relaxed to OI ≥20 on a case-by-case basis. While echocardiography confirms the presence of PPHN, the absence of echocardiographic findings or the inability to perform it should not preclude the initiation of NO therapy (Fig. 9.1). The presence or absence of echocardiographic evidence of PPHN does not seem to affect response to NO.[6]

**Dosage:** NO is started at 20 parts per million (ppm) when OI is approximately 20, and the response is demonstrated by an increase in the $PaO_2$ of 20 mm Hg or more (20-20-20 rule) (Fig. 9.2). Higher doses (up to 80 ppm) are associated with a greater risk of adverse effects like methemoglobinemia and produce minimal improvement in oxygenation.

**Response:** Up to two-thirds of neonates with PPHN respond and demonstrate an average drop in OI by 15 points within 30 to 60 minutes after initiation of NO therapy. Such a response is sustained for at least 24 hours or longer. Complete responders demonstrate an increase in $PaO_2$ of >20 mm Hg after 30 minutes of NO (at 20 ppm), and partial and non-responders show a $PaO_2$ increment of 10–20 mm Hg and < 10 mm Hg, respectively.

**Poor response:** Almost 40% of infants with PPHN do not respond upfront or fail to sustain a response to NO. These infants require echocardiography to assess LV dysfunction and rule out congenital heart disease (if not done earlier). Lack of adequate lung recruitment may impede NO from reaching the alveoli, thus contributing to poor response. Obtain a CXR, optimize PEEP, and consider using high-frequency ventilation or surfactant in such neonates. If there is still a poor response, one may add other pulmonary vasodilators (see below) if the neonate is hemodynamically stable. ECMO is considered the next therapeutic option, which may be needed in up to 20% of neonates receiving NO therapy.

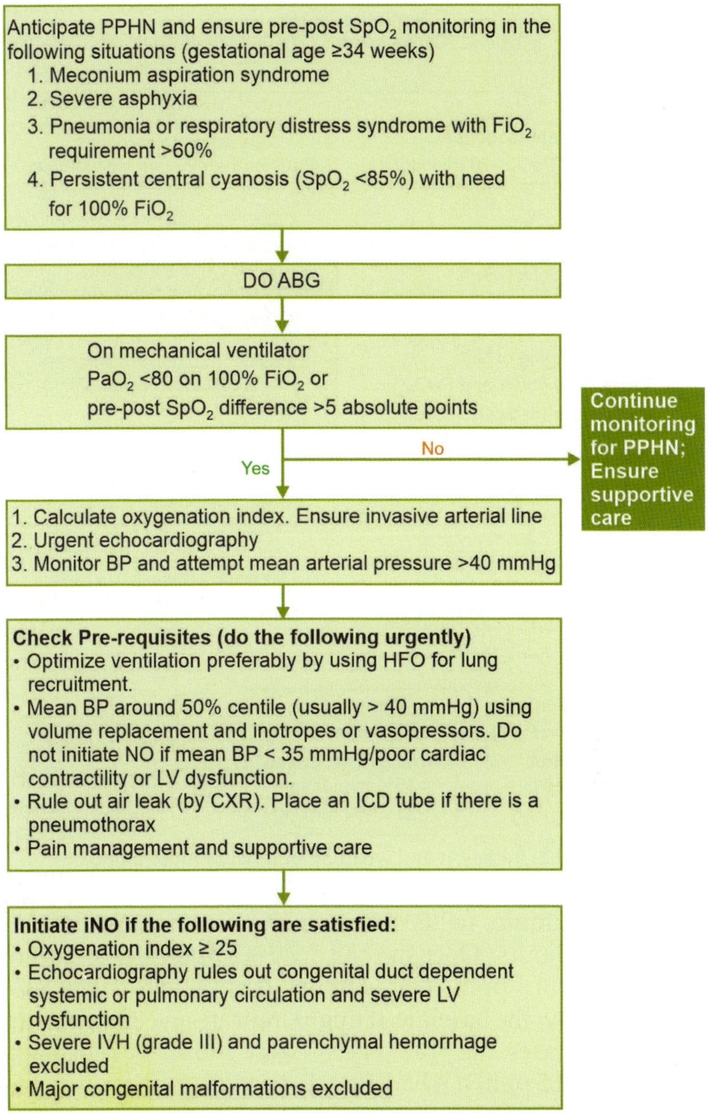


**Fig. 9.1:** Patient selection for INO therapy

**Weaning:** Weaning should be gradual to prevent a rebound increase in pulmonary vasoconstriction associated with the sudden withdrawal of NO therapy. $FiO_2$ is the first to be weaned, and once it is below 60%, NO is weaned only if $PaO_2$ can be maintained at 60 mmHg or higher (corresponding preductal oxygen saturation

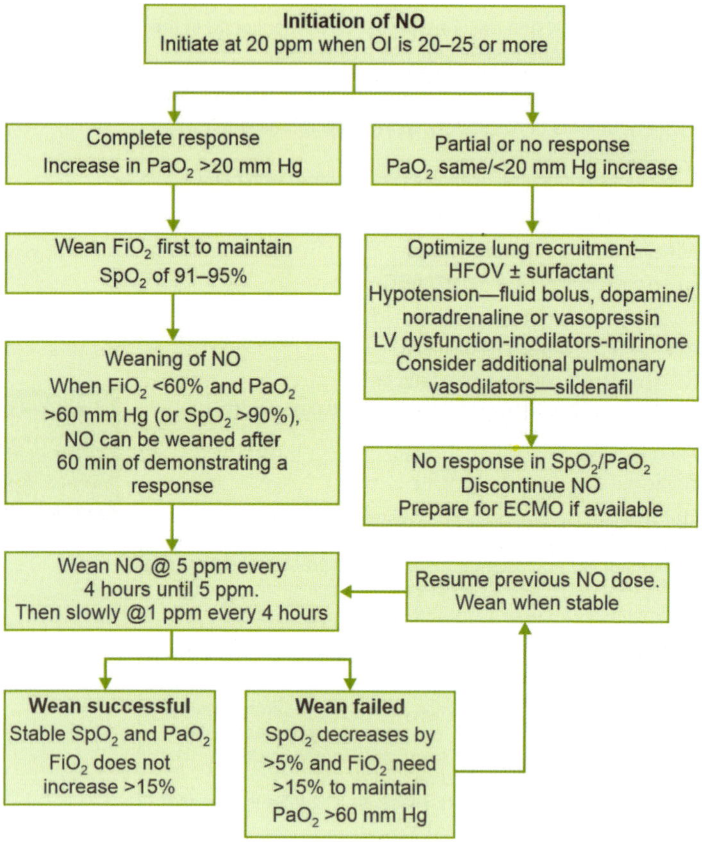


**Fig. 9.2:** Initiation and weaning of inhaled nitric oxide

≥90%) for 60 minutes (60-60-60 rule). NO is weaned at the rate of 5 ppm every 4 hours. Once the NO dose is 5 ppm, further weaning is done slowly at 1 ppm every 4 hours. If $SpO_2$ falls below 85% or drops 10% below the baseline, it might indicate an NO dependency state. In these cases, the previous NO dose should be reinstated or NO restarted at 5 ppm if it had already been discontinued and $FiO_2$ increased by 15%. Subsequent weaning attempts should be slow and not earlier than 4 hours. After two failed weaning attempts, the patient is allowed to stabilize for 12 hours before attempting weaning again.

**Duration of therapy:** The typical duration of NO therapy has been 5 days, which parallels the clinical resolution of PPHN. Sometimes, a longer duration may be required, like in infants with pulmonary hypoplasia. If NO is required for > 5 days, investigations into other causes of pulmonary artery hypertension must be considered, especially if discontinuation results in supra-systemic elevations of pulmonary arterial pressures by echocardiography. The maximum cumulative therapy duration reported in studies is around 14 days.

**Side effects:** These include platelet dysfunction, methemoglobinemia, and the production of toxic byproducts such as nitrates.

- Methemoglobinemia resulting from the reaction of NO with hemoglobin has not been reported at lower doses of NO (< 20 ppm). If the levels are 5%, wean NO by 50%; if levels are > 10%, then NO should be temporarily discontinued. Methemoglobin levels are monitored at 2 hours, 8 hours after initiation, and then once a day during NO therapy.
- NO combines with oxygen to form nitrogen dioxide ($NO_2$), a toxic gas. The safe upper limit of $NO_2$ is 3 ppm. If the levels are more than 3 ppm, the dose of iNO should be reduced by 50%; iNO should be temporarily stopped if $NO_2$ >7 ppm.
- Theoretical risks of platelet dysfunction and bleeding problems. Monitor platelet count.

Nitrogen dioxide and NO levels are continuously monitored by NO delivery apparatus using electrochemical cells, while methemoglobin can be monitored by co-oximetry in blood gas analysers.

**Resource availability:** The American Academy of Pediatrics recommends that centers using NO therapy have expertise and experience in multimodal respiratory support and on-site ECMO capability. Centers offering NO therapy without an ECMO facility should collaborate with an ECMO center for timely transfer (without interruption of NO therapy) in case of treatment failure. Centers should follow a formal protocol approved by the institution, obtain parental consent before initiating therapy, and have a system to collect patient data prospectively. They should also provide long-term neurodevelopmental follow-up and early interventional services.

## OTHER DRUGS

If iNO is ineffective or unavailable, other pulmonary vasodilators such as sildenafil, milrinone, or inhaled/intravenous prostacyclin analogs can be considered. The mechanism of action, indications, dosage, and evidence of two commonly used drugs—sildenafil and milrinone—are summarized in Table 9.1.

**Table 9.1: Mechanism of action, dosage, and indications for sildenafil and milrinone**

| *Drug mechanism of action* | *Dosage* | *Evidence* |
|---|---|---|
| **Sildenafil**<br>Selective phosphodiesterase-5 inhibitor; acting via cGMP, it enhances NO-mediated vascular relaxation.<br>**Indications**<br>• iNO not available.<br>• Stable blood pressure and good ventricular function but hypoxemia persists despite NO.<br>• It can be used as an adjuvant to facilitate the weaning of NO in patients with persistent or rebound pulmonary hypertension. | **Continuous IV infusion**<br>• Loading dose: 0.4 mg/kg administered over 3 hours to minimize the risk of hypotension<br>• Maintenance dose: 1.6 mg/kg/day as continuous IV infusion for up to 7 days<br>Oral: 1–2 mg/kg/dose every 6 hours.<br>Sildenafil is metabolized by the liver and severe hepatic dysfunction may impair its metabolism. | Sildenafil decreases mortality and improves oxygenation in neonates, especially in resource-limited settings where NO and ECMO is unavailable. |
| **Milrinone**<br>Phosphodiesterase-3 inhibitor and acts via cAMP to cause arterial smooth muscle relaxation.<br>It has inotropic and lusitropic effects on myocardium, and improves ventricular function directly and by decreasing afterload.<br>**Indications**<br>PPHN with LV dysfunction (left to right shunt at atrial level but right to left shunt at ductal level). | **Continuous IV infusion**<br>**Dose:** 0.33 to 1 μg/kg/ min.<br>It can cause hypotension and its elimination is impaired in renal impairment requiring dose adjustment. | It has an additive effect with NO therapy. |

## PROGNOSIS

With improved therapy, the mortality for PPHN has been reduced to less than 10% in tertiary care centers. Studies have shown that among PPHN survivors followed up till 18–24 months, 24% and 26% had a hearing and neuro-developmental impairment, respectively. These data demonstrate a need for close follow-up of these infants after discharge.

## REFERENCES

1. Singh Y, Lakshminrusimha S. Pathophysiology and Management of Persistent Pulmonary Hypertension of the Newborn. Clin Perinatol. 2021;48(3):595–618.
2. Chandrasekharan P, Rawat M, Lakshminrusimha S. How Do We Monitor Oxygenation during the Management of PPHN? Alveolar, Arterial, Mixed Venous Oxygen Tension, or Peripheral Saturation? Children (Basel). 2020;7(10):180.
3. Kinsella JP, Truog WE, Walsh WF, Goldberg RN, Bancalari E, Mayock DE, et al. Randomized, multicenter trial of inhaled nitric oxide and high-frequency oscillatory ventilation in severe, persistent pulmonary hypertension of the newborn. J Pediatr. 1997;131(1 Pt 1):55–62.
4. Konduri GG, Sokol GM, Van Meurs KP, Singer J, Ambalavanan N, Lee T et al. Impact of early surfactant and inhaled nitric oxide therapies on outcomes in term/late preterm neonates with moderate hypoxic respiratory failure. J Perinatol. 2013;33(12):944–9.
5. Fuloria M, Aschner JL. Persistent pulmonary hypertension of the newborn. Semin Fetal Neonatal Med. 2017;22(4):220–226.
6. Konduri GG, Kim UO. Advances in the diagnosis and management of persistent pulmonary hypertension of the newborn. Pediatr Clin North Am. 2009;56(3):579–600.
7. Barrington KJ, Finer N, Pennaforte T, Altit G. Nitric oxide for respiratory failure in infants born at or near term. Cochrane Database Syst Rev. 2017;1(1):CD000399.
8. Barrington KJ, Finer N, Pennaforte T. Inhaled nitric oxide for respiratory failure in preterm infants. Cochrane Database Syst Rev. 2017;1(1):CD000509.

Section

5

# Gastrointestinal and Hepatobiliary Tract and Nutrition

CHAPTER

10

# Feeding of Neonates with Umbilical Artery Doppler Abnormalities

Umbilical Doppler flow abnormalities occur in 6% of high-risk pregnancies.[1] Preterm neonates born with abnormalities in the umbilical artery Doppler waveforms, such as absent end-diastolic flow (AEDF) or reversed end-diastolic flow (REDF), are at risk of complications related to enteral feeding, including feed intolerance and necrotizing enterocolitis (NEC).[2] The complications result in undue delay in the initiation and progression of enteral feeds in such infants, thereby prolonging the time to reach full enteral feeds and the hospital stay.

## ENTERAL FEEDING IN INFANTS WITH AREDF

Fetal hypoxia and increased vascular resistance in the mesenteric circulation result in hypoxic-ischemic injury of the intestine before birth, which leads to reduced intestinal wall thickness, villous length and weight, and crypt depth. Such neonates are more vulnerable to intestinal dysbiosis and alteration of the proliferation-apoptosis homeostasis of the gut. This leads to abnormality in the intestine's motor, secretory, and mucosal functions, making it vulnerable to stasis and abnormal colonization and invasion by bacteria.[3]

Moreover, these circulatory changes tend to persist after birth. Baseline blood flow in the superior mesenteric artery (SMA) and celiac axis is significantly reduced after birth and usually normalizes by one week of postnatal age.[2,3] Dynamic changes in SMA flow after feeding is also impaired in infants with AREDF. High metabolic demands associated with enteral feeding in compromised gut perfusion antenatally and postnatally further affect intestinal tissue oxygenation. In addition, intestinal stasis and immunological factors in growth-restricted fetuses also contribute to the development of NEC.

Evidence also shows that the risk of developing NEC is twofold higher in infants with AREDF than in infants with normal umbilical

Doppler flow.[2] Because of these concerns, initiation of enteral feeding is often delayed in infants with AREDF.

## FEEDING STRATEGIES IN INFANTS WITH AREDF

### 1. When to Start Minimal Enteral Nutrition (MEN) in Infants with AREDF?

While the benefits of MEN in stable ELBW neonates are well known, it is controversial if infants with AREDF should be given MEN from the day of birth and for how long MEN is to be continued before considering progressive enteral feeding. Early introduction of MEN may improve nutrition and growth but may increase the risk of feed intolerance and NEC.

Conversely, the late introduction may be detrimental due to a lack of stimulation of the gastrointestinal tract, resulting in villous atrophy and a lack of hormone and enzyme production.

*Among neonates born before 35 weeks of gestation with umbilical artery Doppler flow abnormalities, we initiate MEN on day 1 of life for those weighing 1250 g or more at birth and after 24 hours of life for those weighing less than 1250 g (Fig. 10.1).*

### 2. When to Start Progressive Enteral Feeding?

Delayed initiation of progressive enteral feeding should benefit neonates with AREDF because of the limitations already highlighted—while it could potentially reduce the risk of NEC, it will likely delay the time to reach full enteral feeds and prolong the hospital stay.

In the ADEPT trial, feed volumes were not increased for 2–3 days in neonates with birth weight <1000 g, while it was increased progressively from the second day after initiation of enteral feeds in neonates with birth weight >1000 g.[5] A systematic review found that early feeding decreased the time to reach full feeds and duration of parenteral nutrition (Table 10.1).

| Table 10.1: Time of initiation of enteral feeds: What is the evidence? |
|---|
| A recent meta-analysis, which included six studies involving neonates with Doppler abnormalities, found that early feeding decreased the time to reach full feeds, duration of parenteral nutrition and hospital stay, and rates of hospital-acquired infection. There was a trend toward an increase in rates of feeding intolerance, but the incidence of NEC did not increase. There was no effect on mortality and time to regain birth weight.[4] |

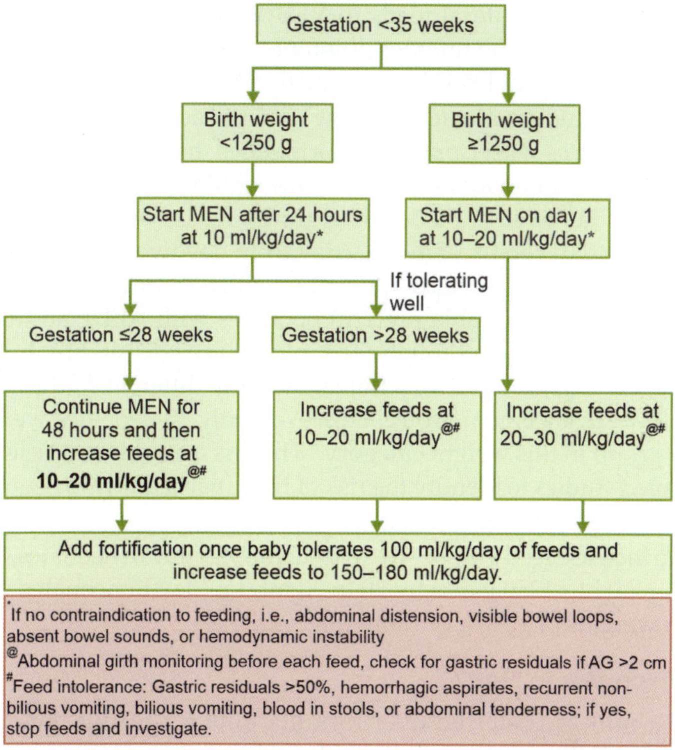


**Fig. 10.1:** Algorithm for feeding infants with AREDF

We increase feed volume the next day after initiating MEN in neonates born after 28 weeks of gestation (provided they tolerated MEN well); we continue MEN for 48 hours and then increase the feed volume in neonates born at or before 28 weeks gestation (Fig. 10.1).

### 3. How to Advance?

There is wide variation in practice in the rate of advancement of feeds. The quantum of increase in the volume is generally 10–20 ml/kg/day in infants less than 1000 g and 20–30 ml/kg/day in infants above 1000 g.

One study that evaluated the effect of slow vs. rapid advancement of enteral feeding in two birth weight groups—<1250 g (20 vs. 30 ml/kg/day) and 1250 g (30 vs. 40 ml/kg/day)—did not find any increase in the incidence of NEC or feed intolerance.[6] The Cochrane review on slow (15–24 ml/kg/day) vs. rapid (30–40 ml/kg/day) advancement of enteral feeds in VLBW infants reported similar results. However, the number of infants with growth restriction or abnormal antenatal Doppler was small in the included studies.[7]

A recent study evaluated the slow vs. rapid advancement of feeds in 83 newborns with Doppler abnormalities. In the <1250 g group, enteral feeds were advanced at 20 ml/kg/day versus 30 ml/kg/day from day two. In the >1250 g group, feeds were advanced at 30 ml/kg/day versus 40 ml/kg/day from day two. The study did not find any increase in feed intolerance with the rapid advancement of enteral feeds in stable preterm neonates with AEDF and birth weight ≥1250 g. Even though feed intolerance was slightly higher in the <1250 g group, it was not statistically different in the rapid vs. slow advancement group. However, only 15 neonates were in each group in this weight category.[6] There is a need for sufficiently powered studies to identify the risk of NEC, particularly in neonates with birth weights of <1250 g.

We increase feed volume by 10 to 20 ml/kg/day in neonates with birth weight <1250 g and by 20 to 30 ml/kg/day in neonates with birth weights of 1250 g or more (Fig. 10.1).

### 4. Which Milk to Start?

Breast milk is preferred over formula milk for feeding preterm infants. Mother's own milk is preferred over human donor milk. NEC has been found to be less if the intake of the mother's milk exceeds 50% of the total intake.[8] Infants fed with exclusive human milk feeding have been found to have decreased incidence of NEC.[9] However, a recent trial found that feed interruptions were not reduced in the human milk-based fortifier group compared to the bovine milk-based fortifier group.[10]

### 5. How to Monitor?

Monitoring for feed intolerance in infants with AREDF is no different from other preterm or LBW neonates. Feed intolerance, if any, is to be managed as per the algorithm in the protocol on 'Feeding of LBW infants.'

### 6. How to Fortify?

Fortification of breast milk is preferably done once the neonate reaches 100 ml/kg/day of feeds. However, in the ADEPT trial, the fortification was started after the infants reached 150 ml/kg/day.

## REFERENCES

1. Barone G, Maggio L, Saracino A, Perri A, Romagnoli C, Zecca E. How to feed small for gestational age newborns. Ital J Pediatr 2013;39:28.
2. Dorling J, Kempley S, Leaf A. Feeding growth restricted preterm infants with abnormal antenatal Doppler results. Arch Dis Child Fetal Neonatal Ed 2005;90:F359–63.
3. Arnon S, Sulam D, Konikoff F, Regev RH, Litmanovitz I, Naftali T. Very early feeding in stable small for gestational age preterm infants: a randomized clinical trial. J Pediatr (Rio J) 2013;89:388–93.
4. Anne RP, Aradhya AS, Murki S. Feeding in preterm neonates with antenatal Doppler abnormalities—a systematic review and meta-analysis. J Pediatr Gastroenterol Nutr. 2022 Jun 1. doi: 10.1097/MPG.0000000000003487. Epub ahead of print. PMID: 35653426.
5. Leaf A, Dorling J, Kempley S, McCormick K, Mannix P, Linsell L, et al. Early or delayed enteral feeding for preterm growth-restricted infants: a randomized trial. Pediatrics 2012;129:e1260–1268.
6. Jain S, Mukhopadhyay K, Jain V, Kumar P. Slow versus rapid enteral feed in preterm neonates with antenatal absent end diastolic flow. J Matern Fetal Neonatal Med 2016;29:2828–33.
7. Oddie SJ, Young L, McGuire W. Slow advancement of enteral feed volumes to prevent necrotising enterocolitis in very low birth weight infants. Cochrane Database Syst Rev. 2017;(8): CD001241.
8. Cacho NT, Parker LA, Neu J. Necrotizing Enterocolitis and Human Milk Feeding: A Systematic Review. Clin Perinatol 2017;44:49–67.
9. Sullivan S, Schanler RJ, Kim JH et al. An exclusively human milk-based diet is associated with a lower rate of necrotizing enterocolitis than a diet of human milk and bovine milk-based products. J Pediatr 2010;156:562–567.
10. O'Connor DL, Kiss A, Tomlinson C et al; OptiMoM Feeding Group. Nutrient enrichment of human milk with human and bovine milk-based fortifiers for infants born weighing <1250 g: a randomized clinical trial. Am J Clin Nutr. 2018 Jul 1;108(1):108–116.

CHAPTER

11

# Neonatal Cholestasis

Cholestasis refers to increased serum conjugated or direct bilirubin and serum bile acids. Accurate estimates of its incidence are not available from India; however, data from the United Kingdom suggests an incidence of 1 in 2500 term infants.[1] Preterm neonates receiving parenteral nutrition for more than two weeks and small-for-gestational age (SGA) infants are at greater risk of cholestasis.

Recognizing cholestasis in neonates is important because unconjugated hyperbilirubinemia is expected at this age and is physiological in most infants; in contrast, cholestatic jaundice is always pathological and warrants evaluation and management.

## DEFINITION

Previously, cholestasis was defined as direct bilirubin (DB) of greater than 1 mg/dl if the total serum bilirubin (TSB) is less than 5 mg/dl or a DB fraction of greater than 20% if the TSB is greater than 5 mg/dl.[2,3,4] The recent guidelines do away with considering the fraction of DB as a percentage of TSB as this is physiologically and clinically complex.[5] Therefore, in the presence of elevated TSB, DB is considered abnormal if values are more than 1 mg/dl, regardless of the level of TSB.

The most used test to measure bilirubin is the Diazo or the van den Bergh method. This does not measure the conjugated bilirubin fraction but rather the direct fraction (conjugated and delta bilirubin, i.e. conjugated bilirubin covalently bound to albumin). There are several fallacies in measuring DB. Due to methodological considerations, the higher the TSB (even if all of it is unconjugated), the higher the DB will be.[2] Because canalicular excretion of bilirubin is a rate-limiting step, even infants with elevated unconjugated bilirubin may retain some conjugated bilirubin.[3]

### When to Suspect?

Hyperbilirubinemia is common in newborns, but this is usually unconjugated and benign[6,7]. The most direct method for establishing cholestasis is measuring the serum total and direct bilirubin. The actual age of the infant at which a direct fraction of bilirubin is to be measured cannot be described. Some guidelines suggest that a healthy breastfed infant with jaundice at two weeks of age having pigmented stools, normal urine color, and normal physical examination may be followed for another week before fractions are measured while a bottle-fed infant with jaundice at two weeks should have direct fraction evaluated immediately. Any infant with jaundice beyond this age should promptly have total and direct bilirubin measured. At any time of presentation, certain important clinical and historical factors should trigger an assessment of cholestasis. These include the presence of persistently pale stools and high-colored urine, which stains diapers or clothing a deep yellow. Any infant at any age with jaundice and a history of cholestasis in siblings or parents, history of fetal loss, cholestasis of pregnancy, acute fatty liver of pregnancy, or maternal infections (TORCH) warrants evaluation.[5]

## EVALUATION

The first step is to establish that there is cholestasis. Although the history of high-colored urine with diaper staining and pale-colored stools helps suspect cholestasis, a definitive diagnosis can only be made by estimating total and direct serum bilirubin. Any value of DB more than 1 mg/dl is suggestive of cholestasis.

The next step consists of carefully evaluating the medical history and conducting a focused physical examination to establish the etiology of cholestasis and determine the general health of the newborn to identify sick neonates.

The etiology of cholestasis may be classified into biliary (obstructive causes) or hepatocellular (membrane transport defects, infective causes, embryogenesis defects, and metabolic). Table 11.1 lists the various etiologies of neonatal cholestasis with critical clinical and laboratory features, imaging findings, and specific therapies, if available.

## HISTORY

Persistently pale stools are an important finding and point towards biliary atresia. The color of the stool should be examined by the

**Table 11.1: Key clinical features, investigations, and treatment of common causes of cholestasis**

| *Condition* | *Key clinical features* | *Key investigations* | *Specific therapy if available* |
|---|---|---|---|
| **Anatomical** | | | |
| Extrahepatic biliary atresia | Cholestasis in an otherwise well baby | Liver biopsy shows portal expansion, portal fibrosis and bile ductular proliferation.<br>Small sized gall bladder (<19 mm) with poor contractility | Kasai portoenterostomy |
| Choledochal cyst | May have abdominal mass | Imaging is characteristic: USG or MRI demonstrates cyst<br>(*Biliary atresia may also have cysts at the porta*) | Surgical excision of cyst and cholodochojejunostomy |
| Inspissated bile duct syndrome | History of phototherapy or exchange transfusions due to indirect hyperbilirubinemia<br>Has been reported after ceftriaxone | USG showing dilated bile ducts with inspissated bile<br>May require intraoperative cholangiogram for diagnosis and treatment | Ursodeoxycholic acid, may require intraoperative flushing of bile ducts |
| Sclerosing cholangitis | | Small duct destruction on liver biopsy<br>Pruning of peripheral small ducts on intraoperative cholangiogram | No specific therapy |
| **Hepatocellular disease** | | | |
| PFIC 1,2 | Diarrhea, deafness, pancreatitis, failure to thrive, pruritus | Low or normal GGT<br>High serum bile acids | Cholestasis regimen |

(*Contd.*)

**Table 11.1: Key clinical features, investigations, and treatment of common causes of cholestasis** (*Contd.*)

| *Condition* | *Key clinical features* | *Key investigations* | *Specific therapy if available* |
|---|---|---|---|
| | | *ATP8B1* gene, *ABCB11* gene, PFIC gene panels | Consider biliary diversion for intractable pruritus, early hepatocellular carcinoma may complicate the course of PFIC2 |
| PFIC 3 | Cholestasis; signs usually do not appear until later in infancy or childhood | Elevated GGT<br>MDR3 immunostaining on liver biopsy<br>*ABCB4* gene, PFIC gene panels | |
| Alpha-1 antitrypsin deficiency | | Alpha-1 antitrypsin level (often falsely low in neonates)<br>Pi type ZZ or SZ<br>Uncommon in India | No specific therapy for liver disease |
| Idiopathic neonatal hepatitis | | This category is shrinking as more identifiable causes of cholestasis are recognized | |
| **Metabolic disease** | | | |
| Galactosemia | Hypoglycemia, coagulopathy, cataract,<br>*E coli* sepsis<br>Neonatal liver failure | Urine for non-glucose reducing substance (baby should be on galactose containing diet at time of testing)<br>Galactose-1-phosphate uridyl (GALT) transferase in red blood cells | Exclude galactose in diet<br>Consider empirically stopping galactose in sick newborns with liver failure |

(*Contd.*)

**Table 11.1: Key clinical features, investigations, and treatment of common causes of cholestasis** (*Contd.*)

| *Condition* | *Key clinical features* | *Key investigations* | *Specific therapy if available* |
|---|---|---|---|
| Tyrosinemia type 1 | Neonatal cholestasis, renal tubular acidosis, neonatal liver failure | Urine succinlyacetone<br>Fumarylacetoacetate (FAH) enzyme deficiency<br>*FAH* gene sequence analysis | Nitisinone with a low phenylalanine/tyrosine formula |
| Ornithine trans-carbamylase deficiency | Lethargy, jitteriness, emesis, encephalopathy, liver failure | Hyperammonemia<br>Low citrulline and high glutamine in blood<br>Orotic acid in urine<br>*OTC* gene sequencing | Treatment of acute hyperammonemia by arginine, sodium benzoate and sodium phenylacetate. May require dialysis.<br>Stop protein in acute episode |
| Fatty acid oxidation defects | Reye's syndrome like illness<br>May have skeletal muscle and cardiac involvement | Hypoketotic hypoglycemia<br>Plasma carnitine and acylcarnitine profiles<br>TMS/GCMS | Supportive measures<br>Carnitine<br>Medium chain triglycerides |
| **Infective etiology** | | | |
| Bacterial sepsis | Sick newborn | Blood cultures | Consider empirical treatment in any sick newborn |
| Urinary tract infections | Sick newborn | Urine cultures | |
| Herpes simplex type 1 and 2 | Neonatal liver failure in 1st week of life | PCR from skin vesicles, blood, conjunctival swab and CSF | Consider empirical therapy in neonatal liver failure—acyclovir |

(*Contd.*)

**Table 11.1: Key clinical features, investigations, and treatment of common causes of cholestasis (*Contd.*)**

| *Condition* | *Key clinical features* | *Key investigations* | *Specific therapy if available* |
|---|---|---|---|
| | Rapidly fatal<br>Skin vesicles in 68% | | |
| Cytomegalovirus | Symptoms vary from isolated hepatitis to generalized disease with chorioretinitis, microcephaly, cerebral calcification, pneumonitis, petechiae and purpura | PCR from urine or blood<br>Cytomegalic cells and inclusion bodies in liver biopsy | Treat only in systemic disease or CMV hepatitis on liver biopsy;<br>Serology alone is not a reliable diagnostic tool and may mislead the diagnosis;<br>IV Ganciclovir for 21 days |
| **Multisystem disorders and others** | | | |
| Alagille syndrome | Syndromic facies, structural heart defects, posterior embryotoxon on eye exam | High GGT, elevated cholesterol, cardiac, eye and vertebral abnormalities<br>PILBD on liver biopsy<br>*JAG 1* and *NOTCH 2* gene sequencing<br>X-ray dorsolateral spine for vertebral fusion abnormalities | Cholestasis regimen<br>Consider biliary diversion for intractable pruritus |
| Non-syndromic paucity of intralobular bile ducts | No specific clinical feature | PILBD on liver biopsy | Variable course<br>No specific therapy |

(*Contd.*)

**Table 11.1: Key clinical features, investigations, and treatment of common causes of cholestasis** *(Contd.)*

| *Condition* | *Key clinical features* | *Key investigations* | *Specific therapy if available* |
|---|---|---|---|
| Panhypopituitarism Or adrenal insufficiency | May mimic sepsis. Hypoglycemia<br>Midline defects like cleft lip or palate, microphallus, Septoptic dysplasia.<br>Ambiguous genitalia | GH, insulin and cortisol at hypoglycemia<br>Testing for adrenal insufficiency. GH stimulation tests<br>MRI brain for pituitary abnormalities | Hormone replacement usually results in resolution of cholestasis |
| Neonatal Hemochromatosis due to gestational alloimmune disease (GALD) | Neonatal liver failure<br>History of previous stillbirths, sibling deaths<br>IUGR, oligohydroamnios, placental edema | High ferritin<br>Low transferrin with transferrin saturation >95%<br>Salivary gland biopsy from lips show iron deposition on Perl's stain<br>T2 weighted MRI show a hepatic siderosis (low signal intensity as compared to skeletal muscle) while the spleen is spared and has comparatively high (bright signal intensity) | IVIG (1 to 3 g/kg used)<br>Double volume exchange transfusion |
| Mitochondrial disorders | Multisystem disorders<br>Unexplained liver disease, cardiac and neurological involvement | Hypoglycemia<br>Lactic acidosis, lactate/pyruvate ratio > 20, ketonemia<br>Hepatic steatosis<br>Gene panels for nuclear and respiratory genes | |

*USG:* Ultrasound; *MRI:* Magnetic resonance imaging; *PFIC:* Progressive familial intrahepatic cholestasis; *PILBD:* Paucity of interlobular bile ducts; *GGT:* Gamma-glutamyl transferase; *UDCA:* Ursodeoxycholic acid; *TMS:* Tandem mass spectroscopy; *GCMS:* Gas chromatography-mass spectroscopy; *PCR:* Polymerase chain reaction; *IUGR:* Intrauterine growth retardation; IVIG: Intravenous immunoglobulin

physician, as there is a significant disparity in the color reported by parents. The onset of jaundice and high-colored urine should be determined. Prenatal history may have important clues. Repeated fetal loss or early sibling deaths may point towards neonatal hemochromatosis due to gestational alloimmune liver disease (NH–GALD). Consanguinity and other affected siblings indicate a genetic/metabolic disease. SGA may point to neonatal hepatitis. The source of nutrition and the onset of jaundice are important, especially in preterm neonates on parenteral nutrition who may develop parenteral nutrition-related cholestasis, which may confound the diagnosis. Cholestasis of pregnancy or acute fatty liver of pregnancy in the mother may point to progressive familial cholestasis (PFIC) or a mitochondrial disorder, while acute fatty liver of pregnancy suggests fatty acid oxidation defects in the newborn. Maternal history of fever or adenopathy may suggest congenital infections (TORCH).

## EXAMINATION

The general condition of the baby should be elicited. A dull, lethargic baby with vomiting and irritability may have sepsis or a metabolic disorder. Multiple stool samples should always be examined to determine if they are pale. The size and consistency of the liver should also be evaluated. An otherwise healthy baby with pale stools and a firm liver is likely to have biliary atresia. Storage disorders should be considered if the spleen is larger than the liver. The early appearance of splenomegaly (in the first few weeks of life) and ascites indicates severe liver damage. It should point to NH-GALD or other causes of severe liver dysfunction, especially metabolic liver disease such as galactosemia (Fig. 11.1).

Extrahepatic features should be closely examined. Cataracts may be seen in galactosemia or congenital infection. Skin rash may be present in hemophagocytic lymphohistiocytosis (HLH), while a vesicular eruption, easily missed, may be the only clue to a HSV infection. Dysmorphic facies points to a genetic syndrome such as Alagilles. Cardiac examination for congenital heart disease and especially for peripheral pulmonic stenosis (seen in Alagilles) may be contributory. The general tone and neurological status may indicate encephalopathy or a multisystem disorder. Hypoplastic genitalia may be seen in hypopituitarism.

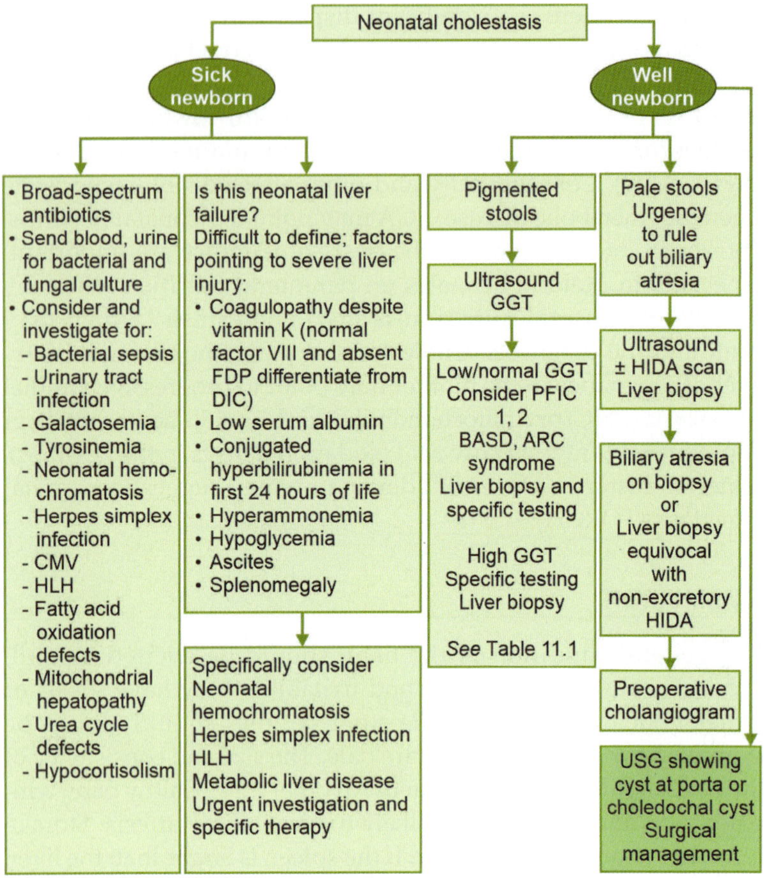


*CMV:* Cytomegalovirus; *HLH:* Hemophagocytic lymphohistiocytosis; *DIC:* Disseminated intravascular coagulation; *GGT:* Gamma-glutamyl transferase; *PFIC:* Progressive familial intrahepatic cholestasis; *BASD:* Bile acid synthetic defect; *HIDA:* Hepatobiliary scintigraphy

**Fig. 11.1:** Diagnostic approach to neonatal cholestasis

## INVESTIGATIONS

A total and differential serum bilirubin establishes the diagnosis of cholestasis. The prothrombin time (PT) and the international normalized ratio (INR) are dynamic markers of liver synthetic function because the relevant clotting factors are produced by the liver and have short half-lives. PT is the single most helpful test to determine the degree of hepatocyte dysfunction. Severe coagulopathy unresponsive to vitamin K may indicate NH-GALD, metabolic liver disease, or sepsis. Although helpful in suggesting hepatobiliary disease, the total serum bilirubin and liver enzymes (AST, ALT, and ALP) do not accurately reflect the degree of hepatocyte dysfunction. Alkaline phosphatase (ALP) is generally not helpful as it varies widely. Gamma-glutamyl transferase (GGT) is usually higher in neonates than older children but is more elevated in those with cholestasis. A normal or low GGT in the presence of cholestasis is seen in progressive familial intrahepatic cholestasis (PFIC) type 1 and 2, bile acid synthetic defects (BASD), and tight junction protein type 2 defect. PFIC will have high serum bile acids while BASD will have low serum bile acids (these should be performed with the patient off ursodeoxycholic acid).

A fasting ultrasound of the abdomen is helpful to suspect biliary atresia and other surgical etiologies such as a choledochal cyst. Findings suggesting biliary atresia include the triangular cord sign, an echogenic tubular structure at the porta, small irregular gall bladder (<19 mm) with poor contractility, among others. Biliary atresia may have non-communicating cystic structures at the porta, which should not be misdiagnosed as a choledochal cyst, and such cases should be urgently referred for surgical management. It is imperative to remember that a normal ultrasound does not rule out biliary atresia.

The hepatobiliary iminodiacetic acid (HIDA) scan is of limited value in evaluating neonatal cholestasis. While an excretory scan rules out biliary atresia, a non-excretory scan may also be seen in hepatocellular causes of cholestasis. The scan requires five days of priming with phenobarbitone or ursodeoxycholic acid, which may delay the diagnosis of biliary atresia. In any case, the HIDA scan should not delay a liver biopsy. The scan may be helpful in cases of ambiguously colored stools and a non-diagnostic liver biopsy and to diagnose conditions such as spontaneous perforations of the bile duct.

Magnetic resonance cholangiopancreatography (MRCP), endoscopic retrograde cholangiopancreatography (ERCP), and percutaneous transhepatic cholecysto-cholangiography (PTCC) are of limited value in the diagnosis of biliary atresia.

Liver biopsy remains the cornerstone of management in the diagnosis of neonatal cholestasis and will provide an accurate diagnosis in 90–95% of cases.[8,9] Features that are diagnostic of biliary obstruction are bile duct proliferation, portal expansion, and portal fibrosis. Neonatal hepatitis shows lobular disarray and inflammatory cells in the porta and giant cell transformation with a little or no change to the bile ducts. Giant cells may also be seen in biliary atresia. In biopsies performed early, the features of biliary atresia may not be apparent as obstructive features develop in a time dependent manner.

An intraoperative cholangiogram is the gold standard for diagnosing biliary atresia and may be followed by a portoenterostomy or Kasai procedure to establish biliary flow. Alagilles syndrome and cystic fibrosis are conditions where a hypoplastic biliary tree may mimic biliary atresia on intraoperative cholangiogram.[10]

Inborn errors of metabolism should be suspected in any sick baby or with coagulopathy out of proportion to liver disease. Evaluation should include blood and urine cultures, blood sugar, blood gas, ammonia, uric acid, electrolytes, lactic acid, pyruvic acid, lactate to pyruvate ratio, ketone bodies in blood and urine for non-glucose reducing substances, succinylacetone, ketone bodies, ketoacids, acylglycines, pH and sulfites.

Cytomegalovirus (CMV) infection is the most common congenital neonatal infection and is mostly asymptomatic but may present with low birth weight, periventricular calcification, chorioretinitis, deafness, hepatosplenomegaly, and jaundice. It is important to remember that IgM serology is not helpful for diagnosis. Considering the prevalence of CMV infection, it may just be a "red herring" and not the cause of cholestasis. PCR from blood, urine, saliva or nasopharyngeal secretions may isolate the virus, but to prove CMV as the cause of cholestasis, cytopathic changes on liver biopsy should be demonstrated. The diagnosis of biliary atresia should not be missed just because the IgM serology for CMV is positive.

Neonatal hemochromatosis due to gestational alloimmune liver disease (NH-GALD) is the most common cause of neonatal liver failure. A high serum ferritin (>800 µg/L), low transferrin but with a high transferrin saturation (>95%), anemia, thrombocytopenia with mildly raised transaminases, and uncorrectable coagulopathy are suggestive of NH-GALD. A lip biopsy will show iron deposition in the salivary gland by Perls stain. The procedure is safe under local anesthetic, even with coagulopathy, and does not usually require fresh frozen plasma or factor VII. T2 weighted MRI might show hepatic siderosis (low signal intensity compared to skeletal muscle) while the spleen is spared and has comparatively high (bright) signal intensity. If a liver biopsy is possible or in the case of death due to suspected GALD, the liver tissue should be stained for iron deposition and immunohistochemistry for C5b-9. The diagnosis of NH-GALD is important as subsequent pregnancies have a 90% risk of recurrence, and this can be prevented by intravenous immunoglobulin infusion to the mother during pregnancy.[11] Table 11.2 outlines the investigation of a neonate with cholestasis.

| Table 11.2: Investigation in a child with cholestasis |
|---|
| **Baseline investigations after establishing cholestasis**<br>Hemogram with differential leucocyte count<br>Complete liver function test *including GGT* and PT/INR<br>Blood glucose<br>Thyroid function test<br>Urine: Microscopy, culture, and non-glucose reducing substance<br>Urine and blood cultures in sick neonates<br>Fasting ultrasound abdomen<br>Eye exam |
| **2nd line investigations for specific etiologies**<br>*Metabolic disorder*<br>Ammonia<br>Blood glucose<br>Blood pH and lactate<br>Triglycerides and cholesterol<br>GALT assay<br>Urine succinyl acetone<br>TMS/GCMS from blood and urine<br>*Infections*<br>PCRs for HSV, CMV<br>Urine and blood cultures<br>Serum triglyceride and cholesterol<br>Consider serum bile acids *off UDCA* in low GGT cholestasis<br>Serum ferritin, and transferrin saturation (if considering hemochromatosis)<br>Alpha one antitrypsin levels and Pi type<br>Sweat chloride if indicated |
| *Consultations to obtain*<br>Ophthalmology: Cataract, posterior embryotoxon, fundus exam for storage disorders and retinitis<br>Genetics: consider gene panels or whole exome sequencing after discussion<br>Critical to involve pediatric surgery early if stools are persistently pale |

*(Contd.)*

| Table 11.2: Investigation in a child with cholestasis *(Contd.)* |
|---|
| *Imaging*<br>Fasting ultrasound<br>HIDA scan, if stool ambiguous in color or biopsy is not conclusive<br>Echocardiography<br>Chest X-ray and X-ray dorsolateral spine for butterfly vertebrae<br>Intraoperative cholangiography |
| *Histopathology*<br>Liver biopsy: In consultation with pediatric gastroenterologist<br>Lip biopsy if considering hemochromatosis (may be done even in infants with coagulopathy)<br>Bone marrow if indicated |

*GGT:* Gamma-glutamyl transpeptidase; *PT:* Prothrombin time; *INR:* International normalized ratio; *GALT:* Galactose-1-phosphate uridyl transferase; *TMS:* Tandem mass spectrometry; *GCMS:* Gas chromatography-mass spectrometry; *UDCA:* Ursodeoxycholic acid; *PCR:* Polymerase chain reaction; *HSV:* Herpes simplex virus; *CMV:* Cytomegalovirus; *HIDA scan:* Hepatobiliary nuclear scan

## Management

### General Management

This consists of meeting the nutritional needs of a neonate with cholestasis and supplementing fat-soluble vitamins. These children should receive 125% of the recommended dietary allowance (RDA) based on ideal body weight.[12,13] Formulas high in medium chain triglycerides (MCT) should be used, although these are not readily available in India. MCT oil may be added to the standard formula or expressed breast milk at 1–2 ml/kg/day in 2–4 divided doses.[13,14] Table 11.3 lists the vitamin and mineral requirements of these babies. Ideally, vitamin levels should be monitored, and supplementation (Table 11.3) tailored according to levels, but vitamin level estimation

**Table 11.3: Daily vitamin and mineral requirements in neonatal cholestasis**

| | |
|---|---|
| Vitamin A | 5000–25000 IU orally daily |
| Vitamin D | 400–1200 IU orally daily |
| Vitamin E | 50–400 IU orally daily |
| Vitamin K | 2.5 mg/biweekly to 5 mg/day orally<br>2.5–5 mg 4 weekly parenterally |
| Water soluble vitamins | Twice daily requirement |
| Calcium | 20–100 mg/kg/day |
| Zinc | 1 mg/kg/day orally |

*Modified from reference 14*

is expensive and cannot be performed in all cases. Vitamin K 5 mg IM must be administered upon diagnosis of cholestasis to prevent complications from vitamin K deficiency coagulopathy. Ursodeoxycholic acid (20–30 mg/kg/day in 2–3 divided doses), a choleretic agent, is often prescribed. It also helps control pruritus in PFIC. Rifampicin (10 mg/kg/day) and cholestyramine may also be prescribed to manage pruritus.

An initial empirical management plan may be initiated while being investigated for different diagnoses in sick neonates with significant coagulopathy despite vitamin K administration. Broad-spectrum antibiotics and antifungals after cultures should be administered. Consideration to the treatment of herpes simplex virus should be given. The formula may be changed to a lactose-free preparation (thus eliminating galactose) while testing of galactosemia is pursued. If other metabolic disorders are suspected, the infant may be kept NPO and put on intravenous fluids.

### *Specific Management*

Specific therapy may be initiated for some disorders. Biliary atresia will require portoenterostomy (Kasai's procedure). Extrahepatic biliary atresia, if operated early (<60 days of age), has much better outcomes in terms of achieving biliary drainage[15] as opposed to surgery at a later age (> 60 days). After a successful biliary drainage procedure, native liver survival is about 28% at 15 years of follow-up.[16] Early surgery improves the chances of a successful biliary drainage procedure and long-term native liver survival. Hence biliary atresia must be suspected and treated early. NH-GALD may require intravenous immunoglobulin at 1–3 mg/kg/day and exchange transfusions. Nitisinone is the specific therapy for tyrosinemia. Chemotherapy should be initiated in hemophagocytic lymphohistiocytosis while treating the triggering bacterial or viral infection. A complete list of specific treatments is provided in Table 11.1. Liver transplantation remains the only option for children with decompensated liver disease.

## REFERENCES

1. Dick MC, Mowat AP. Hepatitis syndrome in infancy--an epidemiological survey with 10-year follow up. Arch Dis Child 1985, Jun;60(6):512–6.
2. Lo SF, Doumas BT. The status of bilirubin measurements in U.S. Laboratories: Why is accuracy elusive? Semin Perinatol 2011, Jun;35(3):141–7.

3. Rosenthal P, Blanckaert N, Kabra PM, Thaler MM. Formation of bilirubin conjugates in human newborns. Pediatr Res 1986, Oct;20(10):947–50.
4. Moyer V, Freese DK, Whitington PF, Olson AD, Brewer F, Colletti RB, Heyman MB. Guideline for the evaluation of cholestatic jaundice in infants: Recommendations of the North American Society for Pediatric Gastroenterology, Hepatology and Nutrition. J Pediatr Gastroenterol Nutr 2004, Aug;39(2):115.
5. Fawaz R, Baumann U, Ekong U, Fischler B, Hadzic N, Mack CL, et al. Guideline for the evaluation of cholestatic jaundice in infants: Joint recommendations of the North American Society for Pediatric Gastroenterology, Hepatology, and Nutrition and the European Society for Pediatric Gastroenterology, Hepatology, and Nutrition. J Pediatr Gastroenterol Nutr 2017, Jan;64(1):154–68.
6. Kelly DA, Stanton A. Jaundice in babies: Implications for community screening for biliary atresia. BMJ 1995, May 6;310(6988):1172–3.
7. Winfield CR, MacFaul R. Clinical study of prolonged jaundice in breast- and bottle-fed babies. Arch Dis Child 1978, Jun;53(6):506–7.
8. Russo P, Magee JC, Boitnott J, Bove KE, Raghunathan T, Finegold M, et al. Design and validation of the biliary atresia research consortium histologic assessment system for cholestasis in infancy. Clin Gastroenterol Hepatol 2011, Apr;9(4):357–362.e2.
9. Morotti RA, Jain D. Pediatric cholestatic disorders: Approach to pathologic diagnosis. Surg Pathol Clin 2013, Jun;6(2):205–25.
10. Altman RP, Abramson S. Potential errors in the diagnosis and surgical management of neonatal jaundice. J Pediatr Surg 1985, Oct;20(5):529–34.
11. Feldman AG, Whitington PF. Neonatal hemochromatosis. J Clin Exp Hepatol 2013, Dec;3(4):313–20.
12. Suchy FJ. Neonatal cholestasis. Pediatr Rev 2004, Nov;25(11):388–96.
13. da Silva FV, Ferri PM, Nascentes Queiroz TC, de Souza Haueisen Barbosa P, Cassiano de Oliveira MC, de Melo Pereira LJ, et al. Nutritional evaluation of children with chronic cholestatic disease. J Pediatr (Rio J) 2016;92(2):197–205.
14. Bhatia V, Bavdekar A, Matthai J, Waikar Y, Sibal A. Management of neonatal cholestasis: Consensus statement of the pediatric gastroenterology chapter of Indian academy of pediatrics. Indian Pediatr 2014, Mar;51(3):203–10.
15. Lally KP, Kanegaye J, Matsumura M, Rosenthal P, Sinatra F, Atkinson JB. Perioperative factors affecting the outcome following repair of biliary atresia. Pediatrics 1989, May;83(5):723–6.
16. Serinet MO, Wildhaber BE, Broué P, Lachaux A, Sarles J, Jacquemin E, et al. Impact of age at Kasai operation on its results in late childhood and adolescence: A rational basis for biliary atresia screening. Pediatrics 2009, May;123(5):1280–6.

CHAPTER

12

# Intestinal Obstruction

Neonatal intestinal obstruction (NIO) is a common neonatal emergency with an incidence of 1 in 2000 live births (Table 13.1). The cornerstone of management in these neonates lies in timely diagnosis.

The common causes of NIO are listed in Table 12.1.

## COMMON CAUSES

**Gastric outlet obstruction** secondary to pyloric atresia accounts for <1% of all congenital NIOs. It is often associated with heterotaxia syndromes and with epidermolysis bullosa.

**Duodenal obstruction** can either result from duodenal atresia (DA) or malrotation. DA occurs once in 5000 to 10,000 live births. About one-third of neonates with DA may have trisomy 21. Associated cardiac anomalies are also common. Gray and Skandalakis have classified DA into three main types:[1]

**Type I (92%):** An obstructing web (of mucosa and submucosa) with intact mesentery.

**Table 12.1: Common causes of neonatal intestinal obstruction based on the site of obstruction**

| | | |
|---|---|---|
| 1. | Foregut | Pyloric atresia/stenosis<br>Duodenal atresia/stenosis/webs (with/without annular pancreas) |
| 2. | Midgut | Malrotation with or without volvulus<br>Jejuno-ileal atresia<br>Meconium ileus/complicated meconium cyst<br>Total colonic aganglionosis |
| 3. | Hindgut | Hirschsprung's disease<br>Anorectal malformation<br>Colonic atresia |

**Type II (1%):** A short fibrous cord connects the two ends with intact mesentery.
**Type III (7%):** Both ends are blind with a V-shaped mesenteric defect.

**Malrotation** refers to the abnormal or incomplete intestinal rotation during embryonic development leading to the duodenal-jejunal and ileocecal junctions lying close to each other, resulting in a narrower mesenteric root. This anatomy predisposes the small bowel to twist around its pedicle, leading to "midgut volvulus." Midgut volvulus causes mechanical obstruction and vascular occlusion of the superior mesenteric vessels. If untreated, midgut volvulus can rapidly progress to bowel ischemia and intestinal gangrene.

**The jejunum and ileum** are the commonest sites of intestinal atresia. The jejunal and ileal atresia (JIA) incidence varies from 1: 1500 to 1: 12000 live births.[1] Associated anomalies are relatively uncommon in JIA (compared to DA). About one-third of the cases may have associated abnormalities, including gastrointestinal (biliary atresia, agenesis of the gallbladder), cardiac, renal, and vertebral anomalies.

**Meconium ileus** is obstruction at the level of distal ileum because of abnormally thick, tenacious, and impacted meconium.

**A complicated meconium cyst** results from a sterile chemical reaction resulting from an antenatal bowel perforation (due to volvulus, atresia, or undefined causes) with extravasation and intraperitoneal dissemination of the meconium. This meconium peritonitis can get walled off to form a cystic cavity with a fibrous wall, referred to as cystic-type meconium peritonitis.

**Hirschsprung's disease** is an important cause of functional NIO wherein variable lengths of the colon starting retrogradely from the rectum are devoid of ganglion cells in the submucosal and myenteric plexuses. Involvement can either be a short segment (up to descending colon), a long segment (up to the cecum), or total colonic aganglionosis (up to the distal ileum). The presentation may either be as NIO as repeated bouts of enterocolitis or delayed up to infancy and manifesting with failure to thrive and chronic constipation.

**Anorectal malformation** (ARM) is one of the most common neonatal surgical emergencies, with an incidence of 1 in 5000 live births, with about a third being isolated and the remainder being associated with other congenital anomalies, especially those with higher lesions.[2]

The associated anomalies include urogenital (50%), vertebral (30%), cardiac (15%), gastrointestinal (10%), and tracheoesophageal fistula (7%). There is a slight male preponderance, and various familial and genetic alterations have also been linked to their occurrence. The currently used 'Krickenbeck classification' of ARM has simplified and standardized the various anomalies into groups based on their treatment strategies. The most common ARM seen in males is the recto-urethral fistula, while that in females is a recto-vestibular fistula. The conventional terms, high and low type ARM, used in common parlance, were derived from the Wingspread classification in 1984. The ARMs were divided into high and low based on the level of the terminal bowel with respect to the levator ani muscle of the pelvic floor. Broadly, a low ARM can be managed with a perineal surgery in the neonatal period itself, whereas a high ARM is best managed with an initial colostomy followed by a definitive procedure after 3–6 months.[3]

## APPROACH TO A NEONATE WITH SUSPECTED INTESTINAL OBSTRUCTION

### History and Examination

Unless proven otherwise, any bilious vomiting with or without abdominal distension in a neonate is due to a surgical cause. However, it is essential to rule out medical causes like sepsis with associated paralytic ileus or necrotizing enterocolitis (NEC).

Antenatal ultrasonography (USG) should be reviewed to look for the presence of polyhydramnios. A double-bubble appearance should raise the suspicion of a DA.[4] In JIA, polyhydramnios is associated with a dilated loop of the bowel, which may be hyperechoic. The routine fetal anomaly USG scan has a low sensitivity to detect intestinal atresia because the sonographic signs of obstruction typically do not become evident until the late 2nd trimester. Overall, the sensitivity falls further as the site of obstruction becomes more distal, from 50% for DA to 40% for JIA and 30% for colonic obstructions.[5]

A thorough history and clinical examination can provide important clues (Table 12.2).

Neonates with ARM usually present with an absent normal anal opening, diagnosed on routine assessment at birth. When missed, they are brought to attention after 24–48 hours once abdominal distension develops, in addition to the failure to pass meconium. An exception to this rule is rectal atresia, an ARM with a normal

**Table 12.2: Common surgical conditions and their salient features**

| | *Antenatal USG findings* | *Vomiting* | *Delayed passage of meconium* | *Abnormal anal opening* | *Other anomalies* | *Dehy-dration* | *Hemody-namic instability* | *Abdominal distension* | *Abdominal signs* |
|---|---|---|---|---|---|---|---|---|---|
| Pyloric atresia | Polyhydramnios, single bubble appearance | +++ (Non-bilious) | – | – | +[*] | + | – | – | Visible gastric peristalsis |
| Duodenal atresia | Polyhydramnios, double bubble appearance | +++ (Bilious; rarely non-bilious) | – | – | ++[†] | + | – | – | None/ epigastric fullness |
| Malrotation and mid-gut volvulus | +/– | +++ (Bilious) | – | – | – | +/– | +++ | Tensely distended | Tenderness +/– erythema |
| Jejunoileal atresia | Polyhydramnios, hyperechoic bowel | +++ (Bilious) | – | – | – | +/– | – | Upper abdominal distension +/– | Visible intestinal loops/ peristalsis |
| Meconium ileus | Polyhydramnios, with echogenic dilated bowel | + | – | – | Cystic fibrosis should be ruled out | +/– | – | + | Abdominal distension develops after birth |

(*Contd.*)

**Table 12.2: Common surgical conditions and their salient features** *(Contd.)*

| | *Antenatal USG findings* | *Vomiting* | *Delayed passage of meconium* | *Abnormal anal opening* | *Other anomalies* | *Dehydration* | *Hemodynamic instability* | *Abdominal distension* | *Abdominal signs* |
|---|---|---|---|---|---|---|---|---|---|
| Meconium peritonitis | Polyhydramnios, bowel dilatation, ascites, and pseudocyst | + | – | – | – | +/– | – | + | Abdominal distension present at birth |
| Colonic atresia | – | Late feature | +/– | – | – | Late feature | – | + | Visible intestinal loops/ peristalsis |
| Hirschsprung's disease | – | Late feature | +/– | – | +[‡] | Late feature | – | + | Abdominal distension develops after birth |
| Total colonic aganglionosis | – | Late feature | +/– | – | – | Late feature | – | + | Abdominal distension develops after birth |

*(Contd.)*

**Table 12.2: Common surgical conditions and their salient features (*Contd.*)**

| | *Antenatal USG findings* | *Vomiting* | *Delayed passage of meconium* | *Abnormal anal opening* | *Other anomalies* | *Dehydration* | *Hemodynamic instability* | *Abdominal distension* | *Abdominal signs* |
|---|---|---|---|---|---|---|---|---|---|
| Anorectal Malformation | –[#] | Late feature | Non-passage of meconium[§] | + | +[**] | Late feature | – | + | Abdominal distension develops after birth |

[*]Epidermolysis bullosa

[†]Down's syndrome, congenital cardiac defects, tracheoesophageal atresia, anorectal malformation (part of VACTER)

[‡]Down's syndrome, Waardenburg syndrome, Congenital Central Hypoventilation, Mowat-Wilson, MEN2, Shah-Waardenburg, Bardet-Biedl, cartilage-hair hypoplasia, Goldberg-Shprintzen syndrome, etc.

[#]In persistent cloaca, indirect clues, as evidenced by a megacystis or hydronephrosis, single umbilical artery, ascites and oligohydramnios, may indicate cloacae.

[§]Low male ARM and most female ARM neonates may demonstrate the passage of meconium from an abnormal site.

[**]Associations (example: VACTERL [vertebral defects, anorectal malformation, cardiac defects, tracheoesophageal fistula, renal and limb anomalies], MURCS [Müllerian duct aplasia, Renal aplasia, Cervicothoracic Somite dysplasia], and OEIS [Omphalocele, Exstrophy, Imperforate anus and Spinal defects], etc.), Chromosomal anomalies (example: Trisomy 13, 18, and 21, etc.) and syndromes (example: Cat-eye, caudal regression, Currarino triad, Down's, Feingold, fetal alcohol, Kabuki, Opitz, Pallister-Hall, Rieger, Townes-Brocks, etc.)

anal opening but atresia high up in the rectum that can only be diagnosed by probing with a stiff catheter.

A decompressing vestibular or perineal fistula may be present in females, delaying the diagnosis. History suggestive of pneumaturia or meconuria (suggesting a genito-urinary communication) should be enquired. Presence or absence of anal, vaginal, and urethral openings, site of any fistula in the perineum (low anomaly), site of the anal dimple, gluteal cleft (poorly developed in high anomaly), and scrotum (bifid or associated with hypospadias in high anomaly) should be examined.

Any meconium-staining or meconium pearls in the perineum or perineal skin tags (low anomaly) should be noted (Fig. 12.1). The examination findings of the perineum in males and females with the most common type of anomaly are depicted in Fig. 12.2. In the cloaca, the urinary tract, the vagina, and the terminal bowel communicate with a common channel of variable length. On examination, the perineum will have only a single opening (Fig. 12.3). Additionally, any associated system anomalies and syndromes should be looked for on general physical examination. The clinical findings are summarised in Table 12.2.

## Investigations

A plain X-ray abdomen in the erect posture is mandatory and usually sufficient in suspected NIO. The bowel gas pattern and dilatation provide a clue to the underlying level of obstruction.

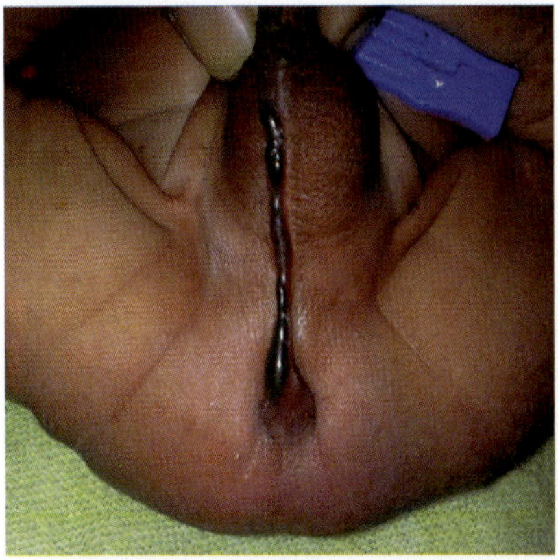

**Fig. 12.1:** Perineal findings in a male neonate with a low type of anomaly diagnosed by the presence of meconium in a subepithelial track (meconium pearls) reaching up to the scrotal raphe

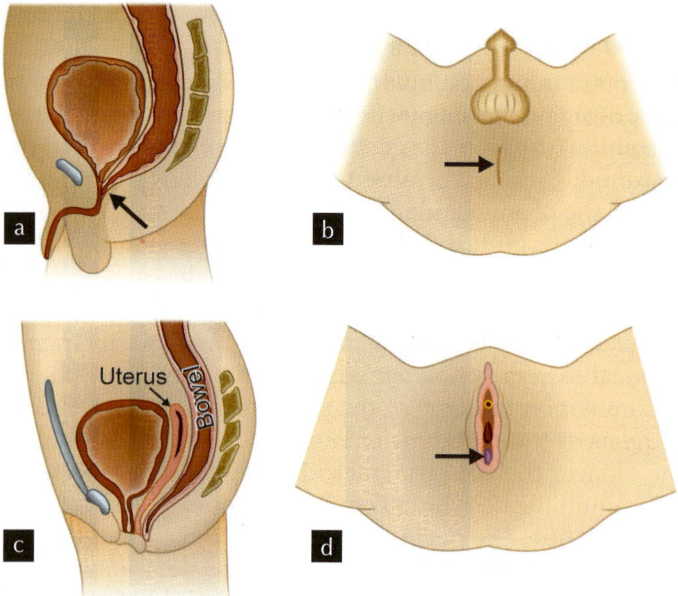


**Fig. 12.2:** (a) Perineal examination in a male child with rectourethral fistula (arrow) will have an absent anal opening with flat perineum. (b) There might be some hyperpigmentation at the supposed anal opening site (arrow), but may be featureless. (c) The most common anatomy in a female child is a vestibular fistula with the terminal bowel opening in the vestibule just posterior to the introitus (arrow). (d) On perineal examination, all three openings should be visible (the arrow shows the vestibular fistula posterior to the urethra and the vaginal opening).

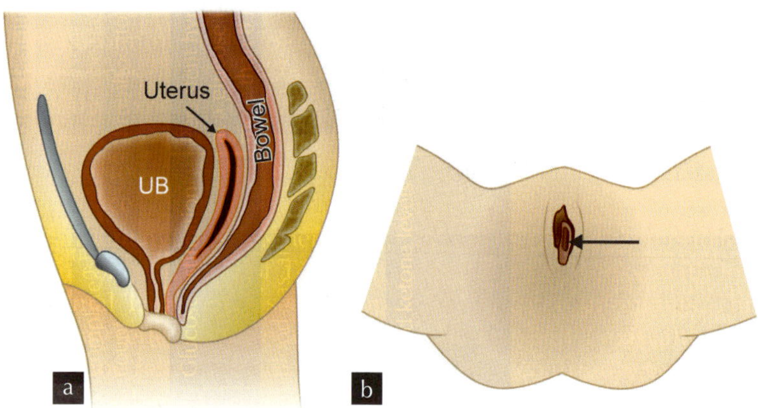


**Fig. 12.3:** (a) The common channel (cloaca) receiving the urethra, vagina, and bowel; (b) Single perineal opening (arrow)

In evolving or doubtful cases, 30 ml of air should be pushed into the stomach with a nasogastric tube before the radiograph. The salient radiographic findings of NIO are also summarised in Table 12.3. The following points are to be noted for diagnosis of ARM:

- If the clinical examination cannot categorize the type of ARM, an 'invertogram' or a 'cross table prone lateral' radiograph of the baby is necessary to determine the level of termination of bowel

**Table 12.3: Summary of salient radiologic findings of neonatal intestinal obstruction**

| | *Plain X-ray* | *Contrast study* |
|---|---|---|
| Pyloric atresia | Single bubble with absent distal air | Upper GI study—non-passage of contrast beyond the pylorus |
| Duodenal atresia | Double bubble (Fig. 12.4) with absent distal air | Not required |
| Malrotation and mid-gut volvulus | Double bubble-like appearance with a paucity of abdominal gas/ground glass appearance | Upper GI study - displaced duodenojejunal junction and "corkscrew" appearance (Fig. 12.5) |
| Jejunoileal atresia | Triple bubble appearance/ multiple air-fluid levels with a cut-off of bowel gas (Fig. 12.4) | Not required for jejunal atresia but when performed for ileal atresia shows microcolon |
| Meconium ileus | Dilated bowel loops with a soap-bubble appearance in the right lower abdomen and no or minimal air-fluid levels | Contrast enema—colon studded with meconium pellets appearing as intraluminal filling defects |
| Meconium peritonitis | Dilated bowel loops +/– air-fluid levels and calcifications | Contrast enema—microcolon |
| Colonic atresia | Dilated bowel loops with multiple air-fluid levels | Contrast enema—microcolon beyond the site of atresia |
| Hirschsprung's disease | Dilated bowel loops and absence of rectal gas shadow | Contrast enema—collapsed rectum with transition zone and proximal dilated bowel |
| Total colonic aganglionosis | Dilated bowel loops with multiple air-fluid levels | Contrast enema—microcolon with typical "?" mark configuration |
| Anorectal malformation | Dilated bowel loops Invertogram: high/intermediate or level of ARM | Not required in the neonatal period |

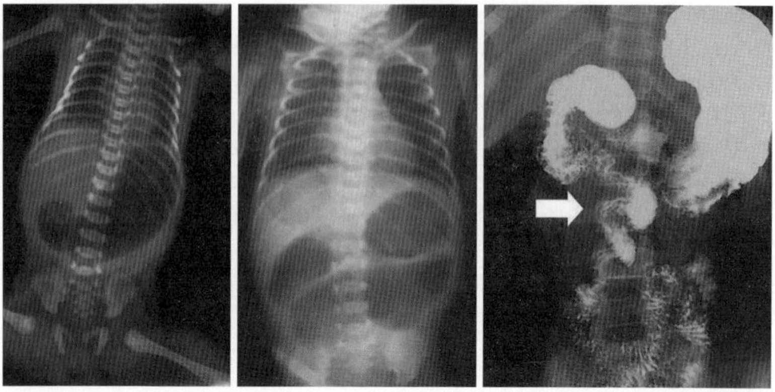

**Fig. 12.4:** Typical double-bubble appearance in DA (left), multiple dilated bowel loops in JIA (center), and "corkscrew" appearance on contrast study in a case of malrotation with volvulus (right; arrow)

in the pelvis in relation to the bone shadows. This is subject to the development of high intraluminal pressure of meconium and a time interval of at least 24 hours after birth for it to become evident.

- A plain X-ray abdomen in the erect posture showing a single large air-fluid level occupying more than half of the width of the abdomen represents a congenital pouch colon (CPC) (Fig. 12.5).

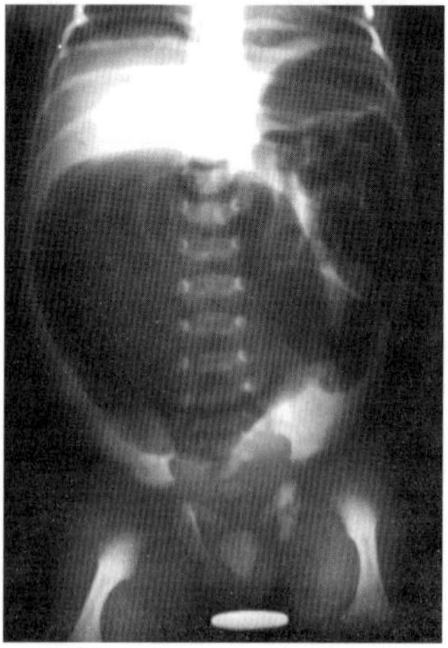

**Fig. 12.5:** Plain X-ray abdomen of a newborn with ARM. The prominently dilated bowel shadow occupying more than 50% of the transverse diameter of the abdomen suggests a possible CPC as the pathology.

In this condition, all or part of the colon is replaced by a pouch-like dilatation, which communicates distally with the urogenital tract via a large fistula. In females, generally, a decompressing fistula is present.

- Diagnosis is based on careful clinical examination noting the number of openings in the perineum and their relative positions (Figs 12.2d and 12.3b).

Rule out associated anomalies, including echocardiography and ultrasonogram of kidneys, and look for bony anomalies, cardiac shadow, and vertebral anomalies on the X-ray.

## MANAGEMENT

### How to Suspect

NIO should be considered when a neonate develops symptoms of intestinal obstruction during the first few hours or days of life. These include abdominal distension, vomiting (usually bilious), and occasionally failing to pass meconium. If the antenatal USG suggests features of NIO, then the neonate should be observed and investigated before ruling out NIO.

Optimizing the condition of neonates before undertaking any procedure is essential by ensuring normothermia, normal urine output, and normal electrolyte status. A naso/oro-gastric tube should be inserted and kept on free drainage. A urinary catheter is inserted only in hemodynamically unstable neonates. Often a central venous line needs to be established because these neonates may require prolonged intravenous fluids, antibiotics, and total parenteral nutrition in the postoperative period.

### How to Investigate

Most cases of NIO are not true surgical emergencies, *the notable exception being midgut volvulus*. Given that the vitality of the midgut is at stake in midgut volvulus, it is crucial *not to lose time on unnecessary investigations before undertaking an exploratory laparotomy*. In most other cases, a careful examination and an abdomen X-ray or a contrast radiograph are enough to arrive at a correct diagnosis. An algorithm (Fig 12.6) depicts the diagnostic workup in cases of suspected NIO.

### Surgical Management

Once a provisional diagnosis is reached, and other congenital anomalies are ruled out or taken care of, the neonate is posted for

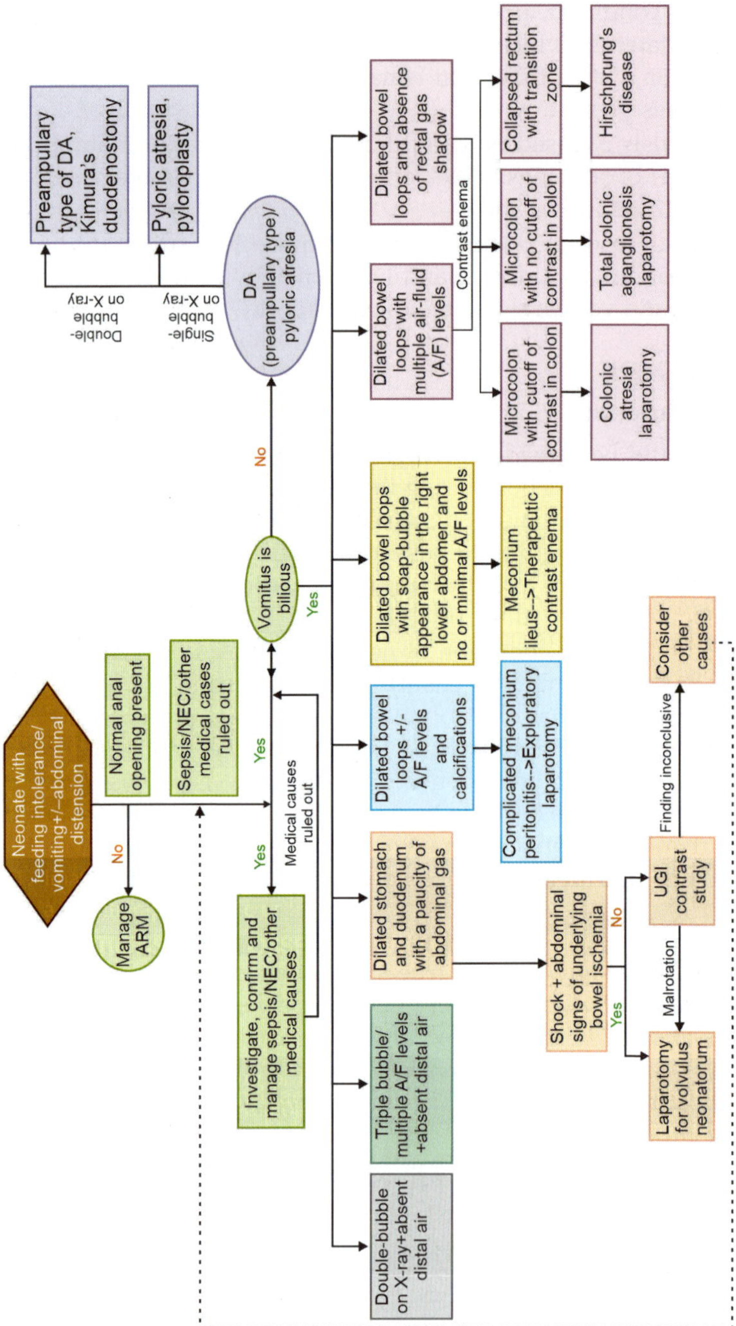


**Fig. 12.6:** Flowchart depicting the diagnostic workup and management of a neonate with suspected neonatal intestinal obstruction

surgical correction. Usually, a right upper transverse incision is given for most procedures (Fig 12.6).

- Heineke-Mikulicz pyloroplasty is done in gastric outlet obstruction where a longitudinal incision is given over the stenosed segment and sutured transversely. In case of complete obstruction, gastro-jejunostomy may be done.
- The surgical procedure performed for DA is Kimura's procedure. A diamond-shaped anastomosis is performed between the dilated proximal duodenum and collapsed distal duodenum.
- In the case of JIA, the large bulbous segment of the intestine is first excised, and then the proximal bowel is anastomosed to the narrow distal bowel in an "end-to-back" fashion.
- In malrotation, Ladd's procedure is done, which involves evisceration of the bowel, detorsion of the volvulus, division of Ladd's bands, straightening of C-loop of the duodenum, widening of the base of the mesentery, and appendicectomy. In the case of gangrenous bowel, a resection with anastomosis of the residual healthy ends may be required.
- In meconium ileus, an enterotomy is made in the distal ileum, the bowel decompressed, and the enterotomy closed or made into a Bishop-Koop stoma where the ileum is transected, a distal loop made as a stoma and proximal end anastomosed in an end-side fashion with the distal loop. With the help of a feeding tube in the stoma, distal bowel washes may be given.
- In Hirschsprung's disease, the transition zone is identified, and a proximal diverting stoma is made. To confirm the diagnosis, a seromuscular biopsy is taken distal to the transition zone. Another biopsy proximal to this level will identify normal ganglionated bowel for a future pull-through procedure.
- In ARM, once the level of the terminal pouch is established (clinically or radiologically), the decision regarding a diverting colostomy or a primary definite procedure is made. A diverting colostomy is performed in the neonatal period for male ARMs (high-type) and females with persistent cloacae. Later after 3–4 months, accurate anatomic information is obtained by a contrast colostogram or genitoscopy (for persistent cloacae), and posterior sagittal anorectoplasty (PSARP) or a posterior sagittal ano-recto urethro vaginoplasty (for persistent cloacae) is undertaken. Stoma reversal is done after 3–4 months after the definitive reconstruction. For boys with a "low type" of malformation, a single-stage perineal procedure like anoplasty

is usually sufficient. Females with ano/recto vestibular fistulas can be observed if they can decompress the bowel and pass stools normally. An elective single-stage limited PSARP can be performed around 3–4 months of age.

## Postoperative Care

Besides general supportive care, nasogastric tube (NGT) effluent, the drain amount and its nature, and the surgical wound site should be monitored. NG aspirates should be replaced volume by volume with Ringer's Lactate. Antibiotics, including third-generation cephalosporins, aminoglycosides, and metronidazole, should be administered for at least five days. A trans-anastomotic tube, if inserted intra-operatively, may help establish early enteral feeds. Total parenteral nutrition (TPN) is administered till bowel function is restored. Effective peristalsis may not return till the proximal bowel dilatation decreases slowly over the following weeks in the postoperative period. This would also be associated with decreasing trend of NGT tube effluent and a change in color from dark green to almost transparent. Trophic feeds are initiated soon after signs of bowel movement are documented. Feeds are then gradually increased over the next few days. The drain is usually removed after establishing full enteral feeds to ensure no anastomotic leak. The per-urethral catheter should be discontinued as early as possible post-operatively unless the neonate is hemodynamically unstable.

## Outcome

The prognosis for isolated intestinal atresia is usually good. Medical conditions such as prematurity or respiratory distress syndrome, associated anomalies, or complications such as short gut syndrome are primarily responsible for those with poor outcomes.[2] Associated cardiac anomalies constitute a significant cause of morbidity and mortality in patients with duodenal atresia.[6] Complex atresias can also have a poor prognosis with the requirement of prolonged TPN and associated risks of sepsis and liver failure.

## REFERENCES

1. Skandalakais JE, Gray SW, Ricketts R, et al. The small intestines. In: Embryology for Surgeons, 2nd ed, Skandalakis JE, Gray SW (Eds), Lippincott Williams and Wilkins, Baltimore 1994. p.184.

2. Best KE, Tennant PW, Addor MC, et al. Epidemiology of small intestinal atresia in Europe: a register based study. Arch Dis Child Fetal Neonatal Ed 2012;97:F353.
3. Cuschieri A. Descriptive epidemiology of isolated anal anomalies: a survey of 4.6 million births in Europe. Am J Med Genet 2001;103:207–15.
4. Holschneider A, Hutson J, Peña Aet al. Preliminary report on the International Conference for the Development of Standards for the Treatment of Anorectal Malformations. J Pediatr Surg. 2005;40:1521–6.
5. Haeusler MC, Berghold A, Stoll C, Barisic I, Clementi M; EUROSCAN Study Group. Prenatal ultrasonographic detection of gastrointestinal obstruction: results from 18 European congenital anomaly registries. Prenat Diagn. 2002 Jul;22(7):616–23.
6. Choudhry MS, Rahman N, Boyd P, Lakhoo K. Duodenal atresia: associated anomalies, prenatal diagnosis, and outcome. Pediatr Surg Int 2009; 25:727–30.

Section

6

# Infections

13. Fungal Infection in Neonates
14. Sepsis Outbreak in NICU

CHAPTER

13

# Fungal Infection in Neonates

Fungal infections are broadly categorized into mucocutaneous and invasive infections. Invasive fungal infection, caused mainly by Candida species, is associated with increased mortality and long-term neurodevelopmental impairment.

## INVASIVE CANDIDA INFECTION

Invasive Candida infection (ICI) includes Candida bloodstream infection (BSI), urinary tract infection (UTI), meningitis, peritonitis, other sterile site infections, and congenital cutaneous candidiasis. In developed nations, the incidence of ICI is inversely proportional to birth weight—the incidence is 1 to 4% in VLBW, 2 to 8% in ELBW, and up to 20% in neonates with birth weight <750 g or gestation <26 wks.[1] Fungal infection is far more common in referred outborn neonates who have already received broad-spectrum antibiotics than inborn neonates. The Delhi Neonatal Infection Study (DeNIS) collaboration data indicated fungal infections to be rare in inborn neonates; in contrast, about a quarter of sepsis episodes in outborn neonates was caused by *Candida spp*. Almost three-fourths of these infections occurred in neonates born at or after 32 weeks' gestation and about two-thirds in those weighing 1500 g or more at birth.[2] Among infections by candida, *C albicans* is the most commonly isolated species (50%), followed by *C. parapsilosis* (33%), *C. glabrata*, *C. krusei*, *C. tropicalis*, and *C. pseudotropicalis*.

### Risk Factors[1,3,4]

The common risk factors associated with invasive candida infection are enlisted in Table 13.1. Extreme preterm neonates and those with complex gastrointestinal disorders like necrotising enterocolitis (NEC), gastroschisis, and bowel perforation are at the highest risk.

| Table 13.1: Risk factors for invasive Candida infection | |
|---|---|
| Extreme prematurity | Complicated gastrointestinal disease |
| Extremely low birth weight (ELBW) | Lack of enteral feedings |
| Prolonged use of antibiotics >5 days | Parenteral lipid infusion for >7 days |
| Usage of two or more antibiotics | Central venous catheter |
| Bacterial sepsis | Endotracheal intubation and mechanical ventilation |
| Use of H2 blockers (Ranitidine) | Proton pump inhibitors |
| Hyperglycemia | Postnatal steroids |

## Clinical Presentation

Clinical features of candida infections range from localized skin infection in term neonates to disseminated infection in extreme preterm neonates. The severity depends on factors like gestation, birth weight, and invasive procedures. ICI usually presents after two weeks of age and has a smouldering course. The signs and symptoms, which are non-specific and similar to bacterial infections, include:

1. **Most common (> 50%):** Apnea, lethargy, bradycardia, respiratory distress, increased oxygen requirement, increased ventilatory settings, thrombocytopenia, increased CRP, and increased immature neutrophils. Thrombocytopenia is commonly seen, but it lacks sensitivity and specificity for diagnosing invasive candidiasis.
2. **Frequent (approximately 1/3rd of cases):** Abdominal distension, bloody stools, gastric aspirates.
3. **Less common (10 to 20%):** Hyperglycemia, metabolic acidosis, hypotension, and elevated total leucocyte count.

Evaluation for dissemination of infection is warranted in systemic candidiasis. Dissemination can involve the heart, kidneys, liver, eyes, and central nervous system. Evaluation can be done at the presentation or around 5 to 7 days after treatment with antifungal agents. Involvement of various organ systems and their clinical presentation are enlisted below:

A. **Renal:** Urinary tract infection, renal abscess.
B. **CNS:** Meningitis, ventriculitis, abscess.
C. **Gastrointestinal:** Peritonitis, spontaneous intestinal perforation.

D. **Respiratory:** Pneumonia.

E. **End organ dissemination.**

  i. **Eye:** Endophthalmitis, chorioretinitis.

  ii. **Heart:** Endocarditis, thrombi.

  iii. **Bones and joint:** Septic arthritis and osteomyelitis.

### Congenital Cutaneous Candidiasis

Clinical presentation includes diffuse skin involvement and systemic features similar to bloodstream infection. It manifests mainly in preterm neonates with a widespread erythematous maculopapular rash with well-demarcated borders leading to vesicle/pustule formation followed by skin desquamation. The most typical site of involvement is skin folds or intertriginous areas (including palms and soles). White plaques over the umbilical cord can be seen at birth. The infection is acquired either *in-utero* or at delivery. Scraping from the skin lesion demonstrates budding yeast cells or pseudohyphae.

## DIAGNOSIS

A positive fungal culture from a normally sterile site—blood, urine, CSF, bone or joint, peritoneum, pleural space—is diagnostic. In case of suspected catheter-related infection, cultures should be obtained from both peripheral venous blood and indwelling catheters.

1. **Blood culture:** Blood culture remains the gold standard.[5] About 90% of cultures grow fungus within 72 hours. Cultures should be monitored for at least 10 days to ensure the detection of fastidious species. The sensitivity of blood culture varies from 28% to 78%. Most candida species can be identified with aerobic processing on standard blood culture media. Repeat culture, if clinically indicated, increases the likelihood of obtaining positive results.
2. **Urine culture:** Urine should be collected by either suprapubic aspiration or sterile catheterization for culture and microscopy. Candida UTI is defined as $10^4$ CFU/ml in the catheter sample and >1000 CFU in the suprapubic urine sample. Hyphae (true and pseudo) and budding yeast cells are identified by microscopy.
3. CSF examination must be done in all cases of candidial bloodstream infections.
4. Cultures from other sites (peritoneal fluid, pleural fluid, etc.) should be obtained depending on the clinical presentation.

5. Candida spp. isolated from ET aspirate is challenging to interpret because it often represents colonization rather than pulmonary invasion. Endotracheal aspirates may not be helpful for the diagnosis.
6. End organ dissemination (EOD) screening must be done in all confirmed bloodstream infections. This includes eye examination for fungal ophthalmitis or retinitis, renal ultrasound for the fungal balls, echocardiography, and cranial ultrasound/CT/MRI.
7. Newer methods of diagnosis include molecular diagnostic assay using β-1,3-d-Glucan, PCR, and peptide nucleic acid fluorescent *in situ* hybridization Yeast Traffic Light (PNAFISH® YTL) assay. All these newer methods are costly, not readily available, and still need further studies to guide their routine clinical use.

## TREATMENT

Most candida species are susceptible to both fluconazole and amphotericin B except *C. glabrata* and *C. krusei*, which are intrinsically resistant to fluconazole, and *C. lusitaniae*, which is resistant to amphotericin B. Amphotericin B deoxycholate is the first-line drug recommended for systemic candidiasis including meningitis based on its efficacy, safety, and cost (Table 13.2).

Before starting treatment with amphotericin B, the following baseline investigations should be done: Hemoglobin, total leucocyte count and absolute neutrophil count, blood urea, serum creatinine, electrolytes, bilirubin, and liver enzymes.

Intravenous or oral fluconazole is an alternative to amphotericin B in neonates who had not received fluconazole prophylaxis. Lipid formulation amphotericin B should be used cautiously because it may not be effective in urinary tract infections (tissue concentration of liposomal amphotericin B is lower in kidneys and lungs). If there is a 2 to 3-fold rise in creatinine level (due to renal tubular dysfunction) with amphotericin B deoxycholate, one might switch to liposomal amphotericin B preparations. Adding 25 mg/kg of flucytosine four times daily may be considered for salvage therapy in meningitis and conditions with inadequate clinical response to amphotericin B therapy. Echinocandins are used to treat fungal infections unresponsive or resistant to amphotericin B and fluconazole.

The usual time of clearance of bloodstream infections is 3 days after appropriate antifungal therapy. The recommended duration of treatment is 2 weeks (3 weeks for meningitis) after documented clearance of candida from the bloodstream.[6]

| Table 13.2: Drugs used in the treatment of invasive fungal infection | | | |
|---|---|---|---|
| *Drug* | *Dose and route* | *Toxicity* | *Monitoring* |
| Amphotericin B deoxycholate | 1 mg/kg/d IV every 24 hours; Infuse over 2–4 hours | Renal, hematologic, hepatic | Urine output, creatinine, potassium, magnesium, liver enzymes |
| Lipid formulation amphotericin B | 3–5 mg/kg/d IV every 24 hours | Similar to amphotericin B, but decreased renal toxicity | Similar to amphotericin B |
| Fluconazole | 12 mg/kg/d oral/ IV every 24 hours | Hepatic, gastrointestinal | Liver enzymes |
| Micafungin (Echinocandin) | 4–10 mg/kg/d IV every 24 hours | Renal, hepatic (minimal) | Creatinine, urine output, liver enzymes |

1. Infusion-related toxicity of Amphotericin B is not seen in neonates; a "Lower test" dosage is not required.
2. Not enough evidence supports using liposomal or lipid formulation Amphotericin B over the deoxycholate form.
3. Primary concern with the use of fluconazole is the emergence of resistance. *C. krusei* and *C. glabrata* are resistant to fluconazole.

In neonates with bloodstream fungal infections and a central venous catheter (CVC) in place:

- Administer a dose of antifungal through the 'old' CVC (for diagnostic purposes, perform a blood culture from CVC before the antifungal therapy).
- Place a peripheral IV line.
- Remove the CVC and send the tip of the CVC for culture.
- Place a new CVC in a site other than the previous at least 36–48 h after CVC removal (if required).

## PREVENTION

Preventive strategies include the following:

1. Antifungal prophylaxis in NICUs with moderate (5–10%) to high (>10%) rates of invasive candidiasis: Intravenous or oral fluconazole prophylaxis, 3–6 mg/kg twice weekly for 6 weeks in all ELBW neonates.[6]
2. Antibiotic stewardship initiatives such as:
   a. Avoiding the use of broad-spectrum antibiotics for empirical antibiotic therapy.

   b. Early stoppage of antibiotics based on the clinical course and culture reports.
   c. Not using more than two antibiotics simultaneously.
3. Avoid the use of proton pump inhibitors or H2 blockers.
4. Early extubation to CPAP.
5. Early enteral feeding, limiting the exposure to parenteral nutrition, and early removal of central venous catheter.
6. Bundle care to prevent CLABSI and VAP.
7. Infection control measures to prevent bloodstream infections and NEC.
8. Restricting postnatal steroid usage.

| **Prophylactic antifungal therapy: What is the evidence?[7]** |
|---|
| Prophylactic systemic antifungal therapy compared to placebo/no therapy in VLBW neonates reduced incidence of invasive fungal infection (RR 0.43; 95% CI 0.31 to 0.59). No significant adverse effects have been noted with fluconazole prophylaxis [*studies done in NICUs with high incidence of invasive candidiasis* (*Cochrane* 2015)]. |

## PROGNOSIS

The mortality rate attributable to invasive candida infection in extreme preterm neonates varies from 13% to 20%. Mortality rates are higher with meningitis or disseminated infection (up to 50%). The risk of neurodevelopmental impairment in extreme preterm infants with invasive candida infection is twofold than in noninfected infants. Duration of hospital stay is also significantly prolonged in them with increased cost implications.

## REFERENCES

1. Saiman L, Ludington E, Pfaller M, Rangel-Frausto S, Wiblin RT, Dawson J, et al. Risk factors for candidemia in Neonatal Intensive Care Unit patients. The National Epidemiology of Mycosis Survey study group. Pediatr Infect Dis J. 2000 Apr;19(4):319–24.
2. Investigators of the Delhi Neonatal Infection Study (DeNIS) collaboration. Characterisation and antimicrobial resistance of sepsis pathogens in neonates born in tertiary care centres in Delhi, India: a cohort study. Lancet Glob Health. 2016 Oct;4(10):e752-60.
3. Barton M, O'Brien K, Robinson JL, Davies DH, Simpson K, Asztalos E, et al. Invasive candidiasis in low birth weight preterm infants: risk factors, clinical course and outcome in a prospective multicenter study of cases and their matched controls. BMC Infect Dis. 2014;14:327.

4. Benjamin DK, Stoll BJ, Gantz MG, Walsh MC, Sanchez PJ, Das A, et al. Neonatal Candidiasis: Epidemiology, Risk Factors, and Clinical Judgment. Pediatrics. 2010 Oct;126(4):e865–73.
5. Invasive fungal infections during the neonatal period: diagnosis, treatment and prophylaxis. Tezer H, Canpolat FE, Dilmen U. Expert Opin Pharmacother. 2012 Feb;13(2):193–205.
6. Pappas PG, Kauffman CA, Andes DR, Clancy CJ, Marr KA, Ostrosky-Zeichner L, et al. Clinical Practice Guideline for the Management of Candidiasis: 2016 Update by the Infectious Diseases Society of America. Clin Infect Dis. 2016 Feb 15;62(4):e1–50.
7. Cleminson J, Austin N, McGuire W. Prophylactic systemic antifungal agents to prevent mortality and morbidity in very low birth weight infants. Cochrane Database Syst Rev. 2015 Oct 24;(10):CD003850.
8. Austin N, Cleminson J, Darlow BA, McGuire W. Prophylactic oral/topical non-absorbed antifungal agents to prevent invasive fungal infection in very low birth weight infants. Cochrane Database Syst Rev. 2015 Oct 24;(10):CD003478.

CHAPTER

# 14

# Sepsis Outbreak in NICU

An outbreak can be defined as the occurrence of new cases of a condition in a given population that substantially exceeds the usual incidence. In the context of NICU, it is said to occur when two or more sterile site isolates of the same species are found, with the same antibiogram, from different neonates (not twins), within a space of 2 weeks. However, even a single case of a rare or multidrug-resistant (MDR) organism should trigger a prompt investigation and response.

NICUs are relatively prone to sepsis outbreaks because of the vulnerable population, reliance on equipment and invasive devices, and prolonged stay of admitted neonates. Such outbreaks lead to significant neonatal morbidity and mortality, hamper patient care, and increase hospital costs. Stringent infection control practices and periodic surveillance are essential to prevent such outbreaks.

**Burden: Evidence**

A review of the reported outbreaks (n=753) from ICUs found that NICUs were the most common to report outbreaks (37.9% of all ICU outbreaks)[1]. *Enterobacteriaceae* group was the most common causative agent of NICU outbreaks (52.9%), with *Klebsiella* being the single most common organism, followed by *Staphylococcus* spp. and *Serratia*. In 48.6% of NICU outbreaks, no cause could be identified. However, substantial measures to curb the outbreak (hand hygiene reinforcement, patient screening, isolation, personal protective equipment [PPE]) were instituted significantly more frequently in NICUs than non-NICUs.

## CAUSATIVE AGENTS AND RISK FACTORS

Some common bacterial and fungal agents responsible for sepsis outbreaks in NICU and their associated risk factors have been enlisted in Table 14.1.

**Table 14.1: Risk factors associated with outbreaks in NICU for some common pathogens**

| *Organism* | *Risk factors associated with outbreak* | *Remarks* |
|---|---|---|
| *Klebsiella pneumoniae*[2] | • Low birth weight<br>• Prolonged hospital stays<br>• Empirical antibiotic treatment<br>• Nasopharyngeal or rectal colonization | • Primary reservoirs: patients (49%), healthcare workers (HCW) (25%), contaminated sinks (14%)<br>• Higher propensity for spread than *E. coli* |
| Methicillin-resistant *Staphylococcus aureus* (MRSA)[3] | • Prolonged hospitalization<br>• Prior antibiotic exposure<br>• Exposure to other patients colonized with MRSA<br>• Overcrowding, understaffing | • Colonization of skin and anterior nares may be seen in up to 30% of patients and HCW.<br>• Outbreaks may necessitate decolonization with topical mupirocin or oral rifampicin. |
| *Pseudomonas aeruginosa*[4] | • Antibiotics use<br>• IV fluids<br>• Blood product transfusion<br>• Use of humidity in incubators<br>• Overcrowding, understaffing<br>• Use of multiple-dose medications | • Potential to form biofilms<br>• May colonize in the hands of HCW (risk factors: Age, use of artificial nails) |
| *Enterobacter cloacae*[5] | • Overcrowding, understaffing<br>• Use of multiple-dose medications | Enteral feeding may be protective against *E. cloacae*. |
| *Serratia marcescens*[6] | • Colonized hands of HCW<br>• Contaminated stock solutions | Tendency for rapid spread |
| Candida species[7] | • VLBW, prematurity<br>• Central venous catheter use<br>• Necrotizing enterocolitis<br>• Receipt of TPN<br>• Prior or prolonged broad-spectrum antibacterial drug use | • Mortality may approach 32–46%<br>• Overall, *Candida albicans* infections are most common, but *C. parapsilosis* outbreaks are being reported |

## VIRAL OUTBREAKS IN NICU

Viral outbreaks account for around 10% of all outbreaks in the NICU.[8] The most commonly implicated viruses include rotavirus, respiratory syncytial virus, enterovirus, hepatitis A virus, and adenovirus. Gastrointestinal symptoms are most frequently encountered (55%), closely followed by lower respiratory symptoms (50%).

The advent of the COVID-19 pandemic has further demonstrated the devastating effect of viral infections. Overall, viral outbreaks in NICU have been shown to have a mortality rate of 7.2%, similar to bacterial outbreaks (6.4%). Hence, it is essential to keep a high index of suspicion for viral pathogens, especially in the presence of predominant gastrointestinal and respiratory symptoms.

Investigations include testing patient samples (stool, nasopharyngeal swab, BAL) for viral antigens by RT-PCR or ELISA. Control measures remain similar to those employed in other outbreaks, including strict hand hygiene, screening of patients, isolation, cohorting, and use of PPE.

### Investigation of the Outbreak

If an outbreak is suspected in the neonatal unit, it is prudent to conduct a thorough investigation to determine the factors responsible for the outbreak at the earliest so that adequate control measures may be instituted.

The general steps for organizing such an investigation include the following:

1. **Confirm and compare:** The first step is to confirm that the outbreak has occurred by comparing the current infection rate with the previous surveillance data, especially from similar settings, such as that with the same patient profile, exact time of the year, etc. In cases of rare infections, such as emerging viral infections or opportunistic bacterial infections, such a comparison may not be necessary.
2. **Team approach:** A multidisciplinary team, including neonatologists, microbiologists, hospital infection control team members, and epidemiologists, must be formed to investigate. The involvement of hospital administration and nursing team is desirable.
3. **Case definition:** The next step is to develop a working case definition that specifies the details in terms of place, person, and time and indicates the clinical features or laboratory tests

necessary for inclusion—for example, "any baby admitted in NICU with *Klebsiella pneumoniae* isolated from any site from 1st Feb to 28th Feb". With increasing understanding, the definition can be made more precise, such as specifying the CFU of cultures or titers of antibodies.

4. **Immediate measures:** Even before the formal investigation is begun, which is often dynamic in nature, the team should plan immediate measures to curb the spread, which may include isolation or cohorting of the presumed cases or exposed population until the investigation is complete. This may occasionally require temporarily stopping new admissions in the NICU.
5. **Literature search:** A thorough literature search should be done to understand the microbiologic features of the suspected organism, the common modes of spread and ecological niche, and measures for treatment and control. For example, while Staphylococcus often colonizes the skin and nasal cavities, Pseudomonas is more often cultured from objects with moisture, and Aspergillus usually inhabits air handling units and AC ducts. Previous reports of outbreaks of the same organism can provide tremendous insights.
6. **Case-based analysis:** The next step is to list out the names and clinical characteristics of the neonates meeting the case definition, including details of:
    a. Chronology of appearance of clinical features.
    b. Location within the NICU.
    c. Details of transport or referral of the neonate to some other unit/OT/radiology suite.
    d. Everyday items for the affected neonates, including equipment like stethoscopes, phototherapy units, BP cuffs, and common medication vials/formula/donor milk sources.
    e. Physicians and nursing staff who have handled the baby.
    f. Similar symptoms in mothers who have handled the baby.
    g. Recent reports from surveillance data, including surface swab cultures.

    Such findings may be tabulated to help establish a common factor among the affected neonates. An "epidemic curve" and a "spot map" can provide a graphical representation of the same in terms of time and place, respectively.

7. **Relevant microbiological investigations:** Liberal microbiological samples should be processed based on clinical suspicion, including one or more of the following:
   a. **Samples from the affected neonates:** Blood C/S, urine C/S (especially in fungal outbreaks), skin surface swab cultures (e.g. Staphylococcus, *Candida auris*, CLABSI), stool C/S and viral PCR.

      Table 14.2 lists the common viruses to be tested for in case of suspected viral outbreaks.
   b. Sending surface cultures from equipment like incubators, warmers, and phototherapy units.
   c. Sending cultures from implicated formula powder/PDHM/medication bottles/parenteral nutrition products.
   d. In case of suspected respiratory or contact-related infections, cultures of healthcare workers and parents need to be sent.

      Leadership involvement, discretion, and confidentiality are paramount when interviewing and sampling healthcare workers.
8. **Establish clonality:** Genotyping of the isolated strains is recommended to attribute the outbreak to a single pathogen conclusively. Typical methods include pulsed-field gel electrophoresis (PFGE) and multilocus sequence typing (MLST).[9] Other methods are random amplification of polymorphic DNA (RAPD), plasmid profiling, and VNTR analysis with high-resolution melting curve (HRMC)[4] analysis. However, in resource-limited settings, isolating an organism with precisely a similar antibiotic susceptibility profile may reasonably indicate an outbreak.

**Table 14.2: Common viruses causing NICU outbreaks**

| *Symptom complex in a suspected viral outbreak* | *Common viruses to be tested for* |
|---|---|
| Gastrointestinal (diarrhea, vomiting, feed intolerance, abdominal distension) | Rotavirus, Norovirus, Adenovirus, Enterovirus, Coxsackie virus, Astrovirus, Cytomegalovirus, Hepatitis A |
| Respiratory (fast breathing, chest retractions, wheezing, desaturation, typical hyperinflation with some perihilar infiltrates on chest radiograph) | RSV, influenza, parainfluenza, rhinovirus, human metapneumovirus, SARS-CoV-2, adenovirus, parechovirus, enterovirus |

9. **Association and causality:** In the case of large outbreaks with multiple suspected causative exposures, a case-control study design may help determine the likely causality and its contribution to the outbreak. Controls in such cases should preferably be conclusively free of infection but otherwise as similar in characteristics to the cases as possible to ensure good matching. A retrospective cohort design can also be employed for such an investigation.
10. **Communicate and publish:** Once the investigation findings are known, it is vital to communicate the results and proposed control measures to the clinical, hospital administration, and microbiology teams. Publishing the findings of a successful outbreak investigation can help investigators worldwide prevent and manage a similar outbreak in their unit.

## SURVEILLANCE

Surveillance is the cornerstone of a well-functioning infection control program in a NICU. It provides reliable information on the background incidence rate of infection to identify an outbreak promptly. It also includes information on the prevailing organisms in the NICU, which can guide empirical antibiotics and control measures. The following components of a surveillance program need to be considered:[10]

A. Standard definitions must be adopted for common healthcare-associated infections, such as those proposed by CDC. Such definitions for central line-associated bloodstream infections (CLABSI), ventilator-associated pneumonia (VAP), catheter-associated urinary tract infection (CAUTI), and surgical site infections (SSIs) help maintain uniformity of data.
B. Denominator: Various denominators are used to quantify background infection/colonization rates, e.g. no. of cases per 100 patient days, no. of CLABSI per 1000 catheter days, and no. of SSIs per 1000 procedures.
C. Case finding may be done based on microbiology reports, surveillance through antibiotic usage, periodic chart reviews, or a combination of these. The microbiology team is often the first to suspect an outbreak of rare or MDR organisms, underscoring the need to communicate well with the microbiology team.
D. Periodic culturing of surface swabs from NICU surfaces, equipment, and patient paraphernalia is recommended to

assess the adequacy of routine housekeeping and disinfection practices. In our unit, such surface swab cultures are sent every month.

E. Routine body surface surveillance culturing from the skin, nasal cavity, stool of patients, and hands and nasopharynx of healthcare workers is not recommended but may be mandated during outbreaks.

F. Record keeping, preferably electronic, of such culture reports should be done, along with periodic data auditing.

## Outbreak Control Measures

Sepsis outbreak prevention and control is an ongoing process that needs to be periodically reinforced and audited to ensure compliance. Measures to prevent and control such an outbreak are listed below:

1. Strict hand hygiene, contact precautions, and barrier nursing.
2. Strict sterilization and disinfection measures and rigid compliance to appropriate housekeeping practices.
3. Use of evidence-proven measures to prevent HAIs, e.g. CLABSI bundle and VAP bundle.
4. **Isolation and cohorting:** Isolation refers to the selective placement of the patients in a separate room with separate handwashing facilities. In case of unavailability of sufficient isolation rooms, patients colonized or infected with the same organism, as in an outbreak, can be cohorted together in a separate room. In around 16% of NICU outbreaks, closure of the NICU to new admissions was required to control the outbreak.[1]
5. Use of personal protective equipment, the extent of which may vary based on the transmission risk of the outbreak pathogen.
6. Screening of patients and healthcare workers during periods of outbreak.
7. Decolonization: Usually, in case of an MRSA outbreak, nasal mupirocin (2%) twice a day for 5 days (ideally twice a month for 6 months) plus daily antimicrobial soap bathing (4% chlorhexidine) and chlorhexidine (0.12%) mouthwash twice daily[11] are recommended for the colonized HCW.
8. Ensuring adequate patient–staff ratio and preventing overcrowding.

9. Continuous education of HCW and updating the HCW about unit-specific rates of target infection.
10. Antibiotic stewardship, including:
    a. Preparation of unit-specific antibiogram.
    b. Antibiotic use monitoring.
    c. Timely de-escalation of antibiotic therapy.

Thus, neonatologists must stay vigilant in recognizing possible outbreaks and, once identified, conduct a thorough investigation, including a comprehensive microbiological evaluation. Irrespective of the causative pathogen, general preventive measures remain effective in curtailing the impact of such outbreaks. Finally, a formal reporting of such outbreaks is necessary to learn meaningful lessons in their management.

## REFERENCES


1. Gastmeier P, Loui A, Stamm-Balderjahn S, Hansen S, Zuschneid I, Sohr D, et al. Outbreaks in neonatal intensive care units - they are not like others. Am J Infect Control. 2007 Apr;35(3):172–6.
2. Baek E-H, Kim S-E, Kim S, Lee S, Cho O-H, In Hong S, et al. Successful control of an extended-spectrum beta-lactamase-producing *Klebsiella pneumoniae* ST307 outbreak in a neonatal intensive care unit. BMC Infect Dis. 2020 Feb 22;20(1):166.
3. Nambiar S, Herwaldt LA, Singh N. Outbreak of invasive disease caused by methicillin-resistant *Staphylococcus aureus* in neonates and prevalence in the neonatal intensive care unit. Pediatr Crit Care Med J Soc Crit Care Med World Fed Pediatr Intensive Crit Care Soc. 2003 Apr;4(2):220–6.
4. Jefferies JMC, Cooper T, Yam T, Clarke SC. *Pseudomonas aeruginosa* outbreaks in the neonatal intensive care unit--a systematic review of risk factors and environmental sources. J Med Microbiol. 2012 Aug;61(Pt 8):1052–61.
5. Dalben M, Varkulja G, Basso M, Krebs VLJ, Gibelli MA, van der Heijden I, et al. Investigation of an outbreak of *Enterobacter cloacae* in a neonatal unit and review of the literature. J Hosp Infect. 2008 Sep;70(1):7–14.
6. van Ogtrop ML, van Zoeren-Grobben D, Verbakel-Salomons EM, van Boven CP. *Serratia marcescens* infections in neonatal departments: description of an outbreak and review of the literature. J Hosp Infect. 1997 Jun;36(2):95–103.
7. van Schalkwyk E, Iyaloo S, Naicker SD, Maphanga TG, Mpembe RS, Zulu TG, et al. Large Outbreaks of Fungal and Bacterial Bloodstream Infections in a Neonatal Unit, South Africa, 2012-2016. Emerg Infect Dis. 2018 Jul;24(7):1204–12.
8. Civardi E, Tzialla C, Baldanti F, Strocchio L, Manzoni P, Stronati M. Viral outbreaks in neonatal intensive care units: what we do not know. Am J Infect Control. 2013 Oct;41(10):854–6.

9. Al-Dorzi HM, Arabi YM. Outbreaks in the adult ICUs. Curr Opin Infect Dis. 2017 Aug;30(4):432–9.
10. Haas JP, Trezza LA. Outbreak investigation in a neonatal intensive care unit. Semin Perinatol. 2002 Oct;26(5):367–78.
11. Huang SS, Singh R, McKinnell JA, Park S, Gombosev A, Eells SJ, et al. Decolonization to Reduce Postdischarge Infection Risk among MRSA Carriers. N Engl J Med. 2019 Feb 14;380(7):638–50.

Section

# 7

# Metabolic, Hematological, Immunological, Genetics and Endocrine Disorders

CHAPTER

15

# Inborn Errors of Metabolism

Inborn errors of metabolism (IEM) are disorders having a block in the normal metabolic pathway caused by a genetic defect of a specific enzyme. Almost 700 in number, these disorders are rare individually, but collectively they are not that uncommon. The incidence of IEM varies widely across geographical locations and can be as high as 1 in 800. The prevalence of IEM in the Indian population is still unknown. A population-based study from Goa (NeoGen, Heel to heal program; 27, 578 neonates) reported positive tests in 0.5% of the neonates. A panel of more than 50 IEM disorders was tested. A three-year data (2008–2011) demonstrated that the incidence of fatty acid oxidation defects was highest (1:480), followed by G6PD deficiency (1:840), organic aciduria (1:2300), congenital hypothyroidism (1:3440) and congenital adrenal hyperplasia (1:13800). However, this data may not represent true prevalence in India, as this program was prematurely terminated, and data on follow-up and management of screen-positive neonates was unavailable.

## CLINICAL PRESENTATION

Regardless of the underlying cause, severe illness in the newborn tends to manifest with non-specific findings, such as poor feeding, drowsiness, lethargy, hypotonia, and failure to thrive. IEM should be considered in the differential diagnosis of any sick neonate presenting with one or more of these features, along with more common causes such as sepsis, hypoxic-ischemic encephalopathy, duct-dependent cardiac lesions, congenital adrenal hyperplasia, and congenital infections (Table 15.1).

IEM disorders can manifest with different clinical presentations in the neonatal period. Various examination findings may explain the underlying IEM (Table 15.2).

The patterns of presentation include:

**Table 15.1: Clinical pointers for IEM**

- Deterioration after a period of apparent normalcy.
- Parental consanguinity.
- Family history of neonatal deaths.
- Rapidly progressive encephalopathy and seizures of unexplained cause.
- Severe metabolic acidosis.
- Persistent vomiting.
- Peculiar odor.
- Acute fatty liver or HELLP (hemolysis, elevated liver enzymes and low platelet counts) during pregnancy: Seen in women carrying fetuses with long-chain-3-hydroxy acyl-coenzyme dehydrogenase deficiency (LCHAD).

## Encephalopathy With/Without Metabolic Acidosis

Encephalopathy, seizures, and tone abnormalities are dominant presenting features of organic acidemias, urea cycle defects, and congenital lactic acidosis. Intractable seizures are prominent in pyridoxine dependency, nonketotic hyperglycinemia, molybdenum cofactor defect, and folinic-acid responsive seizures.

## Acute Liver Disease

Acute liver disease can manifest as jaundice, hepatic failure, cholestasis, or hypoglycemia:

- **Jaundice (as the only feature):** Gilbert syndrome, Crigler-Najjar syndrome.
- **Hepatic failure (jaundice, ascites, hypoglycemia, coagulopathy):** Tyrosinemia, galactosemia, neonatal hemochromatosis, glycogen storage disease type IV.
- **Neonatal cholestasis:** alpha-1 antitrypsin deficiency, Niemann-Pick disease type C.
- **Hypoglycemia:** Persistent and severe hypoglycemia may indicate an underlying IEM. Hypoglycemia is a feature of galactosemia, fatty acid oxidation defects, organic acidemias, glycogen storage disorders, and disorders of gluconeogenesis.

## Dysmorphic Features

- Dysmorphic features are seen in peroxisomal disorders, pyruvate dehydrogenase deficiency, congenital disorders of glycosylation (CDG), and lysosomal storage diseases. Some IEMs may present with nonimmune hydrops fetalis; these include lysosomal storage disorders and CDG (Table 15.2).

**Table 15.2: Clinical pointers toward specific IEM**

| *Clinical finding* | *Disorder* |
|---|---|
| Coarse facies | Lysosomal disorders |
| Cataract | Galactosemia, Zellweger syndrome |
| Retinitis pigmentosa | Mitochondrial disorders |
| Cherry red spot | Sphingolipidosis |
| Hepatomegaly | Storage disorders, urea cycle defects |
| Renal enlargement | Zellweger syndrome, glycogen storage disorder type I |
| Eczema/alopecia | Biotinidase deficiency |
| Abnormal kinky hair | Menke's disease |
| Decreased pigmentation | Phenylketonuria |

### Cardiac Disease

- Cardiomyopathy is a prominent feature in some IEMs, including fatty acid oxidation defects, glycogen storage disease type II, and mitochondrial electron transport chain defects.

## INVESTIGATIONS

Metabolic investigations should be initiated as soon as the possibility is considered. The outcome of treatment of many IEMs, especially those associated with hyperammonemia, is directly related to the rapidity with which problems are detected and appropriate management is instituted.

Urea cycle defects cause hyperammonemia without acidosis. Table 15.3 summarizes the tests performed on all babies with suspected IEM. The disease categories can be diagnosed based on blood ammonia, blood gas analysis, and urine ketone testing (Fig. 15.1).

Metabolic acidosis with or without hyperammonemia is a feature of organic acidemias and fatty acid oxidation defects. The presence of a non-glucose-reducing substance in urine suggests galactosemia. Ketonuria without a reducing substance in urine means glycogen storage diseases, gluconeogenic defects, or organic acidemias. In contrast, no ketonuria would indicate fatty acid oxidative defects, ketogenesis defects or hyperinsulinism.

**Table 15.3: List of first-line investigations to be performed in all babies with suspected IEM**

| *S. No.* | *First line investigations* | *Usual findings* | *IEM disorders* |
|---|---|---|---|
| 1. | Complete blood count | Neutropenia and thrombocytopenia | • Organic acidemia<br>• Glycogen storage disorder type 1b<br>• Mitochondrial disorders |
| 2. | Glucose estimation | Persistent hypoglycemia even at a glucose infusion rate of more than 8 mg/kg/min | FAOD, gluconeogenesis disorders, glycogen storage disease, organic acidemias |
| 3. | Blood gas and anion gap analysis | • Severe metabolic acidosis with a high anion gap<br>• Respiratory alkalosis<br>• Metabolic alkalosis | • Acidosis: Organic acidemia; Mitochondrial disorders; FAOD; Gluconeogenesis disorders<br>• Respiratory alkalosis: UCD<br>• Metabolic alkalosis: Steroid biosynthetic enzymatic defects |
| 4. | Blood ketone levels | Increased α-hydroxybutyrate and acetoacetate levels | Gluconeogenesis defects<br>Glycogen storage defects<br>Organic acidemias<br>Mitochondrial disorders |
| 5. | Plasma ammonia | Hyperammonemia (first line investigation in suspect IEM.)<br>Typical values in newborns: 90–150 μg/dl or 64–107 μmol/L | FAOD, mitochondrial disorders, gluconeogenesis defects, organic acidemias<br>UCD |

*(Contd.)*

**Table 15.3: List of first-line investigations to be performed in all babies with suspected IEM** *(Contd.)*

| *S. No.* | *First line investigations* | *Usual findings* | *IEM disorders* |
|---|---|---|---|
| 6. | Plasma lactate | Persistently high lactate of more than 3 mmol/L in the absence of hypoxia, critical cyanotic heart disease, sepsis, or seizures. | Pyruvate dehydrogenase deficiency FAOD, coenzyme Q defects |
| 7. | Liver function tests | Varying degrees of liver dysfunction and cholestasis | Tyrosinemia, galactosemia<br>Neonatal Hemochromatosis<br>FAOD, mitochondrial defects, UCD |
| 8. | Urine<br>• pH<br>• Reducing sugar<br>• Ketones | a. Urine pH <5 in the setting of metabolic acidosis<br>b. Presence of urine non-glucose reducing sugars<br>c. Positive urine ketone test in a neonate is always pathological | • Same as metabolic acidosis<br>• Galactosemia; Fructosemia; Tyrosinemia type 1<br>• Same as disorders of increased ketones in the blood |

**FAOD:* Fatty acid oxidation defects; *UCD:* Urea cycle defects

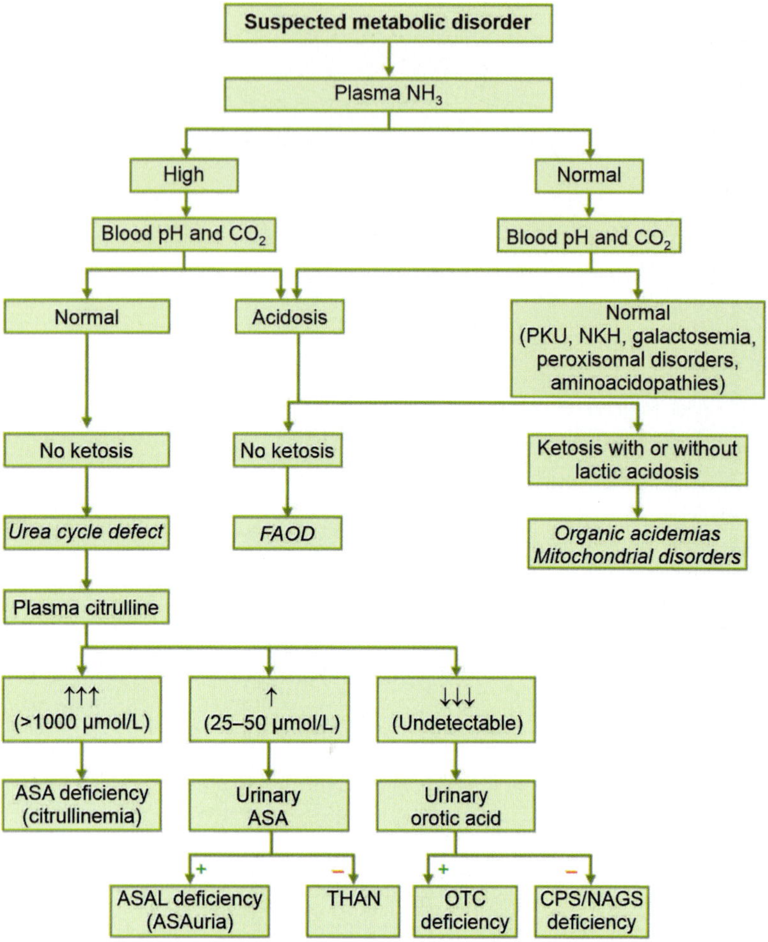


*PKU:* Phenylketonuria; *NKH:* Non-ketotic hyperglycinemia; *ASA:* Argininosuccinic aciduria; *ASAL:* Arginosuccinic acid lyase; *OTC:* Ornithine transcarbamylase; *CPS/NGAS:* Carbamoylphosphate synthetase/N-acetylglutamate synthase; *THAN:* Transient hyperammonemia of the newborn

**Fig. 15.1:** Approach to a newborn with suspected metabolic disorder

Table 15.4 lists the categorization of IEM based on simple metabolic screening tests.

## Second-line Investigations (Ancillary and Confirmatory Tests)

The following tests need to be performed in a targeted manner based on the presumptive diagnosis reached after first-line investigations:

**Table 15.4: Categorization of neonatal IEM using metabolic screening tests**

| *Acidosis* | *Ketosis* | *↑Lactate* | *↑Ammonia* | *Diagnosis* |
|---|---|---|---|---|
| – | + | – | – | Maple syrup urine disease |
| + | +/– | – | +/– | Organic aciduria |
| + | +/– | + | – | Lactic acidosis |
| – | - | – | + | Urea cycle defects |
| – | – | – | – | Nonketotic hyperglycinemia, sulfite oxidase deficiency, peroxisomal disorders, phenylketonuria, galactosemia |

1. **Gas chromatography-mass spectrometry (GCMS) of urine:** For diagnosis of organic acidemias.
2. **Plasma amino acids and acylcarnitine profile by tandem mass spectrometry (TMS):** For diagnosis of organic acidemias, urea cycle defects, aminoacidopathies, and fatty acid oxidation defects.
3. **High-performance liquid chromatography (HPLC):** for quantitative analysis of amino acids in blood and urine; required for diagnosis of organic acidemias and aminoacidopathies.
4. **Lactate/pyruvate ratio:** In cases with elevated lactate.
5. **Urinary orotic acid:** In cases with hyperammonemia for classification of urea cycle defect.
6. **Enzyme assay:** This is required for a definitive diagnosis but is unavailable for most IEMs. Functional enzyme assays include biotinidase assay in cases with suspected biotinidase deficiency (intractable seizures, seborrheic rash, alopecia); and GALT (galactose 1-phosphate uridyl transferase) assay in patients with suspected galactosemia (hypoglycemia, cataracts, reducing sugars in urine).
7. **Genetic testing:** Molecular genetic analysis is now increasingly being used for the definitive diagnosis of medium-chain acyl-CoA dehydrogenase (MCAD) deficiency and mitochondrial disorders. Gene panels using next generation sequencing (NGS) are now available for multiple IEM conditions associated with systemic complications like uncontrolled neonatal seizures, cholestatic liver disease, cardiomyopathy, resistant hypoglycemia and hyperammonemia.

8. **Neuroimaging:** MRI may provide helpful pointers toward etiology. Some IEM may be associated with structural malformations, e.g. Zellweger syndrome has diffuse cortical migration and sulcation abnormalities. Agenesis of the corpus callosum has been reported in Menke's disease, pyruvate decarboxylase deficiency and nonketotic hyperglycinemia. Examples of other neuroimaging findings in IEM include:
   - **Maple syrup urine disease (MSUD):** Brainstem and cerebellar edema.
   - **Propionic and methylmalonic acidemia:** Basal ganglia signal change.
   - **Glutaric aciduria:** Frontotemporal atrophy, subdural hematomas.
9. **Magnetic resonance spectroscopy (MRS):** May be helpful in selected disorders, e.g., lactate peak elevated in mitochondrial disorders, glycine peak in nonketotic hyperglycinemia, leucine peak elevated in MSUD.
10. **Electroencephalography (EEG):** Some EEG abnormalities may suggest particular IEM, e.g. comb-like rhythm in MSUD, burst suppression in NKH, and holocarboxylase synthetase deficiency.
11. **Plasma very long chain fatty acid (VLCFA) levels:** Elevated in peroxisomal disorders
12. **Mutation analysis, when available**.
13. **CSF amino acid analysis:** CSF glycine levels are elevated in NKH, and serine levels are low in serine biosynthesis disorders.

## PRECAUTIONS TO BE OBSERVED WHILE COLLECTING SAMPLES

1. It should be collected before specific treatment is started or feeds are stopped, as the levels may be falsely normal if the child is off feeds.
2. Blood ammonia and lactate samples should be transported in ice and immediately tested. The lactate sample should be arterial and collected after 2-hour fasting in a pre-heparinized syringe. An ammonia sample is to be collected approximately after 2 hours of fasting in an EDTA vacutainer. Avoid air mixing. The sample should be free-flowing.
3. Detailed history, including drug details, should be provided to the lab (sodium valproate therapy may increase ammonia levels).

## SAMPLES WHICH ARE TO BE OBTAINED IN INFANTS WITH SUSPECTED IEM WHEN THE DIAGNOSIS IS UNCERTAIN, AND DEATH SEEMS INEVITABLE (METABOLIC AUTOPSY)

1. Blood: 5–10 ml; frozen at –20°C; both heparinized (for chromosomal studies) and EDTA (for DNA studies) sample to be taken.
2. Urine: Frozen at –20°C.
3. CSF: Store at –20°C.
4. Skin biopsy: Including dermis in culture medium or saline with glucose. Store at 4–8°C. Do not freeze.
5. Liver, muscle, kidney, and heart biopsy: As indicated.
6. Clinical photograph (in cases with dysmorphism).
7. Infantogram (in cases with peroxisomal disorders and storage disorders with skeletal abnormalities).

In case of death of an infant with suspected IEM, a medical autopsy is performed within 4 hours of death (preferably within 2 hours) after a one-to-one discussion with the parents. This urgency is to take tissue samples before post-mortem oxidative damage to the tissue metabolites and enzyme system.

## TREATMENT

In most cases, treatment must be instituted empirically without a specific diagnosis. The metabolic screen helps to broadly categorize the patient's IEM (e.g. urea cycle defect, organic academia, congenital lactic acidosis, etc.) based on which empirical treatment can be instituted.

### Aims of Treatment

1. To reduce the formation of toxic metabolites by decreasing substrate availability (by stopping feeds and preventing endogenous catabolism).
2. To provide adequate calories.
3. To enhance the excretion of toxic metabolites.
4. To institute cofactor therapy for specific disease and also empirically if diagnosis not established.
5. Supportive care—treatment of seizures (avoid sodium valproate—may increase ammonia levels), ensure euglycemia and normothermia, maintain fluid, electrolyte, and acid–base balance, and appropriate treatment of infections and mechanical ventilation, if required.

## Management of Hyperammonemia

1. Discontinue all feeds. Provide adequate calories by intravenous glucose and lipids. Maintain glucose infusion rate of 8–10 mg/kg/min. Start intravenous lipid at 0.5 g/kg/day (increase to 3 g/kg/day). After stabilization, gradually add protein at 0.25 g/kg/day and increase till 1.5 g/kg/day.
2. Dialysis is the only means for rapid removal of ammonia, and hemodialysis is more effective and faster than peritoneal dialysis; however, peritoneal dialysis is more widely available and feasible in most units. Exchange transfusion is helpful but should be done with fresh blood because ammonia levels tend to increase in the stored blood.
3. Alternative pathways for nitrogen excretion:
   - **Sodium benzoate (IV or oral):** Loading dose 250 mg/kg followed by 250–400 mg/kg/day in 4 divided doses (intravenous preparation is unavailable in India).
   - **Sodium phenylbutyrate (unavailable in India):** Loading dose 250 mg/kg followed by 250–500 mg/kg/day.
   - **L-arginine (oral or IV):** 300 mg/kg/day (intravenous preparation not available in India).
   - **L-carnitine (oral or IV):** 200 mg/kg/day.
4. **Supportive care:** Treatment of sepsis, seizures, and ventilation. Avoid sodium valproate.

## Acute Management of a Newborn with Suspected Organic Acidemia[13]

1. Keep nil per oral; provide intravenous glucose infusion.
2. Supportive care: Hydration, treatment of sepsis, seizures, ventilation.
3. Carnitine: 100 mg/kg/day IV or oral.
4. Treat acidosis: Sodium bicarbonate 0.35–0.5 mEq/kg/hr (max 1–2 mEq/kg/hr).
5. Biotin 10 mg/day orally.
6. Vitamin $B_{12}$ (Inj hydroxy-cobalamine) 1000 µg/day I/M (useful in $B_{12}$ responsive forms of methylmalonic acidemias).
7. Thiamine 300 mg/day (useful in thiamine-responsive variants of MSUD).
8. If hyperammonemia is present, treat it as explained above.

## Management of Congenital Lactic Acidosis

1. **Supportive care:** Hydration, treatment of sepsis, seizures, ventilation; avoid sodium valproate.

2. **Treat acidosis:** Sodium bicarbonate 0.35–0.5 mEq/kg/hr (max 1–2 mEq/kg/hr).
3. **Thiamine:** up to 300 mg/day in 4 divided doses.
4. **Riboflavin:** 100 mg/day in 4 divided doses.
5. **Add coenzyme Q:** 5–15 mg/kg/day.
6. **L-carnitine:** 50–100 mg/kg orally.

Treatment of newborn with refractory seizures with no apparent etiology (suspected metabolic etiology).[14]

1. If the neonate persists to have seizures despite 2 or 3 antiepileptic drugs in adequate doses, consider a trial of pyridoxine 100 mg intravenously. If intravenous preparation is unavailable, oral pyridoxine can be given (30 mg/kg/day).
2. If seizures persist despite pyridoxine, give a trial of biotin 10 mg/day and folinic acid 15 mg/day (folinic acid-responsive seizures). A trial of pyridoxal phosphate (15–30 mg/kg/day) should also be given.
3. Rule out glucose transporter defect: Measure CSF and blood glucose. In glucose transporter defect, CSF glucose level is equal to or less than 1/3rd of the blood glucose level. This disorder responds to the ketogenic diet.

## Management of Asymptomatic Newborn with a History of Sibling Death with Suspected IEM

1. The neonate should be kept under observation.
2. One should initiate breastfeeding to keep protein intake @ 0.25 g/kg/d and then gradually increase it to 0.5 g/kg/d.
3. After about 24–48 hours of initiation of feeding, primary metabolic screening, including TMS, should be performed.
4. Urine for GCMS should be collected and stored for further analysis depending on the reports.
5. If the metabolic screen is negative, then establish full feeds over 2–3 days.
6. The infant will need careful observation and follow-up for the first few months, as IEM may present in different age groups in members of the same family.

## Long-term Treatment of IEM

The following modalities are available:

1. **Dietary treatment:** This is the mainstay in phenylketonuria, maple syrup urine disease, homocystinuria, galactosemia, and

glycogen storage disease type I and III. Special diets for PKU and MSUD are commercially available in the West, some of which can also be imported. These special diets are, however, very expensive, and cannot be afforded by most Indian patients. Based on the amino acid content of some common food products available in India, dietary exchanges are calculated and a low phenylalanine diet for PKU and diet low in branched chain amino acids for MSUD are being used in our center. As these are now being manufactured in India and are available at a lower cost, early and appropriate use of special diets in consultation with experts helps improve the long-term outcome. Some disorders like urea cycle disorders and organic acidurias require dietary modification (protein restriction) in addition to other modalities.

2. **Enzyme replacement therapy (ERT)** is now commercially available for some lysosomal storage disorders. However, these disorders do not manifest in the newborn period, an exception being Pompe's disease (glycogen storage disorder Type II) which may present in the newborn period and for which ERT, though very costly, is now available.
3. **Cofactor replacement therapy:** The catalytic properties of many enzymes depend on the participation of non-protein prosthetic groups, such as vitamins and minerals, as obligatory cofactors. The following cofactors may be beneficial in certain IEM:[17]
   - **Thiamine:** Mitochondrial disorders, thiamine-responsive variants of MSUD, PDH deficiency and complex I deficiency.
   - **Riboflavin:** Glutaric aciduria type I, type II, mild variants of electron transfer flavoprotein (ETF), electron transfer flavoprotein-dehydrogenase (ETF-DH), complex I deficiency.
   - **Pyridoxine:** 50% of cases of homocystinuria due to cystathionine β-synthetase deficiency, pyridoxine dependency with seizures, xanthurenic aciduria, primary hyperoxaluria type I, hyperornithemia with gyrate atrophy.
   - **Cobalamin:** Methylmalonic academia (cblA, cblB), homocystinuria, and methylmalonic academia (cblC, cblD, cblF).
   - **Folinic acid:** Hereditary orotic aciduria, methionine synthase deficiency, cerebral folate transporter deficiency, hereditary folate malabsorption, Kearns-Sayre syndrome.
   - **Biotin:** Biotinidase deficiency and holocarboxylase synthetase deficiency.

Table 15.5 enlists a few commercially available preparations of common drugs used for managing IEM:

**Table 15.5: Commercially available preparations of common drugs used for IEM**

| *Cofactor* | *Trade name, formulation* |
|---|---|
| Pyridoxine<br>Pyridoxal phosphate | Tab *Benadon* (40 mg) (Nicholas Piramal), Inj *Vitneurin* (1 ampoule contains 50 mg pyridoxine), Tab *B-long* (100 mg) (Elder)<br>Tab *Tetrofol plus* (contains 25 mg pyridoxal phosphate) |
| Hydroxycobalamin (Vitamin $B_{12}$) | Inj Hydrox-12 (1000 µg/ml; Neon Labs) |
| Thiamine | Tab *Benalgis* (75 mg; Franco India) |
| Riboflavin | Tab *Riboflavin* (5 mg; Shreya) |
| Biotin | Tab *Essvit* (5 mg, 10 mg; Ecopharma) |
| Carnitine | Syrup *L-Carnitor* (5 ml = 500 mg), Tab *L-Carnitor* (500 mg), Inj *carnitor* (1 g/5 ml; Elder) |
| Folinic acid | Tab *Leukorin* (15 mg; Samrath) |
| Sodium benzoate | Sachet (20 g; Hesh Co.) |
| Arginine | ARG-9 Sachet (3 g; Noveau Medicament) |
| Coenzyme Q | Tab *CoQ* (30 mg, 50 mg; Universal Medicare) |

## PREVENTION

1. Genetic counseling and prenatal diagnosis: Most IEMs are single gene defects, inherited in an autosomal recessive manner, with a 25% recurrence risk. Therefore, prenatal diagnosis can be offered wherever available for subsequent pregnancies when the diagnosis is known and confirmed by DNA analysis in the index case. The samples required are chorionic villus tissue or amniotic fluid. Modalities which are available include:[18]
   - **Substrate or metabolite detection:** Useful in phenylketonuria, peroxisomal defects.
   - **Enzyme assay:** Useful in lysosomal storage disorders like Niemann-Pick disease, Gaucher disease.
   - **DNA-based (molecular) diagnosis:** Detection of mutation in proband/carrier parents is a prerequisite.

   DNA-based diagnosis is the gold standard as enzyme assays and metabolite detection needs an expert lab and may have borderline fetal values that may pose a diagnostic dilemma.
2. **Neonatal screening:** Tandem mass spectrometry is used in some countries for neonatal screening for IEM. The cost of

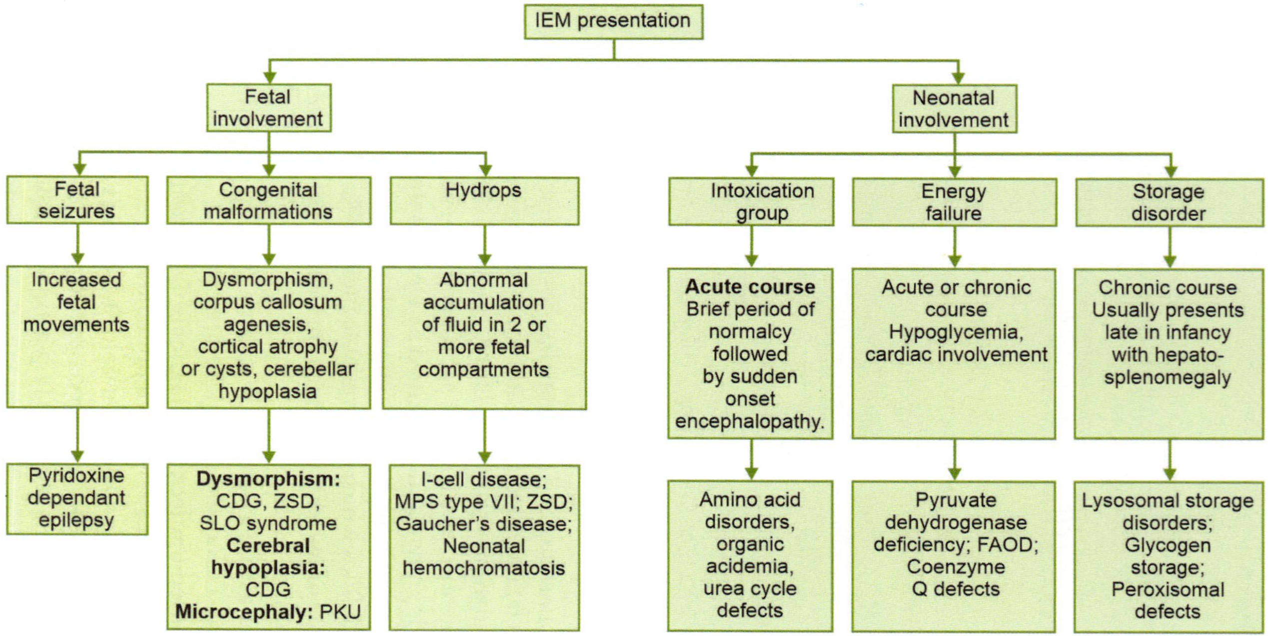


*CDG:* Congenital disorder of glycosylation; *ZSD:* Zellweger spectrum disorder; Smith-Lemli-Opitz syndrome; *PKU:* Phenylketonuria; *MPS:* Mucopolysaccharidosis; FAOD: Fatty acid oxidation defects

**Fig. 15.2:** Clinical presentation of inborn error of metabolism and possible differentials

this procedure is high. Moreover, the test has low specificity (implying many false positives); there are difficulties in interpreting abnormal test results in apparently healthy infants. TMS can detect aminoacidopathies (phenylketonuria, MSUD, homocystinuria, citrullinemia, argininosuccinic aciduria, hepatorenal tyrosinemia), fatty acid oxidation defects, organic acidemias (glutaric aciduria, propionic acidemia, methylmalonic acidemia, isovaleric acidemia).

## OUTCOME

The outcome of IEM diagnosed in the neonatal period depends on the type of IEM (intoxication group or non-intoxication group), as shown in Fig. 15.2, age, and symptoms at presentation. In general, morbidity and mortality are very high in these patients. In a recent retrospective cohort study from India, only seven neonates had intact neurological outcomes in 33 neonates diagnosed with IEM. All three neonates diagnosed by newborn screening had normal outcomes. Mean survival in months was less in the neonates with intoxication type IEM.

## REFERENCES


1. Illsinger S, Das AM. Impact of selected inborn errors of metabolism on prenatal and neonatal development. IUBMB Life. 2010 Jun;62(6):403–13.
2. Sanderson S, Green A, Preece MA, Burton H. The incidence of inherited metabolic disorders in the West Midlands, UK. Arch Dis Child. 2006 Nov;91(11):896–9.
3. Kapoor S, Thelma BK. Status of Newborn Screening and Inborn Errors of Metabolism in India. Indian J Pediatr. 2018 Dec;85(12):1110–7.
4. Sindgikar SP, Shenoy RD. Expanded newborn screening: Guiding principles, concerns, and relevance. Muller J Med Sci Res 2014;5:59–63.
5. Mookken, T. Universal Implementation of Newborn Screening in India. Int. J. Neonatal Screen. 2020,6,24.
6. A Clinical guide to inherited metabolic diseases. JTR Clarke. 3rd Ed (2006), Cambridge University Press, Cambridge.
7. Cataltepe SU, Levy HL. Inborn errors of metabolism. In: Cloherty JP, Eichenwald EC, Stark AR eds. Manual of neonatal care. 6th Edition. Lippincott Williams & Wilkins 2008; Philadelphia: 558–573.
8. Blaser S, Feigenbaum A. A neuroimaging approach to inborn errors of metabolism. Neuroimag Clin N Am 2004;14:307–329.
9. Nordli DR, De Vivo DC. Classification of infantile seizures: Implications for identification and treatment of inborn errors of metabolism. J Child Neurol 2002;17 (Suppl 3):3S3–3S8.

10. Leonard JV, Morris AAM. Diagnosis and early management of inborn errors of metabolism presenting around the time of birth. Acta Pediatrica 2006; 95:6–14.
11. Summar M. Current strategies for the management of neonatal urea cycle disorders. J Pediatr 2001; 38: S30–S39.
12. Leonard JV, Morris AAM. Urea cycle disorders. Semin Neonatol 2002; 7: 27–35.
13. de Baulny HO, Saudubray JM. Branched-chain organic acidurias. Semin Neonatol 2002;7:65–74.
14. Wolf NI, Bast T, Surtees S. Epilepsy in inborn errors of metabolism. Epileptic Disord 2005;7(2):67–81.
15. Kabra M. Dietary management of Inborn errors of metabolism. Indian J Pediatr 2002; 69:421–426.
16. Brady RO, Schiffmann R. Enzyme-replacement therapy for metabolic storage disorders. Lancet Neurol 2004;3:752–756.
17. Saudubray JM, Sedel F, Walter JH. Clinical approach to treatable inborn metabolic diseases: an introduction. J Inherit Metab Dis 2006; 29: 261–274.
18. Elias S, Simpson JL, Shulman LP. Techniques for prenatal diagnosis. In: Rimoin DL, Connor JH, Pyeritz RE, Korf BR eds. Emery and Rimoin's Principles and practice of medical genetics. Churchill-Livingstone, London 2002:802–825.
19. Balakrishnan U, Chandrasekaran A, Amboiram P, Ninan B, Ignatious S. Outcome of Inherited Metabolic Disorders Presenting in the Neonatal Period. Indian J Pediatr. 2021 May;88(5):455–462.

CHAPTER

16

# Neonatal Thrombosis

Thrombosis occurs when more than one of the three components of Virchow's triad is activated, i.e. stasis of flow, injury to the endothelial lining, and hypercoagulability of blood components. Due to physiological differences in procoagulant, anti-coagulant, and fibrinolytic factors, neonates are predisposed to thrombosis, especially with comorbidities like prematurity, perinatal asphyxia, shock, dehydration, sepsis, polycythemia, cyanotic congenital heart disease, and maternal diabetes.

The incidence of thrombosis is 3 to 5 per 100,000 live births and 0.7 to 1.5% of NICU admissions. The commonest sites of thrombosis reported are catheter site-related thrombosis, renal vein thrombosis (RVT), and cerebrosinovenous thrombosis (CST).

## CLINICAL FEATURES

Most thrombotic events in neonates are catheter-related, and the clinical features depend on the anatomical location of the thrombus. Peripheral catheter-related thrombosis can present as limb discoloration, swelling, or gangrene. Thrombosis in some sites, like portal vein thrombosis (PVT), can be asymptomatic in most neonates and is detected on ultrasound surveillance (50 to 75% of cases). Cerebral venous thrombosis (CVT) can present with seizures, abnormal tone, abnormal sensorium, feeding, and respiratory difficulties, while renal vein thrombosis (RVT) can present as a flank mass, haematuria, and thrombocytopenia.

## DIAGNOSIS

Ultrasound Doppler remains the investigation of choice due to its ease of use, non-invasive nature, and bedside availability. Neonates with thrombosis—that is not catheter-related—should be evaluated for coagulation and fibrinolytic factors: Factor V Leiden mutation, prothrombin 20210 mutation, antithrombin deficiency, protein C and protein S deficiency, and antiphospholipid antibodies in mother. It is preferable to delay the analysis of these factors till the infant is at least six weeks of postnatal age unless the clinical condition is severe or recurrent. It is essential to interpret the results of the coagulation factors based on age and gestation-dependent reference values.

## MANAGEMENT

The principles of management of neonatal thrombosis include:

i. Supportive management.
ii. Use of anticoagulation.
iii. Use of thrombolysis or antiplatelet agents, and
iv. Surgical intervention.

Most neonatal thromboses are transient because they have an underlying reversible cause, like indwelling central lines/catheters. Removal of the catheter whenever possible leads to the resolution of thrombosis over the next few days. Given the low recurrence risk of thrombosis in the neonatal period, the primary treatment goals are to reduce the end organ damage and prevent thrombus extension. The main anticoagulant drugs that can be used in neonates are:

i. Unfractionated heparin (UFH).
ii. Low molecular weight heparin (LMWH).
iii. Oral/intravenous vitamin K antagonists (VKAs), and
iv. Thrombolytics and aspirin.

The medications are summarised in Table 16.1.

In addition to the anticoagulant medications mentioned above, fresh frozen plasma (FFP) can also be used in certain instances–for example, in neonates with purpura fulminans if protein C concentrate is unavailable.

The following flowchart depicts the choice between conservative versus initiating antithrombotic therapy in neonatal thrombosis, depending on:

i. The anatomical site of the thrombus.
ii. Symptoms.
iii. Likely etiology, and
iv. Probability of recurrence.

### Monitoring and Therapeutic Endpoints for Anticoagulation

#### *Titration of the Anticoagulant Dose*

The UFH should be titrated with anti-factor Xa (anti-Xa) or aPTT. The target anti-Xa is 0.35 to 0.7 units/ml, while the target aPTT is

**Table 16.1: Common medications used in neonatal thrombosis**

| S. No. | *Class of drug* | *Merits* | *Demerits* | *Dose* |
|---|---|---|---|---|
| 1. | Unfractionated heparin (UFH) | Short half-life and rapid onset and offset of action; Ideal agent for infants with perceived high bleeding risk like post-operative period. | Either aPTT or anti-Xa level may be used for monitoring; Monitoring using anti-Xa has some advantages (fewer tests and dose changes) but is expensive and not easily available. aPTT can be used as an alternative; Long-term use of UFH can cause osteoporosis. | IV bolus of 75 to 100 U per kg followed by infusion of 28 U/kg/hour. |
| 2. | Low molecular weight heparin (LMWH) E.g. Enoxaparin Tinzaparin Dalteparin | Subcutaneous dosing. Low rates of bleeding (0 to 19%) | Low predictability of effect due to the difference in plasma binding; Monitoring can be done only by factor Xa levels; Effect only partially reversible by Protamine. | Enoxaparin 1.5 mg/kg twice daily (therapeutic); 1.5 mg/kg once daily (prophylactic) |
| 3. | Vitamin K antagonists (VKA): Warfarin *(other direct anticoagulants like dabigatran are approved only above 3 months of age).* | Least commonly used antithrombotic agent in neonates | Only available in tablet form; Low predictability of effect because of rapid changes in the physiology of vitamin K-dependent factors in the neonatal period; | Start at 0.1 to 0.2 mg per kg (maximum of 5 mg) |

*(Contd.)*

**Table 16.1: Common medications used in neonatal thrombosis (Contd.)**

| S. No. | *Class of drug* | *Merits* | *Demerits* | *Dose* |
|---|---|---|---|---|
| | | | Breastmilk has low concentrations of vitamin K, hence breastfed infants are sensitive to the effect of vitamin K (antagonist). | |
| 4. | Thrombolytics, e.g. tissue plasminogen activator. | Indicated in case of end-organ or limb damage (*see* management flowchart) | | 0.1 to 0.6 mg/kg/hour |
| 5. | Aspirin | Used in neonates/ infants with recurrent arterial stroke | Helpful in only selected neonates. | 1 to 5 mg/kg/ day |

*APTT:* Activated partial thromboplastin time; *TTR:* Target therapeutic range; *UFH:* Unfractionated heparin; *LMWH:* Low molecular weight heparin; *FFP:* Fresh frozen plasma; *VKA:* Vitamin K antagonists

1.5 to 2 times the normal level. The dose of LMWH is titrated by anti-Xa factor levels.

Vitamin K antagonists (VKA) should be monitored by serial INR measurements (target 2.5, range 2 to 3). INR should be repeated every two weeks, and the dose should be titrated accordingly.

Thrombolytic therapy has a limited role in managing neonatal thrombosis, e.g. if the thrombus occludes a major vessel causing critical compromise of organs or limbs. Before starting thrombolytic therapy, obtaining a D-dimer level and correcting severe coagulopathy is desirable. FFP is given to all neonates before thrombolytic treatment.

### *Therapeutic Endpoints*

Once initiated, anticoagulation therapy should continue for 6 weeks to a maximum of 3 months, depending on the resolution of the thrombus on ultrasound and clinical symptoms. The optimal frequency of serial

**Neonatal thrombosis**

| Anatomical site | Outline of management |
|---|---|
| Cerebral venous thrombus | If without ICH, use LMWH or UFH followed by LMWH.<br>If with ICH, either anticoagulation or supportive management with radiological monitoring for 5–7 days and then anticoagulation if required. |
| Neonatal stroke | First arterial ischemic stroke (AIS) with no ongoing embolic source: Supportive care.<br>First AIS with documented embolic source: Start UFH or LMWH. Recurrent AIS: UFH or aspirin |
| Right atrial thrombus | Remove the central catheter if possible. Treat with LMWH.<br>If cardiac function is compromised, start thrombolytic therapy. |
| Portal vein thrombus | Remove UVC if possible. If thrombosis limited to left portal vein, conservative management, and serial monitoring.<br>Thrombus extending to main portal vein or IVC: Treat with LMWH |
| Renal vein thrombus | Unilateral RVT with no IVC extension: Serial radiological monitoring.<br>Unilateral RVT with IVC extension: Treat with UFH/LMWH<br>Bilateral RVT with renal impairment: Treat with UFH/LMWH or initial thrombolysis followed by UFH |
| Femoral artery thrombus | Treat with UFH or LMWH.<br>Thrombolysis only if limb threatening with proximal extension.<br>Surgical intervention if thrombolysis is contraindicated and organ or limb death is imminent. |
| Central catheter thrombus | LMWH or UFH followed by LMWH<br>Removal of catheter after 3 to 5 days of therapy<br>Thrombolytic therapy only if major vessel occlusion |
| Peripheral catheter-related arterial thrombus | Immediate removal of catheter.<br>If symptomatic, then UFH with or without thrombolysis and microvascular repair. |
| Neonatal purpura fulminans | Initial stabilisation with protein C concentrate 20–60 units/kg or FFP (10–20 mL/kg).<br>Long-term treatment: VKA or LMWH or protein C replacement or liver transplant. |

*ICH:* Intracranial hemorrhage; *UFH:* Unfractionated heparin; *LMWH:* Low molecular weight heparin; *AIS:* Arterial ischaemic stroke; *UVC:* Umbilical venous catheter

**Fig. 16.1:** Management outline for neonatal thrombosis

ultrasound monitoring for neonates on conservative management is unknown and should be based on clinical judgment. Once the clinical symptoms resolve and the thrombus is no longer detected on ultrasound, the therapy can be stopped.

## Prevention of Catheter-related Thrombosis

**Arterial catheters:** To prevent peripheral catheter-related thrombosis, it is preferable to use UFH infusion through the catheters. The appropriate dose is 0.5 to 1 unit/ml of UFH at 1 ml/hour. For umbilical arterial catheters, the dose is 0.25 to 1 unit/ml of UFH. Heplock injection contains 10 IU per ml and is the most commonly used concentration of heparin for flushing intravenous lines. Umbilical arteries should be placed in a 'high' position instead of a 'low' position.

**Cardiothoracic surgeries, neonatal stroke, and cerebral sinus venous thrombus (CSVT):** For most infants with cardiac illness requiring multistage surgeries, thromboprophylaxis with VKA or aspirin is recommended. For neonates with AIS (arterial ischemic stroke), in whom an underlying source of embolus is not ruled out, aspirin prophylaxis is recommended for at least two years.

**Purpura fulminans:** Infants diagnosed with purpura fulminans should be treated indefinitely with either VKA or LMWH, or protein C concentrates to prevent thrombosis.

## Long-term Outcomes and Prognosis

The anatomical location of the thrombus determines the long-term outcomes and prognosis in neonates. Portal vein thrombosis, although initially asymptomatic, can result in portal hypertension later. Similarly, renal vein thrombosis may cause renal hypertension, tubular dysfunction, and renal failure late in life.

## REFERENCES

1. Sirachainan N, Limrungsikul A, Chuansumrit A, et al. Incidences, risk factors, and outcomes of neonatal thromboembolism. J Matern Fetal Neonatal Med 2018; 31:347.
2. Unal S, Gönülal D, Siyah Bilgin B, et al. Experience and Prognosis of Systemic Neonatal Thrombosis at a Level III NICU. J Pediatr Hematol Oncol 2018; 40:e410.
3. Bhat R, Kumar R, Kwon S, et al. Risk Factors for Neonatal Venous and Arterial Thromboembolism in the Neonatal Intensive Care Unit-A Case Control Study. J Pediatr 2018; 195:28.
4. El-Naggar W, Yoon EW, McMillan D, et al. Epidemiology of thrombosis in Canadian neonatal intensive care units. J Perinatol 2020; 40:1083.
5. Barrington KJ. Umbilical artery catheters in the newborn: effects of heparin. Cochrane Database Syst Rev 2000; CD000507.

6. Monagle P, Chan AKC, Goldenberg NA, et al. "Antithrombotic therapy in neonates and children: Antithrombotic Therapy and Prevention of Thrombosis, 9th ed: American College of Chest Physicians Evidence-Based Clinical Practice Guidelines." Chest vol. 141,2 Suppl (2012): e737S-e801S. updated March 2022. Available on https://www.guidelinecentral.com/guideline/9262.
7. Van Ommen CH, Heijboer H, Büller HR, et al. Venous thromboembolism in childhood: a prospective two-year registry in The Netherlands. J Pediatr 2001; 139:676.
8. Shah PS, Shah VS. Continuous heparin infusion to prevent thrombosis and catheter occlusion in neonates with peripherally placed percutaneous central venous catheters. Cochrane Database Syst Rev 2008; CD002772.
9. Cruickshank MK, Levine MN, Hirsh J, et al. A standard heparin nomogram for the management of heparin therapy. Arch Intern Med 1991; 151:333.
10. Klaassen ILM, Sol JJ, Suijker MH, et al. Are low-molecular-weight heparins safe and effective in children? A systematic review. Blood Rev 2019; 33:33.
11. Monagle P, Newall F. Management of thrombosis in children and neonates: practical use of anticoagulants in children. Hematology Am Soc Hematol Educ Program. 2018 Nov 30;2018(1):399–404.
12. Kearon C, Akl EA. Duration of anticoagulant therapy for deep vein thrombosis and pulmonary embolism. Blood. 2014 Mar 20;123(12):1794-801. doi 10.1182/blood-2013-12-512681.
13. Bohnhoff JC, DiSilvio SA, Aneja RK, Shenk JR, Domnina YA, Brozanski BS, Good M. Treatment and follow-up of venous thrombosis in the neonatal intensive care unit: a retrospective study. J Perinatol. 2017 Mar;37(3):306–310.

CHAPTER

# 17

# Inborn Errors of Immunity

Inborn errors of immunity, often referred to as primary immunodeficiency disorders (PID), consist of a heterogeneous group of over 400 disorders characterized by a qualitative or a quantitative defect in the function of the immune system. PIDs typically present with increased susceptibility to infections, but may also be associated with autoimmunity, allergy, and malignancy.[1] Contrary to the usual belief, as a group, PIDs are not uncommon and their estimated incidence is 1 in 1000–5000 in the general population. Table 17.1 summarizes the major categories of primary immunodeficiency disorders.[2] A few of these disorders which may manifest in the neonatal period or early infancy have been enlisted in Table 17.2.

Compared to older children, neonates have a weaker immune system, making them more susceptible to systemic infections. As the maturation of the adaptive immune system (T- and B-cells) depends on antigen stimulation, neonates rely predominantly on the innate immune system. However, neutrophil production as well as function is impaired in them, especially in preterm neonates. Similarly, the cytotoxicity of macrophage and NK cells is lesser as compared to that in adults. Despite a higher number of T-cells in neonates, physiological function is diminished, rendering them susceptible to infection. For humoral immunity, neonates are dependent on maternally transferred antibodies. Since most of these antibodies are transferred in the third trimester, preterm neonates have a significantly smaller pool of antibodies.[3]

## WHEN TO SUSPECT A PID?

The Jeffrey Modell Foundation's 10 warning signs of primary immunodeficiency are widely used to suspect PID. However, many of these signs do not manifest in the neonatal period, necessitating

**Table 17.1: Major categories of primary immunodeficiency disorders**

| *Characters* | *Predominant T cell defect* | *Predominant B cell defect* | *Granulocyte defect* | *Complement defect* |
|---|---|---|---|---|
| Age at the onset of disease | Early onset (2–6 months of age) | Onset after 5–7 months of age (after maternal antibodies get depleted) | Early onset | Onset at any age |
| Specific pathogens involved[#] | Viral and opportunistic organisms (CMV, EBV, Varicella, Mycobacteria, Candida, *Pneumocystis jirovecii*) | Organisms causing mucosal infections (Pneumococcus, Streptococcus, Staphylococcus, Campylobacter, Mycoplasma, Enterovirus Giardia, Cryptosporidia) | Unusual organisms and unusual sites of infections (Staphylococcus, Pseudomonas, Salmonella Candida, Nocardia, Aspergillus) | Encapsulated organisms (Pneumococcus, Neisseria, Hemophilus) |
| Clinical manifestations | • Mucocutaneous candidiasis<br>• Pulmonary infections<br>• Failure to thrive<br>• Chronic diarrhea | • Recurrent sinopulmonary infections<br>• Chronic gastrointestinal symptoms<br>• Enteroviral meningoencephalitis | • Superficial and deep abscess<br>• Suppurative lymphadenitis<br>• Gingivitis, osteomyelitis | • Meningitis<br>• Sepsis<br>• Recurrent sinopulmonary infections |
| Special features | • Graft vs host disease<br>• Postvaccination disseminated BCG/ varicella | • Autoimmunity<br>• Lymphoreticular malignancies<br>• Postvaccination paralytic polio | • Poor wound healing<br>• Delayed separation of umbilical cord | • Autoimmune disorders (glomerulonephritis, SLE, angioedema) |

*CMV:* Cytomegalovirus; *EBV:* Epstein-Barr virus; *SLE:* Systemic lupus erythematosus

[#]In PIDs, infections are more commonly caused by usual pathogenic organisms. However, infections by certain specific organisms may point towards a particular type of defect.

**Table 17.2: Primary immunodeficiency disorders presenting in early infancy**

| *Condition* | *Clinical features* | *Investigations* |
|---|---|---|
| Severe combined immunodeficiency (SCID) | Recurrent life-threatening infections<br>Persistent thrush<br>Failure to thrive<br>Chronic diarrhea<br>Graft versus host disease | Severe lymphopenia<br>Absent thymus on imaging<br>Molecular diagnosis<br>Genetic testing for common gamma chain deficiency |
| 22q11.2 deletion syndrome | Thymic hypoplasia/ aplasia<br>Congenital heart defects (TOF, VSD, truncus arteriosus)<br>Hypocalcemia (tetany, seizures)<br>Abnormal facies<br>Cleft palate | Absent thymic shadow on chest X-ray<br>Low serum calcium levels<br>FISH for 22q11.2 microdeletion |
| X-linked agammaglobulinemia | Recurrent sinopulmonary infections (usually presents after 5–7 months)<br>Absence of tonsillar tissues<br>Poor response to vaccination | Pan hypogammaglobulinemia<br>BTK gene mutation |
| Chronic granulomatous disease (CGD) | Bacterial and fungal infections of skin, lung, lymph nodes with catalase positive organisms: (*Staphylococcus aureus*, Pseudomonas, Candida, Aspergillus, Mycobacterium, Nocardia, Listeria, Serratia, *Escherichia coli*) | Dihydrorhodamine oxidation test (DHR) (preferred)<br>Nitroblue tetrazolium dye reduction test<br>Genetic analysis of Phox genes |

*(Contd.)*

**Table 17.2: Primary immunodeficiency disorders presenting in early infancy** *(Contd.)*

| *Condition* | *Clinical features* | *Investigations* |
|---|---|---|
| Leukocyte adhesion defect (LAD) | Delayed separation of umbilical cord<br>Recurrent bacterial and fungal infections | Neutrophilia<br>Flow cytometry for expression of CD18, CD11a, CD11c on lymphocytes<br>IRGB2 mutation |
| Wiskott-Aldrich syndrome (WAS) (X linked) | Recurrent infections (lymphopenia, impaired T-cell function, hypogammaglobulinemia)<br>Bleeding diathesis<br>Eczema | Thrombocytopenia with small platelet size ($<7$ fL)<br>Flow cytometry for WASp protein |
| Congenital neutropenia | Frequent abscesses, gingivitis, sepsis<br>Aphthous ulcers<br>May be diagnosed incidentally on routine blood counts | Absolute neutrophil count $<500/mm^3$<br>Bone marrow: Maturational arrest of myeloid precursors<br>Mutation in ELANE gene |

**Table 17.3: Warning signs of primary immunodeficiency in childhood and neonatal period**

| *The Jeffrey Modell Foundation's 10 warning signs of immune deficiency* | *Additional warning signs of PID in a neonate* |
|---|---|
| 1. ≥4 new ear infections within 1 year.<br>2. ≥2 serious sinus infections within 1 year.<br>3. ≥2 months on antibiotics with little effect.<br>4. ≥2 pneumonias within 1 year.<br>5. Failure of an infant to gain weight or grow normally*<br>6. Recurrent, deep skin or organ abscesses.<br>7. Persistent thrush in mouth or fungal infection on skin.*<br>8. Need for IV antibiotics to clear infections.<br>9. ≥2 deep-seated infections including septicemia.<br>10. A family history of PID.* | 1. Infections with unusual organisms: Fungi, Mycobacteria, Burkholderia, Serratia, Cryptococcus<br>2. Infections at atypical sites: Deep abscess, omphalitis, encephalitis<br>3. Chronic diarrhea<br>4. History of unexplained deaths in previous siblings/ family members<br>5. Multiple maternal miscarriages<br>6. Eczema, erythroderma |

**Applicable to neonatal period*

a high index of suspicion.[4] Certain warning signs which may point to an underlying PID in a neonate have been enlisted in Table 17.3.

## APPROACH TO A NEONATE WITH SUSPECTED PID

### A. Clinical Examination

A thorough examination can provide important clinical clues to an underlying PID (Table 17.4).

- **Anthropometry:** Failure to thrive is often the first pointer to an underlying PID.
- **General examination:** Pallor, lymphadenopathy, tonsils, umbilicus (discharge/redness/delayed separation of cord), joint swelling, rash.
- **Systemic exam:** Localize the focus of infection.

### B. Investigations

Flowchart 17.1 depicts diagnostic approach in infant with suspected PID.

**Table 17.4: Clinical pointers to specific primary immunodeficiency disorders**

| *Clinical pointers* | *Diagnosis* |
|---|---|
| Hypopigmented hair | Chédiak-Higashi syndrome, Griscelli syndrome |
| Eczema | Wiskott-Aldrich syndrome, hyper-IgE syndrome |
| Petechial lesions | Wiskott-Aldrich syndrome |
| Telangiectasia | Ataxia telangiectasia |
| Absent tonsils/ lymph nodes | Agammaglobulinemia, SCID |
| Aphthous ulcers, gingivitis | Congenital neutropenia, CGD |
| Erythroderma, alopecia | Omenn syndrome |
| Hypertelorism, low set ears, cleft palate, dysmorphism | DiGeorge syndrome or other syndromic PIDs |

*SCID:* Severe combined immunodeficiency; *CGD:* Chronic granulomatous disease

## TREATMENT PRINCIPLES

- Isolation of the patient (home/hospital), with meticulous hand hygiene and asepsis precautions
- Antimicrobial prophylaxis:[6]
  - Antibacterial and *P. jiroveci* prophylaxis is recommended in combined and B-cell defects. Cotrimoxazole (5 mg/kg TMP 3 days/week) is the preferred agent beyond 6 weeks of age. Amoxicillin and Azithromycin are the other commonly used agents.
  - Antifungal prophylaxis: Itraconazole (5 mg/kg once a day) in patients with CGD, Fluconazole (3 mg/kg once a day) in patients with SCID.
- Immunoglobulins: Periodic IVIG are administered in many humoral and combined defects with hypogammaglobulinemia usually at a dose of 400–500 mg/kg/dose every 3–4 weeks. However, it is rarely required in neonatal period.
- Vaccination: Table 17.5.

All standard vaccines can be given to the close contacts of infants with PID, except OPV as there is a risk of infection due to viral shedding is unlikely.[5]

- **Blood products:** Only irradiated leuko-depleted products should be used, to prevent CMV infection and graft versus host disease.
- **Breastfeeding:** In case of severe T-cell deficiency, breastfeeding should ideally be withheld till mother is proven to be CMV negative.

**Flowchart 17.1:** Diagnostic approach in an infant with suspected PID

Infant with suspected PID

↓

**Screening tests**

1. Complete blood count with differential leukocyte count*
   a. Absolute neutrophil counts
      i. ANC <500/mm$^3$ in congenital neutropenia and cyclical neutropenia
      ii. ANC often >20,000/mm$^3$ in LAD
   b. Absolute lymphocyte count (ALC) <2500/mm$^3$, or CD3 count <1500/mm$^3$ in T-cell defects.
   c. Platelet count with platelet size (decreased in WAS)
2. Chest X-ray for thymic shadow
3. HIV testing for the infant and parents; rule out secondary immunodeficiency

↓

Further diagnostic tests based on the suspected PID category

↓

**Suspected T-cell/ combined defect:**

- Flow cytometry for T and B cell markers#
- FISH for 22q11.2 deletion
- Proliferative response to mitogens, antigens, allogenic cells
- Enzyme assays (ADA): SCID

**Suspected B-cell defect:**

Immunoglobulin levels:

a. X-linked agammaglobulinemia: All Ig subclasses low
b. Hyper-IgM syndrome: Normal or elevated IgM; low IgG, IgE, IgA
c. Hyper-IgE syndrome: Highly elevated IgE

Flow cytometry for B cell markers

Suspected phagocytic defect:

- Flow cytometry: CD 11/ CD18 (LAD 1), CD15 (LAD 2)
- Dihydrorhodamine test (DHR) for CGD
- Enzyme assay: NADPH oxidase for CGD

↓

Consider mutation analysis for specific conditions.

↓

**Samples to be taken in:**

- Heparin vial for cell surface markers and DHR testing
- Plain vial for serum Immunoglobulin level

**Note:**

**It is important to use age-specific reference ranges for cell counts.*

*#B-cell markers: CD19, CD20, CD40/ CD40L (hyper-IgM syndrome), CD27 (memory* B cells).

*T-cell markers: CD3, CD4, CD8, CD19/20, CD16/56, CD45 RO (naive)/ RA (memory).*

*Abbreviations: CGD: Chronic granulomatous disease, LAD: Leukocyte adhesion defect, SCID: Severe combined immunodeficiency; WAS: Wiskott-Aldrich syndrome; DHR: Dihydrorhodamine.*

**Table 17.5: Vaccination of infants with suspected or confirmed primary immunodeficiencies[7]**

| *PID category* | *Contraindicated vaccines* | *Risk-specific recommended vaccines* | *Remarks* |
|---|---|---|---|
| B-cell defect (humoral) | OPV<br>BCG<br>MMR<br>Ty21a<br>Smallpox<br>Live influenza vaccine | Pneumococcal<br>*Hemophilus influenzae* type b (Hib) | In severe antibody deficiencies, the effectiveness of any vaccine is uncertain. |
| T-cell defect | All live vaccines | Pneumococcal<br>Meningococcal<br>Hib | Vaccines are likely to be effective |

- **Audiologic evaluation:** A high rate of sensorineural hearing loss has been observed in PIDs. These may be attributable to:
  a. Infection with CMV, enteroviruses.
  b. Persistent inflammation associated with infections.
  c. Frequent use of ototoxic medications such as aminoglycosides.
- Hematopoietic stem cell transplant is curative for many PIDs such as SCID, and the infant should be referred to appropriate centers at the earliest to prevent organ damage.

## AUTOINFLAMMATORY DISORDERS IN INFANCY

Autoinflammatory disorders are characterized by an exaggerated or inappropriate activation of the immune system, resulting in an autonomous production of inflammatory mediators. Such disorders have been included in the umbrella of inborn errors of immunity and typically present with fever, rash, arthritis and organomegaly. Some of these include deficiency of the interleukin-1 receptor antagonist (DIRA), which can present with fever, skin pustules, periostitis of long bones, respiratory distress[1,8]. Other autoinflammatory syndromes which may present in neonatal period include neonatal onset multisystem inflammatory syndrome (NOMID) or chronic infantile neurologic cutaneous and articular (CINCA) syndrome which may present with rash, chronic meningitis, arthropathy, fever and inflammation. The detailed description of these rare disorders is beyond the scope of this chapter, however, one should be aware of these disorders whilst dealing with newborns with aforementioned clinical features.

**Key messages**

- Several inborn errors of immunity can present in early infancy.
- A high index of suspicion is required to diagnose these conditions, and a thorough history, including family history, and examination are pivotal.
- Basic investigations such as complete blood counts, blood smear and chest X-ray might give clues such as lymphopenia, neutropenia, small platelet size and thymic aplasia, towards underlying diagnosis.
- It is advisable to consult a pediatric immunologist for a confirmatory diagnosis. Isolation, antimicrobial prophylaxis, selective vaccination strategies, and timely referral to an expert center is the key to a successful outcome.

## REFERENCES


1. Tangye SG, Al-Herz W, Bousfiha A, Chatila T, Cunningham-Rundles C, Etzioni A, et al. Human Inborn Errors of Immunity: 2019 Update on the Classification from the International Union of Immunological Societies Expert Committee. J Clin Immunol. 2020 Jan;40(1):24–64.
2. Kliegman RM, St. Geme J. Nelson textbook of pediatrics. 21st ed. Philadelphia, Pennsylvania: Elsevier; 2019.
3. Dowling DJ, Levy O. Ontogeny of early life immunity. Trends Immunol. 2014 Jul;35(7):299–310.
4. O'Connell AE. Primary Immunodeficiency in the NICU. NeoReviews. 2019 Feb;20(2):e67–78.
5. Walkovich K, Connelly JA. Primary immunodeficiency in the neonate: Early diagnosis and management. Semin Fetal Neonatal Med. 2016 Feb;21(1):35–43.
6. Papadopoulou-Alataki E, Hassan A, Davies EG. Prevention of infection in children and adolescents with primary immunodeficiency disorders. Asian Pac J Allergy Immunol. 2012 Dec;30(4):249–58.
7. ACIP General Best Practice Guidelines for Immunization | CDC [Internet]. 2023 [cited 2023 Feb 11]. Available from: https://www.cdc.gov/vaccines/hcp/acip-recs/general-recs/index.html.
8. De Rose DU, Coppola M, Gallini F, Maggio L, Vento G, Rigante D. Overview of the rarest causes of fever in newborns: handy hints for the neonatologist. J Perinatol. 2021 Mar;41(3):372–82.

CHAPTER

# 18

# Congenital Hypothyroidism

Congenital hypothyroidism (CH) is a preventable cause of mental retardation. The worldwide incidence of CH is 1: 3000–4000 live births, while the estimated incidence in Indian studies varies from 1: 1200–3400 live births.[1] Thyroid dysgenesis is the commonest cause accounting for 75–80% of all cases of CH.

## PHYSIOLOGY OF THE THYROID IN THE FETUS

Synthesis and secretion of thyroxine (T4) and triiodothyronine (T3) starts from 12 weeks of gestation. Thyrotropin-releasing hormone (TRH) and thyroid stimulating hormone (TSH) are detectable by the end of first trimester but the activity of the hypothalamic-pituitary-thyroid (HPT) axis is still not well developed, with insufficient production of thyroid hormones until 18 to 20 weeks of gestation. Therefore, the fetus depends on the transplacental passage of thyroid hormones during this period. In the second half of pregnancy, fetal T4 and TSH levels increase progressively.

In the hypothyroid fetus, transplacental passage of maternal thyroid hormones and increased conversion of T4 to T3 in the fetal brain by type 2 deiodinase confer neuroprotection, and near normal cognitive outcomes are possible if maternal thyroid function is normal and postnatal therapy is initiated early. In contrast, there is significant neuro-intellectual impairment when both maternal and fetal hypothyroidism are present, as in severe iodine deficiency.

As maternal hypothyroidism (overt as well as subclinical) has an adverse effect on cognitive outcome of the offspring, a brief review of maternal hypothyroidism including pathophysiology as well as management have been provided herewith.

## PHYSIOLOGICAL CHANGES IN THYROID FUNCTION TESTS DURING PREGNANCY

During pregnancy, there is an increase in thyroxine-binding globulin (TBG), and hence in total T4 and T3 levels. Additionally, in high concentration, hCG directly stimulates the thyroid gland (due to structural similarity with TSH), leading to reduction in TSH production, thus decreasing the normal upper and lower limit of TSH by 0.5–1 mU/L and 0.1–0.2 mU/L respectively. Because hCG levels are highest in the 1st trimester, the reduction in TSH is also maximal in the 1st trimester.

## DIAGNOSIS AND MANAGEMENT OF MATERNAL HYPOTHYROIDISM IN PREGNANCY

- **Maternal TSH levels:** The Indian Thyroid Society in its 2019 recommendations suggests a TSH cut-off value of 2.5 mU/L in the 1st trimester and 3 mU/L in the 2nd and 3rd trimesters. American Thyroid Association (ATA) guidelines recommend the use of trimester and population specific TSH cut-offs, in the absence of which an arbitrary cut off of > 4 mU/L is to be taken as the upper limit of reference range (ULRR).[2]
- **Whom to screen:** ATA 2017 guidelines recommend performing first trimester TSH screening only in high-risk pregnancies like women with hypo/hyperthyroidism, thyroid antibody positivity or presence of goitre, history of head and neck radiation, older age (>30 years), autoimmune disorders or family history of such disorders (including type 1 DM), history of pregnancy loss, preterm delivery, infertility, multiple prior pregnancies, morbid obesity, use of drugs known to suppress thyroid function, residence in areas of moderate to severe iodine insufficiency.[2] However Indian Thyroid Society (ITS) recommends universal TSH level screen. In AIIMS Delhi, as our region falls in the moderate iodine deficiency category, and most women are considered high risk, we follow universal screening in the first trimester.
- **Treatment with levothyroxine:** As per NRHM GOI 2014 guideline, starting dose of levothyroxine for subclinical hypothyroidism (TSH: 2.5–10 mU/L, normal FT4) and overt hypothyroidism (TSH >10 mU/L, irrespective of FT4 level) are 25–50 µg/day and 50–100 µg/day, respectively. Once treatment with levothyroxine is initiated, repeat TSH is recommended after 6 weeks to assess the adequacy of treatment.
- **After delivery,** immediate discontinuation of treatment is recommended when thyroxine was initiated for subclinical hypothyroidism (<10 mU/L) during pregnancy at a dose of up to 50 µg/day. A repeat TSH testing is warranted at 6 weeks. If the initial TSH was 10 mU/L or the dose was > 50 µg/day, then thyroxine supplementation may be continued and TSH

reassessed at 6 weeks postpartum. If the mother was already receiving thyroid supplement in pre-pregnancy period, then again, thyroxine supplementation may be continued and TSH reassessed at 6 weeks postpartum.[2,3]

## Neonatal Physiology

As a response to the intrapartum stress and cold ex-utero environment, there is an early postnatal surge of TSH, rising to 60–80 mU/L within 30 to 60 minutes after delivery. The TSH then rapidly falls to about 20 mU/L in the first 24 hours, and further decreases to below 10 mU/L by the end of the first week. T4 levels also increase to peak levels of approximately 17 µg/dl at 24–36 hours, with a gradual decline over 4 to 5 weeks. Preterm infants demonstrate a similar but blunted response.

## Etiology of Congenital Hypothyroidism

CH can be permanent or transient (Table 18.1).

### PERMANENT HYPOTHYROIDISM

**Thyroid dysgenesis** is the commonest cause of permanent CH affecting 1 in 4000 live births. It is usually sporadic with a 2:1 female

| Table 18.1: Etiology of CH |
|---|
| 1. **Permanent hypothyroidism**<br>• Thyroid dysgenesis (aplasia, hypoplasia or ectopia).<br>• Thyroid hormone biosynthetic defects.<br>• Iodine deficiency (endemic cretinism).<br>• Hypothalamic-pituitary hypothyroidism. |
| 2. **Transient hypothyroidism**<br>*Primary*<br>• Endemic iodine deficiency<br>• TSH binding inhibitory immunoglobulins<br>• Exposure to goitrogens (iodides or antithyroid drugs in mother)<br>• Maternal antithyroid medications<br>• DUOX 2 mutation<br>• Isolated hyperthyrotropinemia (normal T4, high TSH)<br>*Secondary or tertiary*<br>• Maternal hyperthyroidism<br>• Transient hypothyroxinemia of prematurity<br>• Drugs: Dopamine, steroids<br>• Sick euthyroid syndrome |

to male preponderance. Some of the genes proposed as operative in dysgenesis have recently been identified as *NKX2-1, NKX2-5, FOXE1, PAX8 and TSHR.*[4]

**Thyroid hormone synthetic defects** account for 10–15% of all cases. These are inherited as autosomal recessive disorders. The defect can lie in iodide trapping or organification, iodotyrosine coupling or deiodination, and thyroglobulin synthesis or secretion. The commonest of these is a defect in the thyroid peroxidase (TPO) activity leading to impaired oxidation and organification of iodide to iodine. These disorders usually result in goitrous hypothyroidism.

Iodine deficiency may be responsible for the observed higher prevalence of CH in Indian newborns. In a study at Kangra, Himachal Pradesh, which is in transition from iodine deficiency to sufficiency, the prevalence of CH was noted to be 4.4% based on cord blood TSH ≥20 mU/L.[5]

**Hypothalamic-pituitary hypothyroidism** is rare and has an estimated incidence of 1 in 50,000. It may be isolated or associated with deficiency of other pituitary hormones. The newborn may have microphallus, midline defects and may present with hypoglycemia or prolonged jaundice in the postnatal period.

## TRANSIENT HYPOTHYROIDISM

Recent studies that have followed up children with CH identified on newborn screening till 2–3 years of age suggest that 17–25% of such children have transient CH.[6] Transient CH due *to transplacental transfer of TSH binding inhibitory immunoglobulins (TBII)* from mothers with autoimmune thyroid disease is seen in 1: 50,000 births. Their effect wanes off by 3 to 6 months in the majority, but may last up to 9 months. Exposure to iodine in sick preterm infants (e.g. application of povidone iodine for skin disinfection—Wolff-Chaikoff effect) or intake of iodine containing expectorants by pregnant mothers can also induce transient hypothyroidism.

Transient hypothyroxinemia of prematurity (THOP) refers to low serum concentration of T4 that may last for 6–8 weeks, with low to normal TSH that is seen in up to 85% of preterm infants. This primarily reflects the underdevelopment of the HPT axis, although low iodine reserves and acute illnesses also contribute to the low T4 levels. The normal levels of fT4 and TSH in preterm infants are presented in Table 18.2.[7] There has been a concern that transient hypothyroxinemia is associated with adverse neurodevelopmental

**Table 18.2: Reference range for TSH and free T4 in preterm infants at day 5–7 of life[7]**

| Gestational age (weeks) | TSH (mU/ml) | | Free T4 (ng/dl) | |
|---|---|---|---|---|
| | Median | Normal range | Median | Normal range |
| 26 – 28 | 2.73 | 0.20 – 13.59 | 0.91 | 0.45 – 1.60 |
| 29 – 29 + 6 | 3.39 | 0.21 – 13.81 | 1.04 | 0.55 – 1.56 |
| 30– 30 + 6 | 2.87 | 0.25 – 15.20 | 1.11 | 0.65 – 1.74 |
| 31 – 31 + 6 | 2.76 | 0.45 – 15.18 | 1.16 | 0.71 – 1.77 |
| 32 – 32 + 6 | 3.10 | 0.44 – 12.50 | 1.20 | 0.80 – 1.86 |
| 33 – 33 + 6 | 3.34 | 0.53 – 11.72 | 1.30 | 0.77 – 2.02 |
| 34 – 34 + 6 | 3.05 | 0.48 – 10.74 | 1.43 | 0.86 – 2.16 |
| 35+ | 3.00 | 0.45 – 11.63 | 1.47 | 0.92 – 2.08 |

outcomes and decreased survival in affected infants. A follow-up study of preterm infants that compared neurodevelopmental outcomes at 19 years of age between those who had and did not have transient hypothyroxinemia found no difference in IQ score and motor function after adjustment for demographic and perinatal characteristics.[8] A recent study analysing the effect of levothyroxine treatment in ELBW babies with THOP weighing < 1000 gm and between 23 and 28 weeks GA did not find any difference in short terms outcome such as mortality and composite morbidity, and long term outcomes such as catch-up growth at 2 years.[9]

**Sick euthyroid syndrome** reflects suppression of the pituitary's response to TRH, with inappropriately low TSH concentrations in the context of low T3 and in the more severe cases, low total T4 concentrations. In addition to the suppression of the hypothalamo-pituitary-thyroid (HPT) axis, medications, low thyroid binding globulin and decreased peripheral conversion of T4 to T3 are implicated in the etiology of sick euthyroid syndrome.

## Diagnosis

**Newborn screening:** Universal newborn screening using either cord blood or venous sample on day 3–5 is currently being done in many parts of the world and should be ideally commenced in India as well.[10,11] Although venous sample at day 3–5 of life provides additional advantage of screening for other inborn errors of metabolism, it inflicts pain to the baby and is more likely to yield false positive results if done early (<48 hours). However, if any baby is planned for early discharge, then the test may be preponed to 48 hours.

Similar to all term neonates, screening for preterm and/or sick neonates should be performed either in cord blood or day 3–5 venous blood. However, a repeat venous sample is mandated after 1–2 weeks in sick babies, and 2–4 weeks in preterm babies, as the first screen may be falsely negative due to physiological suppression of TSH in sickness and prematurity.

Every unit should have their individual policy to screen either cord sample or postnatal venous sample. Three approaches are being used for screening:

1. Primary TSH, back up T4.
2. Primary T4, back up TSH.
3. Concomitant T4 and TSH.

The advantages and disadvantages of these approaches are presented in Table 18.3.

While interpreting TSH results, it is important to note if the sample obtained was whole blood (as in dried blood spot (DBS) obtained on filter paper by heel prick) or serum (cord blood/venous sample). The level in whole blood needs to be multiplied by 2.2 to be equivalent to the level in serum. For example, a TSH of 10 mU/L in whole blood would be equivalent to a TSH of 22 mU/L in serum. AAP as well as ISPAE recommend that the results of DBS should be given as serum units (i.e. by already multiplying by 2.2) by the labs. In the subsequent sections on the steps to be taken based on TSH, we have used serum units for heel prick TSH (Table 18.4).

| Table 18.3: Approaches to screen for CH: Advantages and disadvantages |
|---|
| 1. **Primary TSH, back up T4:** TSH is measured first, and T4 is measured only if TSH is >20 mU/L. This approach is most widely used and cost-effective. It is the most sensitive method for diagnosing primary CH, but likely to miss central hypothyroidism, thyroid binding globulin (TBG) deficiency and hypothyroxinemia with delayed elevation of TSH. |
| 2. **Primary T4, back up TSH :** T4 is checked first and if low, TSH is also checked. This is likely to miss milder/subclinical cases of CH in which T4 is initially normal with elevated TSH. |
| 3. **Concomitant T4 and TSH:** It is the ideal approach but incurs higher costs.[12] |
| 4. Considering all the above facts, the recent Indian Society of Paediatric and Adolescent Endocrinology (ISPAE) guidelines recommend primary TSH assay for screening of congenital hypothyroidism.[11] |

**Table 18.4: Subsequent management based on results of cord blood or heel prick TSH[10,11]**

| *Cord blood/heel prick TSH* | *Inference and action to be taken* |
|---|---|
| ≤ 20 mU/L (or <34 mU/L in 24–48 hr sample) | • Normal.<br>• No further testing is required. |
| > 20 – 40 mU/L | • Considered as borderline screen value.<br>• Repeat TSH, T4/FT4 to be done at 7–10 days of life. |
| > 40 – 80 mU/L | • Obtain venous sample for repeat TSH, FT4/T4 at 72 hours.<br>• Initiate treatment if repeat venous TSH, FT4/T4 is abnormal (according to the age specific reference range given in Tables 18.2 and 18.3) |
| > 80 mU/L | • Obtain venous sample for repeat TSH, FT4/T4 at 72 hours before starting treatment but do not wait for repeat test results to initiate treatment.<br>• Initiate treatment immediately. |

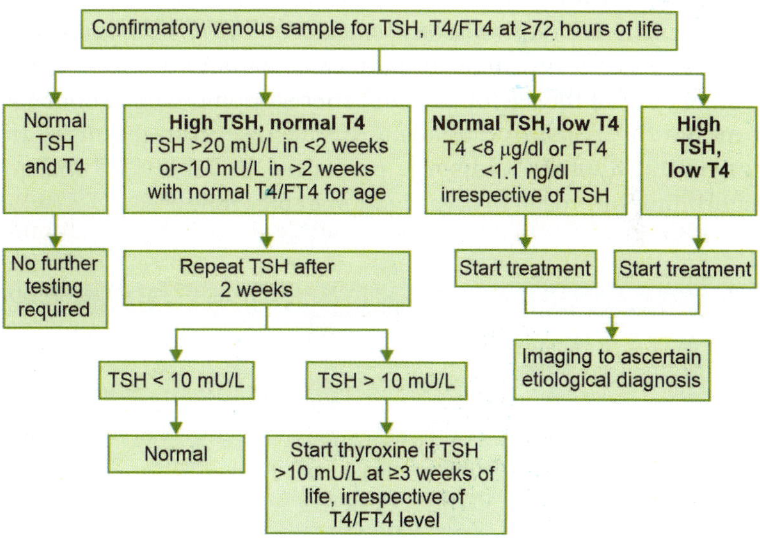


In the absence of facility for universal screening, newborns with the following indications should be screened:

1. Family history of CH.
2. History of thyroid disease or anti-thyroid medicine intake in mother.
3. Presence of other conditions like Down syndrome, trisomy 18, neural tube defects, congenital heart disease, metabolic disorders,

familial autoimmune disorders and Pierre-Robin syndrome which are associated with higher prevalence of CH.

Thyroid function should be tested in any infant with signs and symptoms of hypothyroidism such as postmaturity, macrosomia, wide open posterior fontanel at birth, prolonged jaundice, constipation, poor feeding, hypotonia, hoarse cry, umbilical hernia, macroglossia, hypothermia, or dry edematous skin in infancy. The tests should be performed even in infants who have had a normal newborn screening report.

Once the diagnosis is established, further investigations to determine the etiology should be done, whenever feasible. Ideally if facilities are available then all cases of congenital hypothyroidism should undergo both USG of thyroid as well as nuclear scan to confirm the etiology. A nuclear scan using sodium pertechnetate ($^{99m}$Tc) is especially useful in diagnosing true athyrosis or ectopy, as well as goitrous hypothyroidism due to dyshormonogenesis. *However, if the nuclear scan cannot be done immediately, treatment should be initiated*. Nuclear scan can be performed within 7 days of starting treatment or at the age of 3 years, after stopping medications for 1 month.[18,19] A list of diagnostic studies useful in infants with congenital hypothyroidism is presented in Table 18.5 and an algorithmic approach to investigation in Fig. 18.1.

| Table 18.5: Diagnostic studies for evaluation of CH |
|---|
| 1. Imaging Studies: Will determine location and size of thyroid gland.<br>a. Scintigraphy ($^{99m}$Tc or $^{123}$I)<br>b. Sonography |
| 2. Function Studies<br>a. $^{123}$I uptake<br>b. Serum thyroglobulin |
| 3. Suspected inborn error of T4 synthesis<br>a. $^{123}$I uptake and perchlorate discharge |
| 4. Suspected autoimmune thyroid disease<br>a. Maternal and neonatal serum TBII measurement (not routinely available) |
| 5. Suspected iodine exposure or deficiency<br>a. Urinary iodine measurement |
| 6. Ancillary test to determine severity of fetal hypothyroidism<br>a. Radiograph of knee for skeletal maturation |

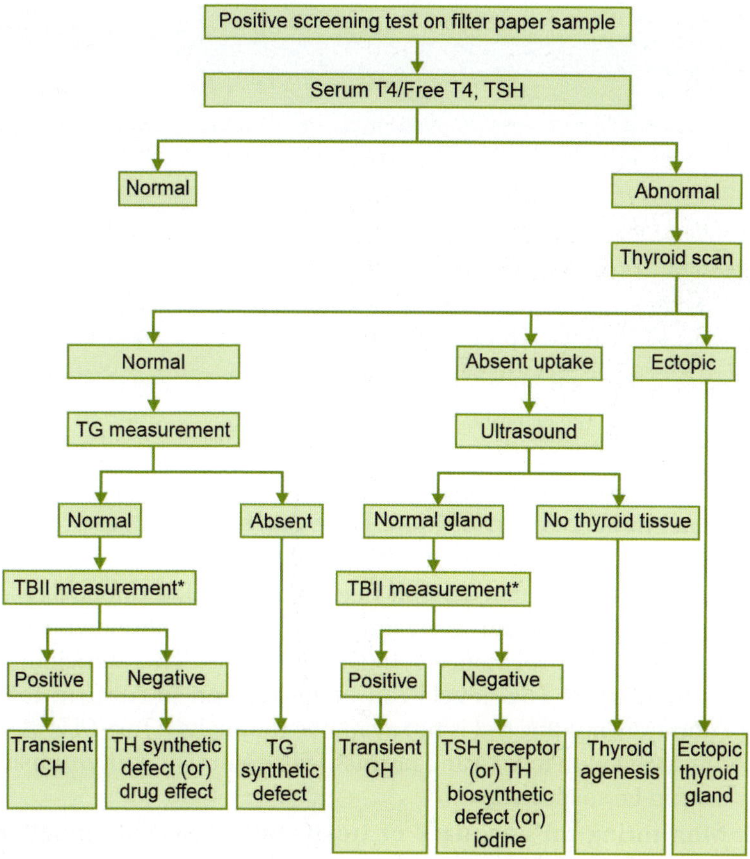


*TBII:* TSH binding inhibitory immunoglobulin (*not routinely available); *TG:* Thyroglobulin (*not routinely available); *TH:* Thyroid hormone

*Adapted from Fisher DA. Management of congenital hypothyroidism. J ClinEndocrinol Metab1991;72:585–8.*

**Fig. 18.1:** Approach to a newborn infant with positive screening test for CH

### *When Should We Ask for Free T4 Levels?*

In most situations, T4 (total) levels are sufficient for diagnosis of hypothyroidism and monitoring treatment, but free T4 can be obtained as a more robust marker of the bioavailable T4, when readily accessible (Table 18.6). When availability or cost is a constraint, free T4 should be definitely estimated in the following situations:[15]

1. **Premature or sick newborns:** T4 (total) values may be low because of abnormal protein binding or low levels of thyroxine

**Table 18.6: Reference ranges for T4, FT4 and TSH in term infants according to postnatal age[13–17]**

| *Age* | *T4 (µg/dl) mean (range)* | *FT4 (ng/dl) mean (SD)/range* | *TSH (mU/L) mean (SD)/ median (range)* |
|---|---|---|---|
| Cord blood | 10.8 (6.6–15) | 13.8 (3.5) | 10.0 (1–20) |
| 1–3 days | 16.5 (11–21.5) | 1.4 (0.04)* | 5.6 (1–10) |
| 4–7 days | 11.3 (0.3)* | 22.3 (3.9) | 6.0 (0.6)* |
| 1–2 weeks | 12.7 (8.2–17.2) | 1.3 (0.03)* | 2.3 (0.5–6.5) |
| 2–4 weeks | 10.1 (0.6)* | 0.9–2.2 | 3.9 (0.4)* |
| 4 weeks to 12 months | 11.1 (5.9–13) | 15.5 (14.0–17.2)** | 2.8 (1.9–4.4)** |

**Data presented as mean (SE); **Data for median (IQR)*

binding globulin (TBG) due to immaturity of liver function, proteinuria or undernutrition. Therefore, free T4 values provide a better estimate of true thyroid function.

2. **Low T4 with normal TSH:** If free T4 is normal, it can be a case of congenital partial (prevalence 1:4000 to 12000 newborns) or complete (prevalence 1:15000 newborns) TBG deficiency. Estimation of TBG levels can be performed to confirm this condition, but this test is not available routinely. If free T4 is also low along with low T4 and normal TSH, central hypothyroidism should be suspected.
3. **Monitoring for adequacy of treatment:** We usually monitor T4 (total) level. This assumes a normal TBG level. This can be confirmed by measuring free T4 or TBG levels once at the time of the first post-treatment T4 measurement.

### *When Should We Ask for a Repeat TSH in Spite of Initial Screen TSH Being Normal?*

If the initial screen TSH was normal, a repeat TSH estimation is recommended in the following clinical scenarios.

1. **Preterm infants born < 32 weeks** should have a repeat TSH done at 2–4 weeks of life. If the second NBS is performed before 36 weeks corrected gestational age, a repeat NBS testing is recommended 4 weeks later (i.e. 6–8 weeks of life) or at 36 weeks corrected gestational age, whichever is earlier.
2. **Infants born with very low birth weight (<1500 gm)** need to have repeat screening at 2–4 weeks.

3. **Acutely ill infants** admitted in the NICU, may have suppressed TSH rise due to sickness, or use of drugs such as dopamine and glucocorticoids that suppress TSH secretion. Thus a normal TSH concentration does not exclude the possibility of congenital hypothyroidism. Thus a repeat thyroid function testing is recommended once the baby is clinically well.
4. **Infants who received a blood or exchange transfusion** prior to initial TSH sample collection need to have thyroid function tests repeated after 2–4 weeks to account for the effect of transfused blood on TSH concentrations.
5. **Monozygotic twins** (or same-sex twin, if zygosity is not known)—the affected twin may have a falsely low TSH due to the subtle intermixing of blood from the normal twin during the fetal period. A repeat TSH is recommended at 2–4 weeks in these infants.

## Treatment of CH

*Term as well as preterm infants with low T4 and elevated TSH* should be started on L-thyroxine as soon as the diagnosis is made. The initial dose of L-thyroxine should be 10–15 µg/kg/day with the aim to normalize the T4 level at the earliest.

Those infants with severe hypothyroidism (very low T4, very high TSH) should be started with the higher dose of 15 µg/kg/day.[18]

### *Monitoring of Therapy*

- T4 should be kept in the upper half of normal range (10 to 16 µg/dl) or free T4 in the 1.4 to 2.3 ng/dl range, with the TSH being maintained in the normal range.
- Blood sample for estimation of T4/FT4 should be collected at least 4 hours after the last dose of thyroxine.[18]
- Clinical follow-up and monitoring of T4 and TSH levels should be planned according to the following schedule:
  - **0 to 6 months:** 1 to 2 weeks after starting thyroxine supplementation, followed by every 2 weeks till TSH has normalized, and then every 2 months till 6 months of age.
  - **6 months to 3 years:** Every 3 months.
  - **Beyond 3 years:** Every 3–6 months.
- Re-check T4 and TSH 4 to 6 weeks after any change in dosage or brand of thyroxine.
- Regular growth monitoring, development assessment and hearing evaluation should be done for all infants with CH.

- After 3 years of treatment, repeat thyroid function test is warranted after stopping thyroid supplement for 4 weeks in cases where treatment was initiated in neonatal period without complete evaluation, in preterm sick neonates, USG suggestive of normal thyroid gland or mild dyshormonogenesis.

## SPECIAL SITUATIONS

1. **Asymptomatic hyperthyrotropinemia (elevated TSH, normal T4)**
   - Can be transient or permanent
   - Perinatal iodine exposure is an important cause of transient elevation of TSH in neonatal period.
   - Other causes include defects in biological activity of TSH or TSH receptor, mild thyroid hormone biosynthesis defect, subtle developmental defects or disturbance in the negative feedback control of TSH.
   - There is controversy regarding the need for treatment in these infants.
   - Persistently elevated TSH>10 mU/L is generally treated. However, in the presence of free T4 levels in the upper half of normal range, expectant management can be followed with repetition of tests after 2 weeks.
   - In case treatment is started, it should be continued till 3 years of age, with monitoring of thyroid function as detailed above. If TSH and T4 have always been within normal limits with no need for escalation of dose during the first 3 years, thyroid function should be re-evaluated after withholding thyroxine for a period of 6 weeks.[12, 18]
2. **Isolated hypothyroxinemia (Low T4 and normal TSH levels)**
   - This clinical situation is commonly seen in preterm infants due to immaturity of HPT axis and is labelled as 'transient hypothyroxinemia of prematurity'. As of now, there is insufficient evidence that early treatment with thyroid hormone leads to improved outcomes.
   - Central (hypothalamic/pituitary) hypothyroidism (incidence 1 in 1,00,000) is also characterized by low T4. However, TSH in these infants may be inappropriately normal or low. In term infants, with low total as well as free T4, this diagnosis should be considered, especially in presence of midline facial abnormalities, hypoglycemia, microphallus, or visual

abnormalities. The infant should undergo testing for other pituitary hormones and MR imaging of hypothalamus and pituitary.

- TBG deficiency (rare) can also present with low T4 and normal TSH. Free T4 is normal and no treatment is required.

3. **Transient hypothyroidism**
   - The causes are listed in Table 18.1.
   - In infants born to mothers with autoimmune thyroiditis, treatment should be started if T4 is low. If presence of TBII is documented in the infant, treatment can be discontinued at 3–6 months.[9,13] However, when TBII estimation is not available, treatment should be continued till the age of 3 years, when T4 and TSH can be tested after withholding thyroxine for 6 weeks.
   - Infants with transient hypothyroidism due to maternal goitrogenic drugs need not be treated unless low T4 and elevated TSH values persist beyond 2 weeks. Therapy can be discontinued after 8–12 weeks. The hyperthyroid mothers can continue intake of antithyroid drugs during breastfeeding because concentration of these drugs is very low in breast milk.[20]

## OUTCOME

The best outcome occurs with L-thyroxine therapy started by 2 weeks of age at 9.5 µg/kg or more per day, compared with lower doses or delayed start of therapy. Residual defects can include impaired visuo-spatial processing, selective memory and sensorimotor defects. More than 80% of infants given replacement therapy before three months of age have an IQ greater than 85 but may show signs of minimal brain damage, including impairment of arithmetic ability, speech, or fine motor coordination in later life. When treatment is started between 3–6 months, the mean IQ is 71 and when delayed to beyond 6 months, the mean IQ drops to 54.[18]

## REFERENCES

1. Gopalakrishnan V, Joshi K, Phadke S, Dabadghao P, Agarwal M, Das V, et al. Newborn screening for congenital hypothyroidism, galactosemia and biotinidase deficiency in Uttar Pradesh, India. IndianPediatr. 2014;51:701–5.
2. Alexander EK, Pearce EN, Brent GA, Brown RS, Chen H, Dosiou C, et al. 2017 Guidelines of the American Thyroid Association for the Diagnosis and

Management of Thyroid Disease During Pregnancy and the Postpartum. Thyroid. 2017 Jan 6;27(3):315–89.

3. National guidelines for screening of hypothyroidism during Pregnancy [Internet]. 2014 [cited 2018 Aug 26]. Available from: http://www.nhm.gov.in/nrhm-components/rmnch-a/maternal-health/guidelines.html.
4. Szinnai G. Clinical genetics of congenital hypothyroidism.Endocr Dev. 2014;26:60–78.
5. Kapil U, Jain V, Kabra M, Pandey RM, Sareen N, Khenduja P. Prevalence of neonatal hypothyroidism in Kangra Valley, Himachal Pradesh. Eur J ClinNutr. 2014;68:748–9.
6. Korzeniewski SJ, Grigorescu V, Kleyn M, Young WI, Birbeck G, Todem D, et al. Transient hypothyroidism at 3-year follow-up among cases of congenital hypothyroidism detected by newborn screening.J Pediatr. 2013;162:177–82.
7. Lin X, Zheng LJ, Li HB, et al. Reference intervals for preterm thyroid function during the fifth to seventh day of life. Clin Biochem 2021.
8. Hollanders JJ, Israëls J, van der Pal SM, Verkerk PH, Rotteveel J, Finken MJ; Dutch POPS-19 Collaborative Study Group. No Association Between Transient Hypothyroxinemia of Prematurity and Neurodevelopmental Outcome in Young Adulthood. J Clin Endocrinol Metab2015;100:4648–53.
9. Yoon SA, Chang YS, Yang M, Ahn SY, Sung SI, et al. Effect of levothyroxine supplementation in extremely low birth weight infants with transient hypothyroxinemia of prematurity. Sci Rep. 2022 Jun 11;12(1):9717.
10. Sudhanshu S, Riaz I, Sharma R, Desai MP, Parikh R, Bhatia V. Newborn Screening Guidelines for Congenital Hypothyroidism in India: Recommendations of the Indian Society for Pediatric and Adolescent Endocrinology (ISPAE) – Part II: Imaging, Treatment and Follow-up. Indian J Pediatr. 2018 Jun;85(6):448–53.
11. Desai MP, Sharma R, Riaz I, Sudhanshu S, Parikh R, Bhatia V. Newborn Screening Guidelines for Congenital Hypothyroidism in India: Recommendations of the Indian Society for Pediatric and Adolescent Endocrinology (ISPAE) – Part I: Screening and Confirmation of Diagnosis. Indian J Pediatr. 2018 Jun;85(6):440–7.
12. American Academy of Pediatrics, Rose SR; Section on Endocrinology and Committee on Genetics, American Thyroid Association, Brown RS; Public Health Committee, Lawson Wilkins Pediatric Endocrine Society, Foley T, Kaplowitz PB, Kaye CI, Sundararajan S, Varma SK. Update of newborn screening and therapy for congenital hypothyroidism. Pediatrics 2006; 117:2290–303.
13. Fisher DA. Disorders of the thyroid in newborns and infants. In Sperling MA, ed. Pediatric Endocrinology, 2nd edition. Philadelphia: Saunders, 2002; 161–86.
14. Soldin OP, Jang M, Guo T, Soldin SJ. Pediatric reference intervals for free thyroxine and free triiodothyronine. Thyroid 2009; 19: 699–702.
15. Fisher DA. Management of congenital hypothyroidism. J Clin Endocrinol Metab1991; 72:525–8.
16. Kapelari, K., Kirchlechner, C., Högler, W. et al. Pediatric reference intervals for thyroid hormone levels from birth to adulthood: a retrospective study. BMC Endocr Disord, (2008).

17. Sheikhbahaei S, Mahdaviani B, Abdollahi A, Nayeri F. Serum thyroid stimulating hormone, total and free T4 during the neonatal period: Establishing regional reference intervals. Indian J Endocrinol Metab. 2014;18(1):39.
18. Léger J, Olivieri A, Donaldson M, Torresani T, Krude H, van Vliet G, ESPE-PES-SLEP-JSPE-APEG-APPES-ISPAE; Congenital Hypothyroidism Consensus Conference Group European Society for Paediatric Endocrinology consensus guidelines on screening, diagnosis, and management of congenital hypothyroidism. J Clin Endocrinol Metab. 2014;99:363-84.
19. Woo HC, Lizarda A, Tucker R, et al: Congenital hypothyroidism with a delayed thyroid-stimulating hormone elevation in very premature infants: incidence and growth and developmental outcomes. J Pediatr 2011;158:538–542.
20. Hudzik B, Zubelewicz-Szkodzinska B. Antithyroid drugs during breastfeeding. Clin Endocrinol (Oxf). 2016 ;85:827–830.

CHAPTER

# 19

# Metabolic Bone Disease

Metabolic bone disease (MBD), formerly known as osteopenia of prematurity. Clinically, it presents between 5 and 11 weeks of postnatal life with poor extra-uterine growth, increased work of breathing and fractures.[1,2] In addition, MBD has long-term consequences, including short stature and osteopenia, in young adulthood.[3]

## Definition

It is best defined as reduction in bone mineral content relative to the expected level of mineralization for an infant of comparable size or gestational age in combination with radiographic and biochemical changes.[4]

## Incidence

16–40% in VLBW and ELBW infants.[5]

## Risk Factors

**Prenatal:** Placental insufficiency, maternal vitamin D deficiency, genetic (high number of TA repeats), male gender.

**Postnatal:** Prematurity, inadequate intake of calcium and phosphate, vitamin D deficiency, immobility, liver disease, renal disease, drugs use such as caffeine, steroids and diuretics.

## Prevention

1. Establishment of early enteral feeding
2. Reduced duration of parenteral nutrition
3. Early fortification of human milk in babies who are at high risk for developing osteopenia.
4. Physical activity like passive range of motion and joint compression can improve bone mineralization.[6]

## How and When to Start Screening?

Figure 19.1 depicts algorithm for screening and monitoring of metabolic bone disease.

**Table 19.1: Diagnosis of metabolic bone disease[7]**

| | | |
|---|---|---|
| 1. | Serum phosphate and ALP levels | < 5.6 mg/dl and > 900 IU/L (sensitivity of 70% and specificity of 100%)[8] |
| 2. | Serum PTH levels | >100 pg/ml |
| 3. | Tubular reabsorption of phosphate | >95% (with low or normal PTH s/o phosphate deficiency). |
| 4. | X-rays | Evident only after 20–40% of bone demineralisation. Koo's score<br>Grade 1: Presence of bone rarefaction<br>Garde 2: Above plus metaphyseal alterations, shadow, and subperiosteal bone formations.<br>Grade 3: Spontaneous fractures. |
| 5. | Dual energy X-ray absorptiometry (DEXA) | BMD >0.068 g/cm$^2$ is considered normal.<br>Target regions in neonates—lumbar spine, the forearm and the calcaneus. |
| 6. | Quantitative ultrasound (QUS)<br>a. Speed of sound<br>b. Bone transmission time | Significant correlation of QUS<br>• With ALP, calcium, phosphate and vitamin D<br>• With gestational age and birth weight |

**Table 19.2: Treatment of metabolic bone disease of prematurity**

| | | *Calcium (mg/kg/day)* | *Phosphorous (mg/kg/day)* | *Vitamin D (IU/day)* |
|---|---|---|---|---|
| 1. | Enteral | 150–220 | 75–140 | 200–1000 |
| 2. | Parenteral | 75–100 | 50–80 | 200–1000 |
| 3. | Treatment | 20–80 | 10–50 | 200–1000 |

As per 2013 AAP report recommended vitamin D intake is 200-400 IU/day[9]; ESPGHAN recommends 800–1000 IU/day of vitamin D[10]; Optimal calcium: phosphorous ratio in parenteral nutrition is 1.7:1[11]

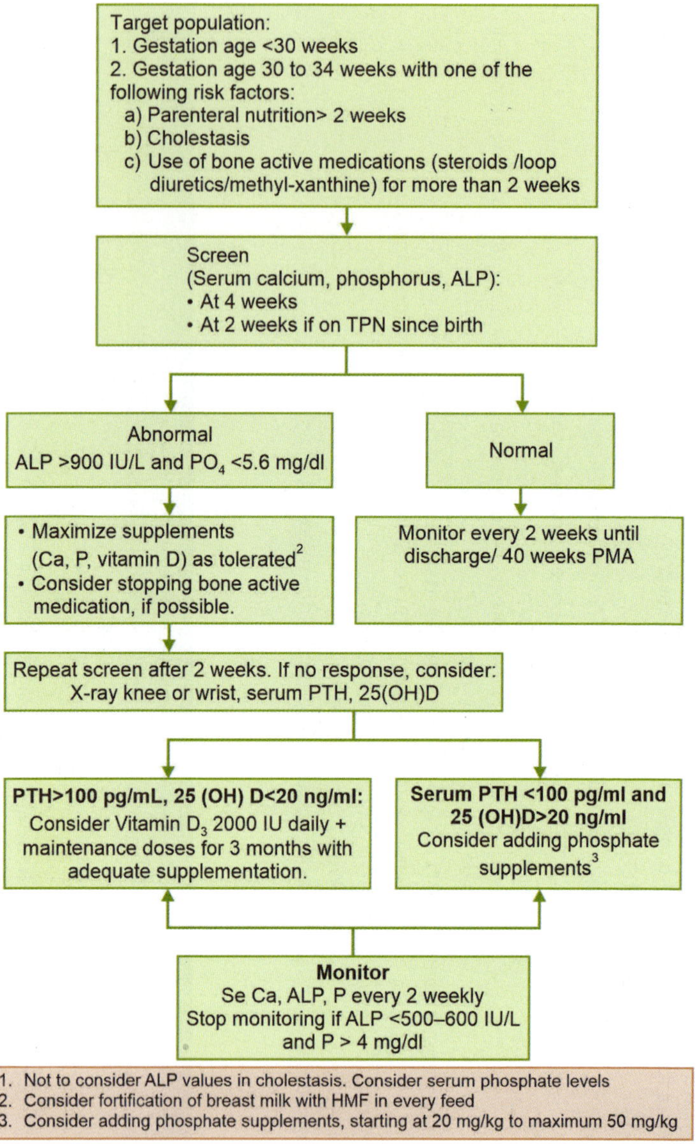


**Fig. 19.1:** Algorithm for screening and monitoring of metabolic bone disease[12]

## REFERENCES

1. Chan AP, Robinson DT, Calkins KL. Hypertriglyceridemia in Preterm Infants. NeoReviews. 2022 Aug 1;23(8):e528–40.

2. Mitchell SM, Rogers SP, Hicks PD, Hawthorne KM, Parker BR, Abrams SA. High frequencies of elevated alkaline phosphatase activity and rickets exist in extremely low birth weight infants despite current nutritional support. BMC Pediatr. 2009 Jul 29;9(1):47.
3. Greer FR. Calcium and Phosphorus and the Preterm Infant. NeoReviews. 2016 Apr 1;17(4):e195–202.
4. Metabolic Bone Disease of Prematurity | Articles | Neoreviews [Internet]. [cited 2017 Jul 6]. Available from: http://neoreviews.aappublications.org/content/10/8/e402?utm_source=TrendMD&utm_medium=TrendMD&utm_campaign=NeoRev_TrendMD_%25SPONSORED%25.
5. Rustico SE, Calabria AC, Garber SJ. Metabolic bone disease of prematurity. J Clin Transl Endocrinol. 2014 Sep 1;1(3):85–91.
6. Stalnaker KA, Poskey GA. Osteopenia of Prematurity: Does Physical Activity Improve Bone Mineralization in Preterm Infants? Neonatal Netw. 2016 Jan 1;35(2):95–104.
7. Faienza MF, D'Amato E, Natale MP, Grano M, Chiarito M, Brunetti G, et al. Metabolic Bone Disease of Prematurity: Diagnosis and Management. Front Pediatr [Internet]. 2019 [cited 2019 Jul 8];7. Available from: https://www.frontiersin.org/articles/10.3389/fped.2019.00143/full.
8. Backström MC, Kouri T, Kuusela AL, Sievänen H, Koivisto AM, Ikonen RS, et al. Bone isoenzyme of serum alkaline phosphatase and serum inorganic phosphate in metabolic bone disease of prematurity. Acta Paediatr Oslo Nor 1992. 2000 Jul;89(7):867–73.
9. Abrams SA, Committee on Nutrition. Calcium and vitamin d requirements of enterally fed preterm infants. Pediatrics. 2013 May;131(5):e1676–1683.
10. Bronsky J, Campoy C, Braegger C, ESPGHAN/ESPEN/ESPR/CSPEN working group on pediatric parenteral nutrition. ESPGHAN/ESPEN/ESPR/CSPEN guidelines on pediatric parenteral nutrition: Vitamins. Clin Nutr Edinb Scotl. 2018 Dec;37(6 Pt B):2366–78.
11. Boullata JI, Gilbert K, Sacks G, Labossiere RJ, Crill C, Goday P, et al. A.S.P.E.N. clinical guidelines: parenteral nutrition ordering, order review, compounding, labeling, and dispensing. JPEN J Parenter Enteral Nutr. 2014;38(3):334–77.
12. Munns CF, Shaw N, Kiely M, Specker BL, Thacher TD, Ozono K, et al. Global Consensus Recommendations on Prevention and Management of Nutritional Rickets. Horm Res Paediatr. 2016;85(2):83–106.

CHAPTER

# 20

# Differences in Sex Development

Differences in sex development (DSD) are an umbrella term encompassing around 50 different disorders. Terms such as pseudohermaphroditism, hermaphroditism, sex reversal, and gender-based diagnostic labels are controversial terminologies and have been replaced by umbrella terminology of DSD. A neonate with suspected DSD at birth is not only a potential medical emergency (salt wasting congenital adrenal hyperplasia [CAH]) but also a social emergency.

### Definition

DSD is defined as congenital conditions in which there is discrepancy in the development of chromosomal, gonadal, and anatomic sex. Table 20.1 describes the normal anatomical genital characteristics of a male and female neonate.[1]

## CLASSIFICATION AND NOMENCLATURE OF THE DSD

Based on the Chicago consensus meeting 2006, the revised nomenclature now broadly classifies DSD as:

| Table 20.1: Essential features of normal male and female genitalia in a newborn[1] |
|---|
| **Female**<br>• Vaginal opening fully visible 3 to 4 mm slit or stellate orifice with heaped up mucosa (i.e. no posterior labial fusion).<br>• Clitoris width 2 to 6 mm.<br>• Absence of gonads in labia majora or inguinal region. |
| **Male**<br>• Urethra at the tip of glans (which may be inferred by a fully developed foreskin).<br>• Penis of normal stretched length (2.5–5 cm) and diameter (0.9–1.3 cm).<br>• Bilateral testes of normal size (8–14 mm) in the scrotal sacs. |

1. **46, XX DSD:** It is further subclassified as:
   i. Disorders of ovarian development.
   ii. Maternal or fetal androgen excess, and
   iii. Syndromic or complex disorders like cloacal exstrophy or vaginal atresias as part of syndromes.
2. **46, XY DSD:** This group has subgroups of:
   i. Disorders of testicular development.
   ii. Disorders of androgen biosynthesis or action (receptor defects or defect in action like androgen insensitivity).
3. **Chromosomal DSD:** Includes DSD as a component of chromosomal anomalies like Turner syndrome, Klinefelter syndrome and mixed gonadal dysgenesis.

### Incidence of DSD Subtypes[2–9]

Overall incidence of DSD varies from 1: 10000 to 100000, depending on the subtype. Amongst the DSD, reported prevalence from India of 46,XX and 46,XY varies between 45% to 47% each, respectively. Amongst 46,XX DSD, CAH accounts for the most common cause (45% to 60%). Amongst the 46, XY DSD, CAH and androgen insensitivity syndrome account for 15% of cases and 5 to 12% are due to 5-alpha reductase deficiency. Approximately, 8 to 10% cases are accounted for by ovotesticular DSD.

## APPROACH TO THE DIAGNOSIS AND INVESTIGATIONS

### Clinical Approach

*1. Pointers Towards DSD*

Meticulous initial physical examination is the first important step (Table 20.2). Micropenis is defined as stretched penile length

**Table 20.2: Clinical examination findings which suggest need for investigations[1, 11, 12]**

**Probable pointers to DSD[1, 11, 12]**

- Overt genital ambiguity (cloacal exostrophy).
- Apparent female genitalia with an enlarged clitoris, posterior labial fusion or an inguinal/labial mass.
- Apparent male genitalia with bilateral undescended testes, micropenis, isolated perineal hypospadias, or mild hypospadias with undescended testis.
- Asymmetry in size, pigmentation or rugation of labioscrotal folds.
- Family history of DSD.
- Discordance between genital appearance and a prenatal karyotype.

below 2.5 standard deviations of the mean for the age.[10] The term micropenis is used when the penis is otherwise normally formed and microphallus is used when micropenis is associated with hypospadias or epispadias.

The degree of virilization of the external genitalia can be assessed as per Prader staging[13] (phenotypically female with mild clitoromegaly as stage 1 and phenotypic male with impalpable testes as stage 5).

Another scoring system used for 46,XY neonates is the external masculinization score[14] (EMS, total score 12) and the internal MS (IMS, total score 10);[14] EMS scoring is based on:

i. Presence or absence of scrotal fusion.
ii. Presence or absence of micropenis.
iii. Location of urethral meatus
iv. Presence or absence of bilateral gonads. IMS requires imaging to see the presence of internal genital structures like uterus, fallopian tubes, epididymis, and vas deferens. Score less than 7 indicate undervirilisation of male genitalia.

## Differential Diagnosis for Possible Subtype of DSD, on Clinical Examination

Based on the clinical examination, possible subtype of DSD can be ascertained (Table 20.3). *However, it is important to remember*

**Table 20.3: Differential diagnosis of various clinical phenotypes**

| *Clinical examination* | *Possible differential diagnosis* |
|---|---|
| Bilateral non-palpable gonads with hyper-pigmentation of genitalia. | Virilised female with CAH |
| Unilateral palpable gonad, asymmetry of the external genitalia. | Gonadal dysgenesis associated with 45, X/46,XY karyotype |
| Midline facial/neural defects/optic nerve hypoplasia in a baby with micropenis, but without asymmetry of genitalia or bifid scrotum. | Pituitary hormone deficiencies |
| Dysmorphic features, skeletal abnormalities, campomelic dysplasia in a baby with underdeveloped labia majora/minora or an under virilized male. | Antley Bixler syndrome, POR deficiency, SOX 9 mutations |
| Cloacal, anorectal malformations, bladder exostrophy epispadias complex anomalies, absence of anal opening. | VATER, VACTERL anomalies |

*that gender assignment should not be made based only on the clinical examination.*

**Investigative approach**[11–12]

1. **First line of investigations:** A provisional diagnosis can be made within the first week based on the first line investigations. Samples for 17-hydroxyprogesterone (17-OHP) and cortisol should be collected before initiating hydrocortisone (in cases of neonates presenting with salt wasting crisis).
   a. Serum electrolytes, random blood sugar.
   b. Karyotyping/FISH or PCR.
   c. Ultrasound to look for Müllerian structures and gonads.
   d. Serum 17-OHP, cortisol.

   **Interpretation of 17-OHP**
   i. Unaffected neonatal concentrations: <15 nmol/L.
   ii. In classical 21-hydroxylase deficiency levels: >300–800 nmol/L
   iii. Non-classical CAH: 15–51 nmol/L; may require synacthen stimulation for further diagnosis.
   iv. In 11-beta hydroxylase and 3-beta hydroxysteroid dehydrogenase deficiency: Modest increase (15–100 nmol/L).
   v. Prematurity, cross-reacting steroids, sampling prior to 48 to 72 hours of age and stressed normal neonates can have 17-OHP as high as 100 nmol/L. Hence, avoid sampling neonates prior to 48 hours of life.

   In other situations of suspected false positives like prematurity and ELBW, although gestation and birth weight specific values are available for interpretation, repeat samples may need to be sent for definitive diagnosis. Urine steroid metabolites and urine mass spectroscopy would also be helpful for diagnosis.

   The results of the first-tier assays usually guide the need for second line of investigations (enumerated below). It is advisable to consult a pediatric endocrinologist for the second tier of investigations, since the normal hormonal levels vary during the initial few months and interpretation and final diagnosis may require more than one test done on more than one occasion.

2. **Second line of investigations**
   a. Serum testosterone, dihydrotestosterone, FSH, LH.
   b. Serum 11 deoxycortisol.
   c. Anti-Müllerian hormone.

d. hCG stimulation test.
e. Synacthen stimulation test.
f. Detailed imaging, genitogram and laparoscopy.

Figure 20.1 summarizes the approach to evaluation of DSD.

## Management Principles in Neonates[11–12]

### *1. Gender Assignment*

It is essential for the physician to be sensitive and empathetic with the family. Till the work up is complete and results of essential investigations are available, use gender-neutral terminologies (baby, newborn).

Explain to the parents regarding the possibility of waiting for gender assignment till later in life, in cases of significant ambiguity.

After the preliminary investigations and karyotype is available, in the neonatal period, broadly.

1. Female assignment is suggested for those with 46, XX and CAH, since 95% develop female gender identity; complete AIS, and 46, XY LH receptor deficiency.
2. Male assignment is recommended for those with 5α-reductase deficiency, since 60% later identify themselves as male, and for 17β-HSD3 deficiency, since >50% later switch to male.

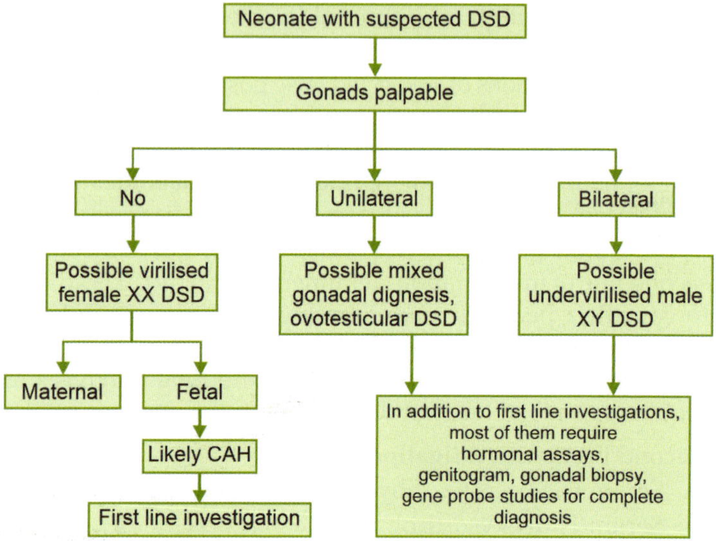


**Fig. 20.1:** Diagnostic approach for DSD

3. For ovotesticular DSD: Difficult to assign gender in the neonatal period, since a multitude of factors have to be taken into account including anticipated quality of sexual function, surgical options/indications/risks, fertility potential and socio-cultural factors.

*2. Medical Management*

The subgroup of neonates with CAH as a cause of DSD needs routine and emergency medical management to be stable. These neonates can present as a medical emergency (salt wasting crisis or adrenal crisis), either within the first week of life or they can present later on, when it is precipitated by intercurrent illnesses like sepsis, diarrhea, vomiting, etc.

i. Neonates who are suspected as CAH at birth (virilised females or males with strong family history): It may take 5 to 14 days, and rarely a month, for salt wasting crisis to manifest, and hence it is important to closely monitor the weight, fluid balance and serial electrolytes for the first few weeks. The management of CAH should begin as soon as the laboratory values of electrolytes are detected to be abnormal, without waiting for 17-OHP results.

   Adrenal crisis during the first weeks should be managed as described below. Once stable, these neonates are discharged on maintenance doses of oral salt (NaCl 1 to 3 gm per day in feeds) and steroid supplementation (Hydrocortisone 10 to 15 mg per $m^2$ per day and Fludrocortisone acetate 0.1 to 0.2 mg per day, available as Floricot, 100 µg tablet manufactured by Samarth pharmaceuticals, INR 10/tablet). Follow-up is done 3 monthly where growth and serum electrolytes are monitored. These neonates are predisposed to present with adrenal crisis later on also, even with minor intercurrent illnesses. The dose of steroids is increased by 2 to 3 times during febrile illnesses and diarrhea.

ii. Neonates not suspected at birth (males, females with minimal virilization) can present with features of salt wasting crisis or adrenal crisis, usually precipitated by some illness, anytime during the neonatal period or infancy. Any neonate or infant presenting with pointers to adrenal crisis like hypoglycemia, hyperpigmentation, electrolyte imbalance and shock unresponsive to fluids and inotropes should receive management described as follows.

**Management of adrenal crisis:** Features of adrenal or salt wasting crisis include shock, hypoglycemia, hyponatremia, hyperkalemia and metabolic acidosis.

1. **Shock and dyselectrolytemia:** Normal saline boluses should be administered as required and salt loss should be replaced initially with intravenous normal saline with glucose added (1.5 times maintenance fluids). The sodium requirement in some cases may be as high as 8 mEq per kg per day. Fluids are continued till the neonate is stable.
2. **Steroid supplementation:**
   a. The neonates presenting with first episode of adrenal crisis (who are not on any maintenance steroid or salt supplementation) should be administered hydrocortisone at 50 to 100 mg/m$^2$/day in divided doses 8 hourly. This stress dose should be continued till 48 to 72 hours, when the neonate becomes stable. The dose of hydrocortisone should be tapered and brought to maintenance dose of 10 to 15 mg/m$^2$/day and Fludrocortisone (0.1 to 0.2 mg per day) is added. Fludrocortisone is not needed when hydrocortisone is given at a dose > 50 mg/m$^2$/day as at higher dose, hydrocortisone has sufficient mineralocorticoid activity.
   b. In neonates who were previously discharged on salt and steroid supplementation, and present with adrenal crisis due to intercurrent illness, the dose of hydrocortisone should be increased to three times the maintenance dose. Fludrocortisone can be restarted once the hydrocortisone is weaned to the maintenance dose.

***Ensure that blood samples are taken for diagnosis of CAH and adrenal crisis (serum electrolytes, 17 OHP, cortisol and renin) prior to initiating the steroid therapy as emergency management.***

*3. Definitive Treatment*

DSD in the newborn period is best managed by a multidisciplinary team consisting of the neonatologist, pediatric endocrinologist, pediatric surgeon, psychologist and social worker.

a. **Hormonal treatment:** In cases of anticipated hormonal treatment (testosterone injections in case of microphallus, pubertal estrogen and progestin in female gender assignment), it is advisable to take the opinion of pediatric endocrinologist.
b. **Surgical treatment:** The definitive surgery should only be considered once the psychosocial factors, the adult gender

identity, the fertility potential; the individual's own preference of sexual activity is ensured and discussed with a reasonable level of surety. The definitive surgery should not be done in haste. Surgical corrections may be required: Correction of chordee, orchidopexy (by one year of age) and hypospadias repair (at 6–18 months of age). In significantly virilized females, surgical correction (vaginoplasty and clitoroplasty) is done at 2–6 months of age.

## PROGNOSIS

The risk of future tumor development and fertility are the two important prognostic factors which decide the quality of life in each case of DSD. The risk of gonadoblastoma, dysgerminoma and seminoma is present in XY intra-abdominal gonads, more so in dysgenetic gonads. Removal of the intra-abdominal gonads, if non-functional or orchidopexy should be done as indicated.

Fertility may be possible utilizing sperm retrieval and ICSI in patients who have functional gonads and do not require testosterone at puberty such as X/XY mosaicism, 5α-reductase deficiency and partial AIS patients. Among females, stimulation of ovulation and embryo transfer using fertilized donated ova have been used, including in females with CAH and Turner syndrome.

## REFERENCES

1. Hughes IA, Houk C, Ahmed SF, Lee PA, Group LC. Consensus statement on management of intersex disorders. Archives of Disease in Childhood. 2006; 91:554–563.
2. R Walia et al. Disorders of sex development: A study of 194 cases Endocrine Connections Publish Ahead of Print, published on January 31, 2018 as doi:10.1530/EC–18–0022.
3. Prasad K et al. Pediatric Disorders of Sex Development. Indian Journal of Pediatrics, Volume 76—September, 2009;956–958.
4. Joshi RR, Rao S, Desai M. Etiology and Clinical Profile of Ambiguous Genitalia - An Overview of 10 Years Experience. Indian Pediatr 2006;43:974–979.
5. Rajendran R, Hariharan S. Profile of intersex children in South India. Indian Pediatr 1995;32:666–671.
6. Ammini AC, Gupta R, Kapoor A et al. Etiology, clinical profile, gender identity and long term follow up of patients with ambiguous genitalia in India. J Pediatr Endocrinol Metab 2002;15:423–430.
7. Göllü G, Yýldýza RV, Bingol-Kologlu M et al. Ambiguous genitalia: an overview of 17 years' experience. J Ped Surg 2007;42:840–844.

8. Nimkarn S, Likitmaskul S, Sangacharoenkit P et al. Ambiguous genitalia: an overview of 22 years experience and the diagnostic approach in the pediatric department, Siriraj Hospital. J Med Assoc Thai 2002;85:496–505.
9. Gupta DK, Menon PSN. Ambiguous Genitalia: Ambiguous Genitalia: An Indian perspective. Indian J Pediatr 1997;64:189–194.
10. Hatipoğlu N, Kurtoğlu S. Micropenis: etiology, diagnosis and treatment approaches J Clin Res Pediatr Endocrinol. 2013;5(4):217–23.
11. H. Nihal et al Micropenis: Etiology, Diagnosis and Treatment Approaches Journal of Clinical Research in Pediatric Endocrinology·December 2013 J Clin Res Pediatr Endocrinol 2013;5(4):217-223 DOI: 10.4274/Jcrpe.1135.
12. Lee P, A, Nordenström A, Houk C, P, Ahmed S, F, Auchus R, Baratz A, Baratz Dalke K, Liao L, -M, Lin-Su K, Looijenga 3rd L, H, J, Mazur T, Meyer-Bahlburg H, F, L, Mouriquand P, Quigley C, A, Sandberg D, E, Vilain E, Witchel S, Global Disorders of Sex Development Update since 2006: Perceptions, Approach and Care. Horm Res Paediatr 2016;85:158–180.
13. Ahmed SF, Achermann JC, Arlt W, Balen AH, Conway G, Edwards ZL, Elford S, Hughes IA, Izatt L, Krone N, Miles HL. UK guidance on the initial evaluation of an infant or an adolescent with a suspected disorder of sex development. Clinical endocrinology 2011 1;75:12–26.
14. Prader, A.Genital findings in the female pseudo-hermaphroditism of the congenital adrenogenital syndrome; morphology, frequency, development and heredity of the different genital forms. Helvetica paediatrica acta 1954, 9(3), pp.231–248.
15. Ahmed, S.F., Khwaja, O. and Hughes, I.A.The role of a clinical score in the assessment of ambiguous genitalia. BJU International 2000, 85: 120–124.

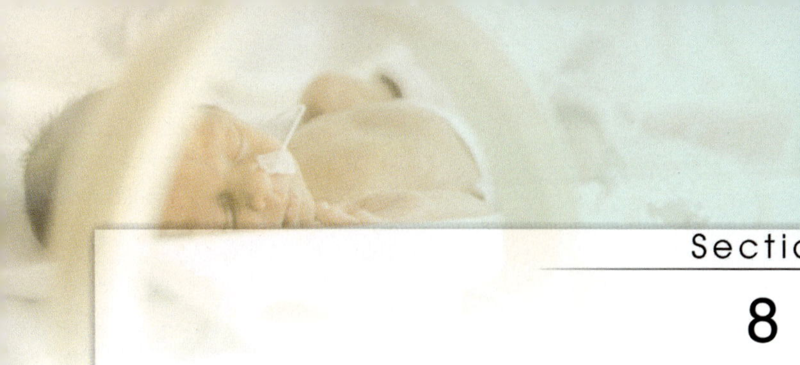

Section

8

# Miscellaneous

CHAPTER

21

# Early Detection and Management of Cerebral Palsy

## INTRODUCTION

Cerebral palsy (CP) is a disorder of movement and posture causing a variable degree of functional limitation. It results from a non-progressive insult to the developing brain and is frequently accompanied by cognitive, behavioral, sensory, and musculoskeletal comorbidities and epilepsy[1,2]. CP is the most common motor disability observed in childhood. The incidence of CP is inversely proportional to gestational age[3,4]. Globally its incidence rate varies between 1–2 per 1000 live births; the incidence is slightly higher in developing than developed countries.[3]

Though most CP cases develop as an aftermath of an antenatal or perinatal insult, the diagnosis may be traditionally made after 1–2 years of life. This leads to the loss of the critical period, where the brain is more sensitive to stimulation and intervention.[5]

Early diagnosis ensures diagnosis-oriented surveillance and early intervention, helps better utilize early neuroplasticity for an improved developmental outcome, helps minimize secondary complications, and allays parental anxiety.

### Whom to Screen?

Any neonate with an antenatal, perinatal risk factor for a brain injury is to be screened.[6] Box 21.1 provides a list of common risk factors associated with the future risk of CP.

### How to Screen?

The diagnosis of CP and early prediction of motor severity in young infants must be based on standardized examination tools as the evolving clinical signs, incomplete development of voluntary motor skills, and brain immaturity may confound clinical observation. Based on the currently available evidence, the following are recommended for early prediction of a high risk of cerebral palsy in young infants.

**Box 21.1: Risk factors associated with cerebral palsy**

**Preconception risk factors:** Stillbirths, abortions, assisted reproductive technology, and advanced maternal age (> 40 years).

**Antenatal risk factors:** Fetal growth restriction; prematurity; birth-defects, chronic maternal disorders such as thyroid disease, pre-eclampsia, and infection; substance abuse; chorioamnionitis; placental abnormalities.

**Perinatal birth risk factors:** Instrumental delivery, low birth weight, birth asphyxia, respiratory distress syndrome, hypoglycemia, hyperbilirubinemia, neonatal encephalopathy, and sepsis.

**Postnatal risks factors:** Stroke, infection, accidental and non-accidental brain injury.

### Age <5 Months of Corrected Age

1. General movements assessment (98% sensitivity).
2. Hammersmith Infant Neurological Examination (HINE) (90% sensitivity).
3. Brain magnetic resonance imaging (MRI) (86–89% sensitivity).[5–7]

### Age > 5 Months of Corrected Age

1. HINE (90% sensitivity).
2. MRI (86–89% sensitivity).
3. Developmental Assessment of Young Children (83% sensitivity).[5, 6]

Abnormal general movement, a low HINE score, and abnormal neuroimaging may predict CP more accurately than a neurological examination or imaging alone (Fig. 21.1).

#### *General Movements*

General movements are the best indicator of functional motor maturity. These are serial gross movements with variability in speed and amplitude that involve all body parts, but the distinctive pattern is lacking.[1,8] These are the first movements to develop in a human fetus, which evolve before isolated limb movement and disappear around five months of corrected age.[10] Based on age-specific characteristics, normal general movements are divided into preterm, writhing, and fidgety general movements (Table 21.1).[8–10] Similarly, abnormal general movements are classified as poor repertoire, cramped-synchronized and chaotic. Prechtl's state-4 (actively awake) is optimal for assessing general movements. It should not be evaluated during crying and non-nutritive sucking.[1]

The predictive power of neurological outcome at 12–15 months of Prechtl's qualitative assessment of general movement is excellent.[11]

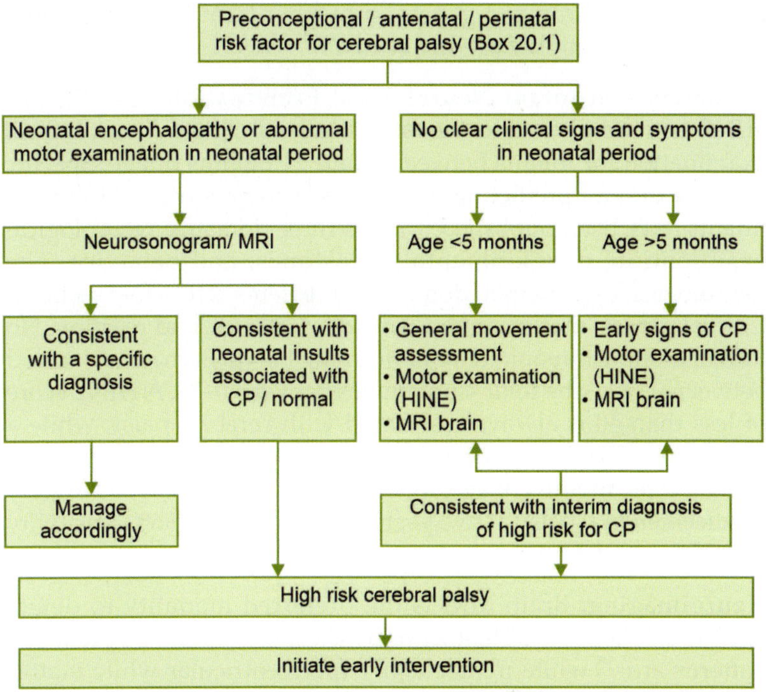


*HINE:* Hammersmith infant neurological examination

**Fig. 21.1:** Algorithm for early diagnosis and management of cerebral palsy

**Table 21.1: Age-specific characteristics of normal general movements**

| *General movement type* | *Postmenstrual age (in weeks)* | *Description of GM* |
|---|---|---|
| Preterm GM | 28 to 36–38 weeks | Variable in quality, pelvic thrust/ tilts, and truncal movement |
| Writhing GM | Term to 8 weeks post-term | Writhing or squirming nature of movements of small to moderate magnitude occurring at a slow to medium speed |
| Fidgety GM | 6–9 weeks post-term | The continuous flow of small irregular movements involves the head, trunk, and limb, with slight amplitude movement superimposed on the larger movement. |

Cramped synchronized general movements and absent fidgety movements are highly predictive of CP[5].

**Hammersmith Infant Neurological Examination (HINE):** The HINE is a simple, scoreable, standardized clinical neurological examination for infants between 2 and 24 months of age. Specific cut-off scores for predicting cerebral palsy in preterm and full-term infants have been published.[12] It has three domains: Neurological examination, developmental milestones, and behavior. The neurological examination domain has 26 items across five sections: Cranial nerves, movement quality, tone, reflexes, and reaction. No formal training is required for performing HINE. Each item is scored between 0–3, so the total score ranges between 0–78. A HINE score of less than 40 is always associated with cerebral palsy, while a score above 73 is not associated with cerebral palsy at two years of age. At three months of age, a HINE score of less than 56 strongly predicts cerebral palsy at two years of corrected age (96% sensitivity and 85% specificity).

**Neuroimaging:** Brain MRI is the preferred modality to detect structural lesions consistent with CP. The most commonly predicted patterns are[5,13] white matter injury (periventricular white matter injury: Periventricular leukomalacia, periventricular infarction) in 56% of cases, cortex and deep gray matter lesions (basal ganglia, thalamus, multicystic encephalomalacia, watershed infarct) in 18%, and cortical malformations in nearly 10% cases. As myelination is incomplete before two years of age, mild white matter lesions may be missed before this age. Normal neuroimaging, however, does not entirely refute a future risk of cerebral palsy. Repeat imaging is recommended if the neurological examination is persistently abnormal on subsequent follow-ups.

## Early and Interim Diagnosis of CP

Early markers of cerebral palsy include poor repertoire, cramped synchronized general movement, head lag or fisting/obligatory grasp persistence, and asymmetric primitive reflexes. The pattern of abnormal general movements, motor examination, and neuroimaging findings differ in various subtypes of CP and, therefore, can be utilized to predict the future CP subtype (Table 21.2).

Early in life, all features may not be present, and despite a high suspicion of cerebral palsy, a confirmed diagnosis may not always be possible. It is now recommended that all such infants should be

**Table 21.2: Common early clinical and radiological findings in various subtypes of cerebral palsy**

| *Unilateral spastic hemiplegia* | *Bilateral spastic diplegia* | *Bilateral spastic quadriplegia* | *Dyskinetic* |
|---|---|---|---|
| **General Movements** | | | |
| • Cramped synchronized GMs<br>• Absent fidgety movements<br>• Asymmetric segmental movements (e.g. wrist or hand). | • Poor repertoire<br>• Absence of fidgety movements | • Early-onset and prolonged cramped synchronized general movements<br>• Absent fidgety movements | • Poor repertoire GMs<br>• Absence of fidgety movements with arm movements in a circular manner and fanning of fingers |
| **Motor Examination** | | | |
| • Decreased hand regard<br>• Persistent obligatory grasp<br>• Early handedness<br>• Difficulty in transiting out of sitting<br>• Asymmetric primitive reflexes<br>• Persistent unidirectional cruises or steps.<br>• Same leading leg constantly<br>• Reduced variability in motor activity | • The hand function is better than the lower limb function and avoids sitting on the floor.<br>• Weight-bearing on toes.<br>• Reduced variability in motor activity | • Persistence of head lag<br>• Sits with support with a rounded back<br>• Bilateral fisting<br>• Poor reach and grasp with either hand<br>• Reduced variability in motor activity | • Twisting of arm or neck on voluntary activity<br>• Difficulty in midline play, prefers toys positioned at shoulder width<br>• Hands-switching while reaching out for objects<br>• Delay in initiating movement<br>• Postural worsening with voluntary movement and emotion (excitability)<br>• Reduced variability in motor behavior |

*(Contd.)*

**Table 21.2: Common early clinical and radiological findings in various subtypes of cerebral palsy** *(Contd.)*

| *Unilateral spastic hemiplegia* | *Bilateral spastic diplegia* | *Bilateral spastic quadriplegia* | *Dyskinetic* |
|---|---|---|---|
| **Neuroimaging** | | | |
| • Vascular insults observed in 24%<br>• Cortical malformations in13%<br>• Unilateral grade IV parenchymal/ventricular hemorrhage with porencephaly<br>• Parietal white matter lesion involving the trigonal area<br>• Middle cerebral artery stroke with asymmetric myelination of the posterior limb of the internal capsule (PLIC) | • Bilateral white matter lesion (31–60%)<br>• Cystic periventricular leukomalacia (Grade II-III) with poorly myelinated PLIC<br>• Moderate to severe white matter injury | • Gray matter injury was observed in 34%<br>• Various cortical malformations were noted in 16%<br>• Grade III cystic PVL with the absence of PLIC myelination<br>• Severe white matter injury ± deep nuclear gray matter involvement | • Gray matter injury with thalamic and lenticular nucleus involvement |

labeled as at a "high risk of cerebral palsy" until a final diagnosis is established. For a diagnosis of high-risk of cerebral palsy, an infant should have motor dysfunction as an essential criterion with one out of two additional criteria (abnormal neuroimaging or presence of risk factor).[7,13] Motor dysfunction is defined as poor quality of general movement, abnormal standard motor examination (suboptimal HINE score), or substantially delayed milestones for chronological age.

## Early Intervention

The early intervention aims to optimize motor, cognition, and communication skills using task-specific active interventions, prevent secondary impairments, minimize complications impairing neurodevelopmental outcomes, and promote parental or caregiver coping and mental health.

A. **Early intervention for optimal motor and cognitive skills:** Motor interventions (physical and occupational therapy) based on daily life-oriented tasks using self-generated high-intensity active movements are recommended. The mechanism of action for these motor interventions is the modulation of neuroplasticity to induce functional improvement. A distinction between unilateral and bilateral CP is required as the management and rehabilitative strategies differ.[14]
   - **Unilateral (hemiplegia) cerebral palsy:** Early constraint-induced movement therapy (CIMT) has been shown to result in better long-term hand function. Daily 30–60 minutes therapist supervised home intervention for at least six weeks is recommended.
   - **All CP subtypes:** Task-specific, goal-directed, infant-initiated motor training (e.g. goal activity motor enrichment (GAME)) have been associated with improved functional outcomes and reduced comorbid complications such as contractures and pain.

   Passive stimulation approaches controlled entirely by the therapist are not recommended.

B. **Interventions targeting secondary impairments and prevention of complications:**[15,16] Table 21.3 lists the various pharmacological agents, their mechanism of action, their dose, and their side effects when given to decrease secondary impairments. Table 21.4 lists the interventions to prevent secondary complications.

**Table 21.3: Pharmacological agents used for tonal abnormality in cerebral palsy[22]**

| | *Used for* | *Mechanism of action* | *Dose* | *Side effects* |
|---|---|---|---|---|
| **Benzodiazepines (Diazepam)** | Spasticity | $GABA_A$ receptor agonist | 0.2–0.8 mg/kg in 3–4 divided doses | Drowsiness, sedation, hypersalivation |
| **Tizanidine** | | Centrally acting alpha-2 adrenergic agonist | Initiate at 1–2 mg/day maximum up to 36 mg/day | Hypotension, sedation, asthenia, dry mouth, dizziness |
| **Baclofen** | | $GABA_B$ receptor agonist | Initiate at 2.5 mg/day titrate maximum up to 20–60 mg/day | Sedation, confusion, dizziness, ataxia, hypotension, paraesthesia |
| **Dantrolene** | | Inhibit calcium release from the sarcoplasmic reticulum | 12 mg/kg/day<br>Initiate at 0.5 mg/kg/dose in three divided doses, increase by 0.5 mg/kg/dose every 5–7 days. | Hepatotoxicity is a primary concern<br>Nausea, vomiting, diarrhea, and paraesthesia |
| **Clonidine** | | Alpha-2 adrenergic agonist | 1–10 µg/kg/day | Sedation, hypotension |
| **Trihexyphenidyl** | Dystonia | Anticholinergic | Initiate at 0.1 mg/kg/day and gradually titrate maximally up to 1–2 mg/kg/day. | Dry mouth, constipation, sleep disturbance |

**Table 21.4: Interventions to prevent complications**

| *Domains* | *Intervention* |
|---|---|
| GI problems (feeding, drooling, constipation) | 1. Soften the food.<br>2. Slight upright or recline position for feeding.<br>3. Sensory motor and functional chewing training.<br>4. Orolingual stimulation for better swallowing coordination.<br>5. Glycopyrrolate and botulinum toxin may be considered for sialorrhea.<br>6. Ensure adequate fluid and fiber intake.<br>7. Use laxative, in case of refractory constipation. anterograde enema can also be used. |
| Vision | 1. Formal vision assessment as early as within 48 hours of life.<br>2. Visual issues should receive intervention at term equivalent age and followed 3 monthly thereafter.<br>3. Surgical correction of strabismus along with exotropia/ esotropia for better alignment and binocular fusion.<br>4. Visual training and attention for stimulation of vision<br>5. High contrast/color stimuli in an interactive fashion for betterment of visual mobility and stimulation (i.e. Illuminating/lightning toys). |
| Sleep | 1. Structured routine bed time in quiet and dark room.<br>2. Avoid vigorous game, screen time prior to sleep.<br>3. Pharmacological intervention to reduce pain and dystonia and improvement of sleep quality.<br>4. Use of melatonin as sleep promoting agent. |
| Musculoskeletal | 1. Routine pelvis X-ray every 6–12 monthly after 1 year of age to early detection and management of hip dislocation.<br>2. Ankle foot orthosis to be worn to maintain dorsiflexion and range of motion.<br>3. Regular use of standing equipment to prevent hip dislocation and maintain hip abduction range of motion.<br>4. Early and moderate contracture application of specially designed cast.<br>5. Prolonged and severe contracture (>20°) combination of cast and surgical correction should be considered. |

(*Contd.*)

**Table 21.4: Interventions to prevent complications** (*Contd.*)

| *Domains* | *Intervention* |
|---|---|
| Tone | Appropriate combination of pharmacological and surgical intervention (botulinum toxin, diazepam, oral and intrathecal baclofen, tizanidine and trihexyphenidyl, selective dorsal rhizotomy) to be considered. |
| Epilepsy | It should be treated with standard pharmacotherapy as per protocol. |
| Undernutrition | • Early identification of undernutrition and signs of vitamin deficiency.<br>• Identify the significant contributors to undernutrition, such as oral motor dysfunction and abnormal sensitivity, gastroesophageal reflux and other gastrointestinal problems, excessive spasticity or dystonia, endocrinopathy, and recurrent infections.<br>• Optimize calorie and protein intake, allow frequent small meals.<br>• Change the consistency of food to a thicker paste-like consistency.<br>• Supplement with vitamins and mineral.<br>• Use adaptive utensils to promote self-feeding. |

C. **Intervention for parental or caregiver mental health and coping skills:**[20] Timely counseling and cognitive and behavioral therapy to alleviate parental anxiety and stress, kangaroo care, and structured musical interaction can promote maternal and neonatal bonding and reduce maternal anxiety.

## REFERENCES


1. Spittle AJ, Morgan C, Olsen JE, Novak I, Cheong JLY. Early Diagnosis and Treatment of Cerebral Palsy in Children with a History of Preterm Birth. Clin Perinatol. 2018 Sep;45(3):409-420. doi 10.1016/j.clp.2018.05.011. Epub 2018 Jul 2. PMID: 30144846.
2. Rosenbaum P, Paneth N, Leviton A, Goldstein M, Bax M, Damiano D, Dan B, Jacobsson B. A report: the definition and classification of cerebral palsy April 2006. Dev Med Child Neurol Suppl. 2007 Feb;109:8-14. Erratum in: Dev Med Child Neurol. 2007 Jun;49(6):480. PMID: 17370477.
3. Himpens E, Van den Broeck C, Oostra A, Calders P, Vanhaesebrouck P. Prevalence, type, distribution, and severity of cerebral palsy in relation to gestational age: a meta-analytic review. Dev Med Child Neurol. 2008 May;50(5):334-40. doi: 10.1111/j.1469-8749.2008.02047.x. Epub 2008 Mar 18. PMID: 18355333.
4. Oskoui M, Coutinho F, Dykeman J, Jetté N, Pringsheim T. An update on the prevalence of cerebral palsy: a systematic review and meta-analysis. Dev Med Child Neurol. 2013 Jun;55(6):509-19. doi 10.1111/dmcn.12080. Epub 2013 Jan 24. Erratum in: Dev Med Child Neurol. 2016 Mar;58(3):316. PMID: 23346889.
5. Bosanquet M, Copeland L, Ware R, Boyd R. A systematic review of tests to predict cerebral palsy in young children. Developmental Medicine and Child Neurology. 2013 May;55(5):418–26.
6. Novak I, Morgan C, Adde L, Blackman J, Boyd RN, Brunstrom-Hernandez J, Cioni G, Damiano D, Darrah J, Eliasson AC, De Vries LS. Early, accurate diagnosis and early intervention in cerebral palsy: advances in diagnosis and treatment. JAMA Pediatrics. 2017 Sep 1;171(9):897–907.
7. Shevell M. Quality standards subcommittee of the American Academy of Neurology; practice committee of the child neurology society. Practice parameter: evaluation of the child with global developmental delay: report of the quality standards subcommittee of the American Academy of Neurology and the practice committee of the child neurology society. Neurology. 2003;60:367–80.
8. Ferrari F, Cioni G, Einspieler C, Roversi MF, Bos AF, Paolicelli PB, Ranzi A, Prechtl HF. Cramped synchronized general movements in preterm infants as an early marker for cerebral palsy. Archives of pediatrics and adolescent medicine. 2002 May 1;156(5):460–7.
9. Guzzetta A, Belmonti V, Battini R, Boldrini A, Paolicelli PB, Cioni G. Does the assessment of general movements without video observation reliably

predicts neurological outcome? European Journal of Paediatric Neurology. 2007 Nov 1;11(6):362–7.

10. Einspieler C, Prechtl HF. Prechtl's assessment of general movements: a diagnostic tool for the functional assessment of the young nervous system. Mental retardation and developmental disabilities research reviews. 2005 Feb;11(1):61–7.
11. Paro-Panjan D, Sustersic B, Neubauer D. Comparison of two methods of neurologic assessment in infants. Pediatric neurology. 2005 Nov 1; 33(5):317–24.
12. Haataja L, Mercuri E, Regev R, Cowan F, Rutherford M, Dubowitz V, Dubowitz L. Optimality score for the neurologic examination of the infant at 12 and 18 months of age. The Journal of Pediatrics. 1999 Aug 1;135(2): 153–61.
13. Ment LR, Bada HS, Barnes P, et al. Practice parameter: neuroimaging of the neonate: report of the Quality Standards Subcommittee of the American Academy of Neurology and the Practice Committee of the Child Neurology Society. Neurology.
14. Morgan C, Fetters L, Adde L, Badawi N, Bancale A, Boyd RN, Chorna O, Cioni G, Damiano DL, Darrah J, De Vries LS. Early intervention for children aged 0 to 2 years with or at high risk of cerebral palsy: international clinical practice guideline based on systematic reviews. JAMA Pediatrics. 2021 Aug 1;175(8):846–58.
15. Trivić I, Hojsak I. Evaluation and treatment of malnutrition and associated gastrointestinal complications in children with cerebral palsy. Pediatric Gastroenterology, Hepatology and Nutrition. 2019 Mar 1;22(2):122–31.
16. Chung CY, Chen CL, Wong AMK. Pharmacotherapy of Spasticity in Children With Cerebral Palsy. J Formos Med Assoc. 2011 Apr;110(4):215–22.

CHAPTER

22

# Unknown Baby

Abandoned or orphaned infants are admitted to the hospital as 'unknown babies' for care and management till they are rendered fit for discharge.

## CLINICAL EVALUATION[1,2]

- Asymptomatic and well-appearing neonates should be clinically observed till the time of disposition to child welfare units.
- Preterm and symptomatic neonates should be evaluated for sepsis, the need for antibiotic therapy, and other workups.
- All neonates should be tested for congenital syphilis (VDRL or RPR test) and treated if needed.
- The hepatitis B vaccine should be given immediately and hepatitis B immunoglobulin for neonates less than seven days old.
- Evaluating for HIV and need for antiretroviral prophylaxis (nevirapine).
- Tetanus immunoglobulin (250 units IM) should be given if there is any suspicion of cord cut with unsterile technique or unhealthy cord on examination.
- In babies with non-specific symptoms of neonatal abstinence syndrome and concern for drug exposure *in-utero*, urine, and meconium can be tested.[3]

Infants with an uncomplicated course can be followed up in regular pediatric OPD, whereas sick and preterm babies should be followed up in high-risk clinics. At discharge, these babies are handed over to the child care unit or specialized adoption agency as directed by the court/committee. The hospital medical social service officer (MSSO) facilitates the process (Fig. 22.1).

**Admit abandoned neonate till fit for discharge**

1. Triage and stabilisation (check blood sugar)
2. Clinical evaluation (including screening for birth defects, weight, gestational age and postnatal age)
3. Obtain comprehensive maternal and birth history where possible
4. Inj. Vitamin K 0.5–1.0 mg IM
5. Congenital syphilis evaluation
6. Hep B vaccine and immunoglobulin
7. HIV evaluation, nevirapine prophylaxis
8. Routine immunization

**Post-discharge:**

- Well babies in routine pediatric OPD
- Preterm and sick babies in high-risk clinic

1. Register as a medicolegal case (MLC)
2. Inform hospital MSSO
3. Mandatory reporting within 24 hours child line services or the nearest police station/ child welfare committee
4. Social investigation by a social worker/child welfare officer or child welfare police officer (in 15 days)
5. Committee orders disposition of the baby after inquiry

**Fig. 22.1:** For evaluation of abandoned babies

## REFERENCES

1. Guha A, Rai A, Gupta D, Mondal R. Abandoned Babies at Tertiary Care Rural Medical College Hospital: The Indian Scenarios. Indian J Pediatr 2019;86:335–339.
2. World Health Organization. Survive and thrive: transforming care for every small and sick newborn. Geneva: World Health Organization; 2019. https://apps.who.int/iris/handle/10665/326495.
3. Brasher MI, Silverstein A, Moher J. Evaluation and Management of an Abandoned Infant at a Quaternary Care Hospital. J Emerg Med 2022;62(3):e69–e76.

CHAPTER 23

# Developmental Dysplasia of the Hip and Congenital Talipes Equinovarus

Newborns require a thorough examination to detect upper or lower limb deformities, including developmental dysplasia of the hip (DDH) and clubfoot. DDH affects 1–2 in every 1000 births, with a higher incidence in female infants. Early diagnosis is crucial, as delayed treatment can lead to hip osteoarthritis and the need for surgical intervention. Clubfoot, also known as congenital talipes equinovarus (CTEV), is a congenital foot abnormality that affects 1–2 in every 1000 births and is more common in male infants. Its timely diagnosis and prompt treatment through serial plaster cast greatly improve the chance of correction.

## CLINICAL PRESENTATION

The mother should be asked about risk factors, such as family history for DDH and breech presentation. Physical examination should include Ortolani and Barlow's maneuvers to screen for DDH. Barlow's maneuver tries to dislocate the hip by adducting and pushing it posteriorly, while Ortolani attempts to reduce a subluxated hip by abducting and pushing it anteriorly. *Universal ultrasound screening does not help prevent late detection of the condition*. Therefore, USG screening should be offered to infants with abnormal clinical examinations and risk factors. Limitation of hip abduction and asymmetric thigh folds can be signs of DDH in older infants. Clinical screening, however, is not always reliable.

Clubfoot can be identified before birth through routine fetal scans or during routine physical examinations in newborns. The Pirani scoring system (Table 23.1) should be used to assess the severity of clubfoot deformities.[1]

**The clubfoot deformity comprises four components:** Forefoot adduction, midfoot cavus, hindfoot varus, and hindfoot equinus. In a normal foot, the dorsum of the foot can be passively extended to the anterior aspect of the distal leg, but this movement is generally

| Table 23.1: The Pirani scoring system for CTEV | | | | |
|---|---|---|---|---|
| *S. No.* | *Parameter* | *Scoring* | | |
| | | 0 | 0.5 | 1 |
| **Midfoot** | | | | |
| 1. | Medial Crease | Multiple fine creases | 2–3 creases | Single deep crease |
| 2. | Curved lateral border of the foot | Straight lateral border | Curved lateral border at the level of metatarsals | Curved lateral border at the level of calcaneocuboid joint |
| 3. | Lateral head of the talus (on passive correction) | Lateral head of the talus covered by navicular | Lateral head of talus partially covered by navicular | Lateral head of talus uncovered |
| **Hindfoot** | | | | |
| 1. | Posterior Crease | Multiple fine creases | 2–3 creases | Single deep crease |
| 2. | Equinus | Able to reach beyond plantigrade | Reaches till plantigrade | Not able to reach till plantigrade |
| 3. | Empty heel | Calcaneum easily palpable | Calcaneum palpable with a layer of soft tissue in between | Calcaneum not palpable |

not possible in CTEV patients. The examination should also include documentation of posterior and medial skin creases on the foot and an assessment of the foot's flexibility. which can indicate prognosis and potential for nonoperative correction. A general examination of the whole body should be performed, including spine and upper limb examination, to rule out any associated disorders such as secondary clubfoot or arthrogryposis multiplex congenita.

## MANAGEMENT

For babies with an abnormal hip examination, an ultrasound of the hips is the investigation of choice. USG assesses the coverage of the acetabulum, femoral head position, and the joint's stability.

Graf et al. described two angles to evaluate the infant hip joint on ultrasound: (i) The $\alpha$ angle is formed between the acetabular roof and the vertical cortex of the ilium, (ii) the $\beta$ angle is formed between the cartilaginous roof and the vertical cortex of the ilium. The greater the $\alpha$ angle, the more reduced the hip. A hip ultrasound should be performed in all newborns with high-risk factors for DDH (positive family history and breech presentation) before the child is 6 months old. Plain radiographs of the hip are useful after four months of age to assess the acetabular development, femur-acetabulum relationship, and femoral coverage, as well as avascular necrosis of the femoral head.[2]

The goal of the management for DDH is to obtain a concentric reduction of the femoral head into the acetabulum, which subsequently corrects the development of the joint structures by remodeling and biological plasticity. The first step is achieved by closed means. Pavlik harness is used for children till six months of age to maintain the concentric reduction of the hip joint, whereas a hip spica cast is used in older children to maintain a stable reduction. The second step after obtaining and maintaining the concentric reduction is to evaluate the correction of the acetabular dysplasia by getting serial X-rays of the hip as the child ages. The potential of acetabular dysplasia for rectification after obtaining concentric hip reduction decreases significantly after 3–4 years of age.[3,4]

Surgical management is required for patients presenting late and those not responding to conservative treatment for sufficient time. It includes open reduction of the hip with a hip spica cast application, femoral/acetabular osteotomies for maintaining concentric hip reduction, and correcting the acetabular dysplasia.[5]

The diagnosis of CTEV is mainly clinical. The treatment starts with serial manipulation and casting of the foot (Ponseti method), starting soon after the newborn's birth. The serial manipulation and casting are repeated every week: The first cast corrects the cavus with exaggeration of supination, the subsequent casts take care of the forefoot adduction and supination, and the hindfoot equinus is fixed in the last.

In most cases, percutaneous tenotomy of the Achilles tendon is required to correct the residual hindfoot equinus. After fully correcting the deformity, foot abduction orthosis is prescribed to prevent the recurrence of the deformity till 3–4 years of age. These orthoses, which maintain the foot in 10 degrees of dorsiflexion and

70 degrees of external rotation, must be worn 23 hours a day for 3–4 months, followed by night-time use for 3–4 years.[6]

Operative management is required in CTEV cases with failure of conservative management or relapse of the deformity. Even for such patients, the management starts with serial manipulation and casting to make the foot supple, followed by surgical correction of the residual deformity. The operative procedures include various soft tissue releases and bony procedures in the form of medial opening wedge and lateral closing wedge osteotomies. The bony procedures are generally done after the age of 4 years.

## OUTCOMES

The outcome of DDH is fairly good when the condition is diagnosed early, immediately after the newborn's birth. The higher the age at presentation, the worse the outcomes after the interventions. After eight years, the condition is better left untreated till skeletal maturity, as the surgical management complications outweigh the procedure's benefits. Even after prompt diagnosis and management of DDH, total hip replacement is required in many patients after the 3rd–4th decade of life.

The prognosis for CTEV is good with serial manipulation and casting with greater than 90% success rates. However, even after total correction of the deformity, the foot is not entirely normal like the other uninvolved foot. The size of the foot remains small for the whole life, and the calf is also smaller than the contralateral limb. Also, serial clinic-radiological monitoring is required till skeletal maturity to look for and manage relapse of the deformity promptly.[7]

## REFERENCES

1. Sankar WN, Weiss J, Skaggs DL. Orthopedic conditions in the newborn. J Am Acad Orthop Surg. 2009 Feb;17(2):112–22.
2. Vaquero-Picado A, González-Morán G, Garay EG, Moraleda L. Developmental dysplasia of the hip: update of management. EFORT Open Rev. 2019 Sep 17;4(9):548–556.
3. Kotlarsky P, Haber R, Bialik V, Eidelman M. Developmental dysplasia of the hip: What has changed in the last 20 years? World J Orthop. 2015 Dec 18;6(11):886–901.
4. Roposch A, Liu LQ, Protopapa E. Variations in the use of diagnostic criteria for developmental dysplasia of the hip. Clin Orthop Relat Res. 2013 Jun;471(6):1946–54.

5. Mulpuri K, Song KM, Gross RH, Tebor GB, Otsuka NY, Lubicky JP, et al. The American Academy of Orthopaedic Surgeons Evidence-Based Guideline on Detection and Nonoperative Management of Pediatric Developmental Dysplasia of the Hip in Infants up to Six Months of Age. J Bone Joint Surg Am. 2015 Oct 21;97(20):1717–8.
6. Hartofilakidis G, Karachalios T, Stamos KG. Epidemiology, demographics, and natural history of congenital hip disease in adults. Orthopedics. 2000 Aug;23(8):823–7.
7. Ganesan B, Luximon A, Al-Jumaily A, Balasankar SK, Naik GR. Ponseti method in the management of clubfoot under 2 years of age: A systematic review. PLoS One. 2017 Jun 20;12(6):e0178299.

Section

9

# Diagnostic Modalities and Procedures

CHAPTER

24

# Amplitude-integrated EEG (aEEG) in Neonates

Amplitude-integrated EEG (aEEG) is a simpler version of conventional scalp EEG, which depicts amplitudes from 2 or 4 scalp electrodes on a time-compressed semi-logarithmic scale. A 6 cm tracing depicts compressed data of one hour, making it easy to review brain activity for hours and days altogether. The lower border comprises the lowest-detected amplitudes, and the highest amplitudes form the upper border of the tracing. Amplitudes <10 µV are displayed on a linear scale, and those >10 µV are depicted on a logarithmic scale. This differential amplitude representation leads to better detection of minute changes in the lower amplitude range and prevents the higher amplitudes from distorting the trace morphology. A representative trace is depicted in Fig. 24.1. Raw data is displayed alongside the compressed trace.

## ELECTRODES

Recording can be done with four electrodes for a two-channel aEEG and two electrodes for a single-channel aEEG. Usually, the signal is

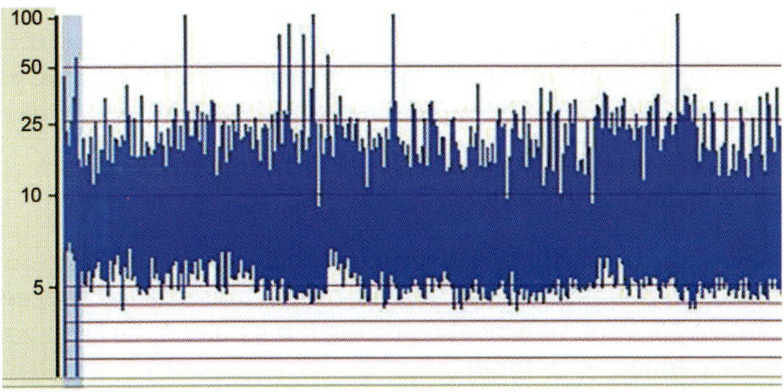


**Fig. 24.1:** A representative aEEG trace showing amplitude depiction in linear followed by logarithmic scale along the Y-axis and time along the X-axis

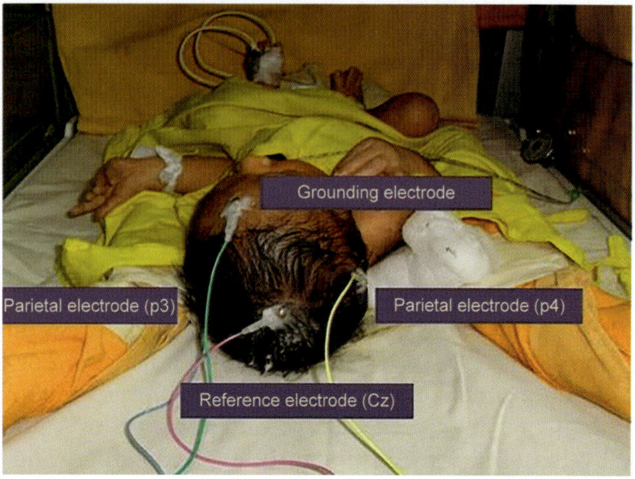


**Fig. 24.2:** Position of bilateral parietal, ground, and reference electrodes in a neonate undergoing aEEG

recorded from two electrodes placed in the biparietal location (P3/P4). A third electrode, acting as a reference electrode, and a fourth one as a ground electrode, are also appropriately placed (Fig. 24.2).

**Three types of electrodes are available:** Cup, needle, and hydrogel. Cup electrodes can be disinfected and reused, while needle and hydrogel electrodes are for one-time use only. The standard disinfection protocol should be followed before the application of the electrodes, and caution should be practiced in extremely premature infants to avoid skin injury. One should always check for electrode dislocation and the resulting electrode artifact. While recording, the behavioral state of the neonate and factors affecting it, like the administration of sedative drugs, should be assessed. Events like handling, apnea, and abnormal movements should be appropriately marked.

## INTERPRETATION[4–8]

The aEEG record is interpreted under the headings of background pattern, sleep-wake cycling (SWC), and the presence or absence of seizure. A convenient way of reporting it is by using the Hellstrom-Westas qualitative method.

Representative background and SWC images are depicted in Fig. 24.3a and b and Fig. 24.4a and b. Some semi-quantitative scoring systems have also been developed for reporting aEEG.

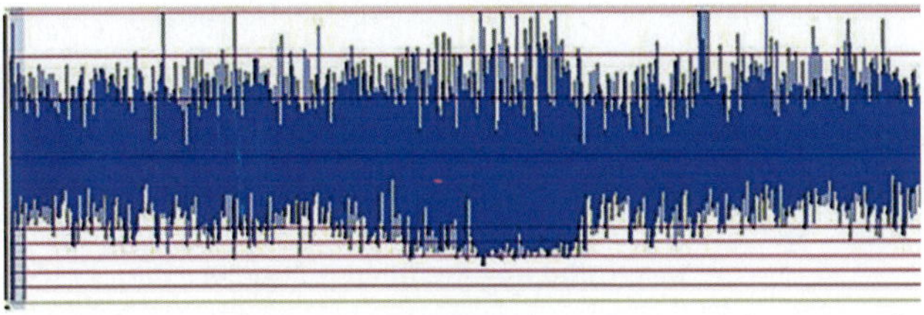

(a) Discontinuous background pattern with minimum amplitudes mostly below 5 μV and maximum above 10 μV

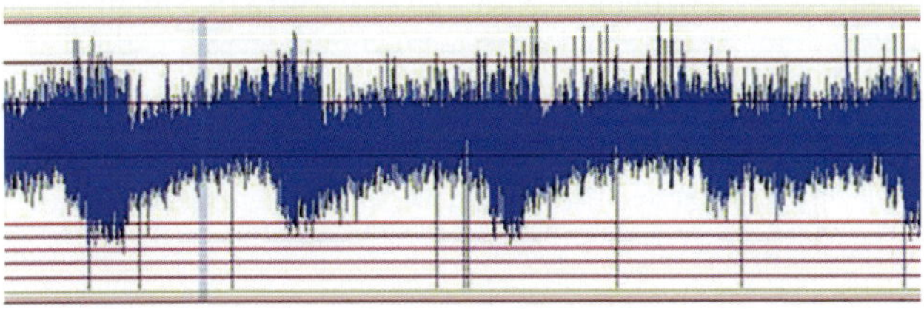

(b) Continuous background pattern with minimum amplitudes mostly between 5–10 μV and maximum around 10–25 μV

**Fig. 24.3:** Amplitude-integrated EEG tracing showing (a) discontinuous (upper border of amplitude above 10 μV and lower below 5 μV) and (b) continuous (upper border of amplitude around 10–25 μV and lower between 5–10 μV) background activity

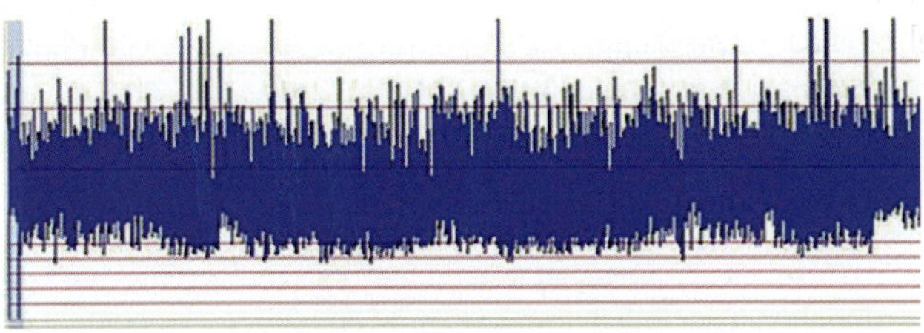

(a) Absent sleep–wake cycling

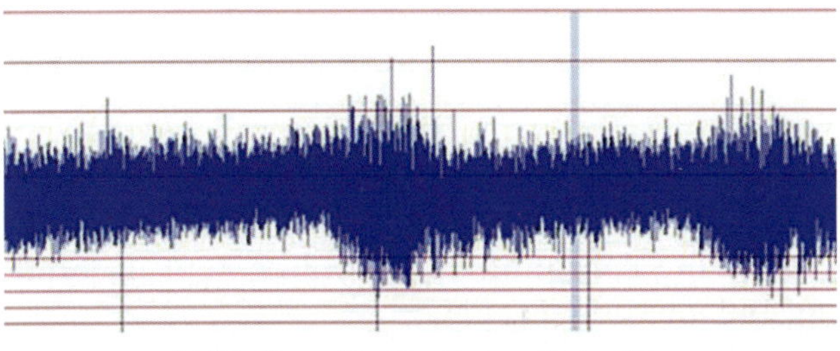

(b) Regular and mature sleep–wake cycling

**Fig. 24.4:** Amplitude-integrated EEG tracing showing (a) absent and (b) mature and regular sleep–wake cycling

| **Table 24.1: Classification of aEEG patterns in term and preterm infants using the Hellström-Westas Method** | |
|---|---|
| **Background pattern:** Describes the dominating type of electrocortical activity in the aEEG trace. | |
| *Continuous* | Continuous activity with a lower amplitude of around 7–10 μV and maximum amplitude of 10 to 25 μV. |
| *Discontinuous* | Discontinuous background with a minimum amplitude below 5 μV and maximum amplitude above 10 μV. |
| *Burst suppression* | Discontinuous background with a minimum amplitude at 0–2 μV and bursts with amplitude >25 μV. |
| *Low voltage* | Continuous background pattern of very low voltage (around or below 5 μV). |
| *Inactive/flat* | Inactive (isoelectric tracing) background below 5 μV. |
| **Sleep–wake cycling (SWC)**<br>The broader bandwidth represents discontinuous background activity during quiet sleep, and the narrower bandwidth corresponds to the more continuous activity during wakefulness and active sleep. | |
| *No SWC* | No cyclic variation of the aEEG background. |
| *Imminent/ immature SWC* | Some, but not fully developed, cyclic variation of the lower amplitude, but not developed as compared with normative gestational age representative data. |
| *Developed SWC* | Clearly identifiable sinusoidal variations between discontinuous and more continuous background activity, with cycle duration >20 minutes. |
| **Seizures**<br>An abrupt rise in the minimum amplitude and a simultaneous rise in the maximum amplitude are often followed by a short period of decreased amplitude. The raw EEG should show concurrent seizure activity, with a gradual build-up and then a decline in frequency and amplitude of repetitive spikes or sharp-wave or activity with a duration of at least 5 to 10 seconds. | |
| *Single seizure* | A solitary seizure |
| *Repetitive seizure* | Single seizures appear more frequently than at 30 minutes intervals. |
| *Status epilepticus* | Continuously ongoing seizure activity for >30 minutes. |

The following confounders should be kept in mind while reporting and interpreting aEEG:

1. Elevated background activity may occur due to the following:
    a. Handling of the baby.
    b. Muscle activity (more for frontal electrodes).

c. High-frequency ventilation.
d. Gasp artifact.
e. ECG artifact.

2. Falsely low amplitude may be due to:[9]
a. Severe scalp edema
b. Deep sedation
c. Leads artifact

## INDICATIONS OF aEEG MONITORING[2,3]

a. **Asphyxiated newborns:** Before the advent of therapeutic hypothermia: An abnormal aEEG within 3–6 hours of life was highly predictive of the adverse outcome when combined with clinical indicators than either individually alone.[10]

**Therapeutic hypothermia era:** A 6-hour-abnormal aEEG is not a good predictor of adverse outcome in a cooled neonate; however, a normal early record is highly predictive of a good outcome, and persistent abnormality beyond 48 hours is highly predictive of poor neurodevelopmental outcome. Absent SWC in the first 72 hours of life is highly predictive of future adverse developmental outcomes.[11]

Hypothermia trials have shown that newborns with moderate encephalopathy (discontinuous pattern) on aEEG showed benefit, whereas those with severe encephalopathy (burst suppression, continuous low voltage, or flat trace) didn't. Amplitude-integrated EEG, in conjunction with the clinical picture, is a valuable tool for assessing the degree of severity in selecting patients for therapeutic hypothermia. However, it should not be used as the sole criterion.

b. **Detection of neonatal seizures:** Studies have shown that the accuracy of aEEG in detecting neonatal seizures varies between 70–80%. Detailed clinical evaluation and conventional EEG recording remain the gold standard for diagnosing neonatal seizures. The presence of seizures on aEEG record of an asphyxiated newborn receiving therapeutic hypothermia is associated with later adverse neurodevelopmental outcomes.

c. **Preterm newborns:** Although not as extensively used as in term neonates, background abnormalities not in sync with gestational age are associated with adverse developmental outcomes in preterm newborns. Extensive intraventricular hemorrhages are associated with lower maximum and minimum amplitudes in the first 72 hours of life and reduced bursts (<130 bursts/hour) on aEEG. These two findings are also associated with poor neurodevelopmental outcomes later.

Advantages of aEEG include its ease of interpretation, guidance in decision-making in real-time in neonatal intensive care units, information about the long-term outcome, improved detection of subclinical seizures, and improvement in newborn care by allowing timely decisions on initiating and tailoring therapy.

Limitations of aEEG include covering a relatively small area of the head (since only 2–4 electrodes are used), with a propensity to miss focal abnormalities and brief episodes of seizures. Additionally, there is limited normative data available for preterm neonates.

## REFERENCES

1. Bruns N, Blumenthal S, Meyer I, Klose-Verschuur S, Felderhoff-Muser U, Muller H. Application of an Amplitude-integrated EEG Monitor (Cerebral Function Monitor) to Neonates. J. Vis. Exp. 2017;127:e55985.
2. Hellstrom-Westas L, Rosen I, Svenningsen NW. Predictive value of early continuous amplitude-integrated EEG recordings on outcome after severe birth asphyxia in full-term infants. Arch Dis Child Fetal Neonatal Ed. 1995;72: F34–8.
3. Olischar M, Klebermass K, Kuhle S, Hulek M, Kohlhauser C, Rücklinger E, et al. Reference values for amplitude-integrated electroencephalographic activity in preterm infants younger than 30 weeks gestational age. Pediatrics. 2004;113:e61–6.
4. Burdjalov VF, Baumgart S, Spitzer AR. Cerebral function monitoring: a new scoring system for evaluating brain maturation in neonates. Pediatrics. 2003;112:855–61.
5. Cerebral Function Monitor, in Neonatal Equipment, everything you want to know. 5th ed., Deorari AK, Paul VK, Sachdeva A, eds. New Delhi, India: CBS Publishers; 2017.
6. Shalak LF, Laptook AR, Velaphi SC, Perlman JM. Amplitude-integrated electroencephalography coupled with an early neurologic examination enhances the prediction of term infants at risk for persistent encephalopathy. Pediatrics. 2003;111:351–7.
7. Thoresen M, Hellstrom-Westas L, Liu X,deVries LS. Effect of hypothermia on amplitude-integrated electroencephalogram in infants with asphyxia. Pediatrics. 2010;126:e131–9.
8. Gluckman PD, Wyatt JS, Azzopardi D, Ballard R, Edwards AD, Ferriero DM, et al. Selective head cooling with mild systemic hypothermia after neonatal encephalopathy: a multicentre randomized trial. Lancet 2005;365:663–70.

9. Shah DK, Mackay MT, Lavery S, Watson S, Harvey AS, Zempel J, et al. Accuracy of bedside electroencephalographic monitoring compared with continuous conventional electroencephalography for seizure detection in term infants. Pediatrics 2008;121:1146–54.
10. Hellström-Westas L, Klette H, Thorngren-Jerneck K, Rosen I. Early prediction of outcome with aEEG in preterm infants with large intraventricular hemorrhages. Neuropediatrics 2001;32:319–24.
11. Glass HC, Wusthoff CJ, Shellhaas RA. Amplitude-integrated electroencephalography: the child neurologist's perspective. J Child Neurol. 2013;28:1342–50.

CHAPTER

# 25 Genetic Diagnosis and Counseling

A successful pregnancy outcome depends upon the timely identification of potential fetal abnormalities through prenatal screening or diagnosis. However, it is not uncommon to encounter abnormal prenatal screening results on history evaluation after birth or to detect infants with genetic conditions for the first time in the neonatal intensive care unit. Prompt confirmation of the diagnosis is essential to guide management, prognosticate, and counsel the family. Improvements in technology and the reduction in the cost of genomic testing have led to its increasing use in the routine care of sick newborns. As a neonatologist, one must acquaint oneself with current prenatal screening practices and various genetic diagnostic strategies that must be applied while evaluating such newborns. It is also vital to apply genetic counseling principles while ordering genetic testing and receiving the genetic test results.

**Prenatal screening** for genetic disorders includes screening the pregnant lady for common chromosomal aneuploidies using blood testing and fetal ultrasonographic evaluation at different times during pregnancy. It comprises information about high-risk situations requiring genetic counseling (Table 25.1).

## FIRST-TRIMESTER SCREENING

This includes maternal serum beta-human chorionic gonadotrophin (free β-HCG) levels along with pregnancy-associated plasma protein-A (PAPP-A), which are analyzed between $10–13^{+6}$ weeks of pregnancy, and after that, age-appropriate multiples of the median (MoMs) calculated. Nuchal translucency (NT) and nasal bone (NB) are important sonographic markers for various aneuploidies and monogenic conditions. NT refers to measuring the subcutaneous accumulation of fluid at the back of the fetal neck. An increased NT (> 99th centile) is an independent risk factor for chromosomal aneuploidies, structural anomalies (e.g. cardiac defects), and single gene defects (e.g. Noonan syndrome) in the fetus.[1,2] Absent nasal

**Table 25.1: Indications for genetic counseling and prenatal testing**

| |
|---|
| **During pregnancy**<br>1. Advance maternal age (>35 years).<br>2. High risk of aneuploidies in screening tests.<br>3. Fetal structural defects/soft markers (e.g. echogenic bowel, ventriculomegaly) detected in antenatal ultrasound. |
| **During periconception period**<br>1. Previous child with a chromosomal abnormality/single gene disorder.<br>2. Family history of chromosomal abnormality, undiagnosed intellectual disability, recurrent abortions, early neonatal deaths, or congenital malformations all?<br>3. Any of the parents is a known carrier of a balanced chromosomal abnormality.<br>4. Parents being a carrier of prevalent autosomal recessive condition such as beta thalassemia. |
| **In newborns**<br>1. Congenital malformations, dysmorphism, growth retardation.<br>2. Unexplained IUGR, skeletal dysplasia.<br>3. Neuromuscular presentation: Floppiness, arthrogryposis, talipes with antenatal polyhydramnios.<br>4. Unexplained sepsis like presentation, encephalopathy, seizures, jaundice, or cardiomyopathy.<br>5. Any metabolic derangement—metabolic acidosis, hypoglycemia, high lactate, hyperammonemia, ketonuria.<br>6. Ambiguous genitalia. |
| **Others**<br>1. Parental consanguinity (3rd degree or more); detailed family history should be taken.<br>2. Maternal illness (e.g. systemic lupus erythematosus).<br>3. Teratogen exposure (e.g. valproate intake/ radiation exposure).<br>4. Bad obstetric history all? (yes, we have to check the history). |

bone increases the risk of chromosomal anomalies.[2] When combining ultrasound parameters (NT and NB)), and other demographic information such as maternal weight, age, ethnicity, and the number of fetuses, a "combined test' risk estimate is generated by automated software for the common trisomies, i.e. trisomy 21, 13 and 18 to identify "at risk" women. It provides a detection rate of 85–90% for trisomy 21, with a false positive rate of about 5%.[1]

## SECOND-TRIMESTER SCREENING

The measurement of serum analytes in the second trimester (quadruple test) is done between 15–22 completed weeks.

It provides a detection rate of about 80% with a false positive rate of 5%. Alpha-fetoprotein (AFP) measurement in the second-trimester screen provides a risk estimate for the fetus' open neural tube and abdominal defects.[3] All the patients should be offered a detailed second-trimester ultrasound to detect fetal structural anomalies and soft markers. "Soft markers" are ultrasound findings more commonly observed in aneuploid fetuses, but are not pathological, e.g. echogenic intracardiac foci, ventriculomegaly, pyelectasis, choroid plexus cysts, etc. The presence of soft markers in isolation or various combinations increases the risk of fetal aneuploidies.[4]

## NON-INVASIVE PRENATAL TESTING (NIPT)

Analysis of cell-free fetal DNA in the maternal circulation is, currently, the most sensitive and specific screening test available for common aneuploidies (trisomy 21, 18, 13 and sex chromosome aneuploidies). It alleviates the risk of miscarriage associated with invasive procedures such as CVS or amniocentesis.

Fetal cell-free DNA is released in maternal circulation by the apoptosis of placental trophoblasts and becomes detectable from about ten weeks of pregnancy till term. Cell-free DNA screening can be done using various molecular methods (targeted massively parallel sequencing or single nucleotide polymorphism based). The basic methodology involves differentiating the fetal DNA, which comprises three copies of a particular chromosome (e.g. chromosome 21), from the maternal DNA with two copies. Next-generation sequencing (NGS) based technology sequences millions of fragments of cell-free DNA (both maternal and fetal) which is then mapped to the human genome and analyzed if a particular chromosome is being over-represented. It provides a sensitivity of 99% for trisomy 21 and 13 and 98% for trisomy 18, with a combined false positive rate of 0.13%.[1] NIPT is not used for vanishing twins, the presence of a malformation on ultrasound, or triplet pregnancy.[5]

While screening tests should be offered to all pregnant women based on their gestational age at presentation, detailed pre-test counseling should be provided, including the detection rates, false positive rates, costs, and requirement of confirmatory testing for the positive screen results. The possibility of incidental detection of maternal mosaicism for a chromosomal aneuploidy or a malignancy should also be explained for NIPT.

## PRENATAL DIAGNOSTIC PROCEDURES

### Amniocentesis

Under ultrasonography guidance, 15–20 ml of amniotic fluid is aspirated from the amniotic fluid pocket, free of fetal parts, using a sterile 20-gauge needle. The sample is centrifuged, and the pelleted cells are grown in a culture medium for about two weeks before they can be used for chromosomal analysis or DNA is extracted for molecular analysis. Rapid diagnostic techniques like quantitative fluorescent polymerase chain reaction (QF-PCR) or fluorescent *in-situ* hybridization (FISH) can also be done directly on the amniotic fluid sample. The risk of procedure-related pregnancy loss (0.1–0.3%) should be informed during the pre-test counseling.[6,7]

### Chorionic Villus Sampling (CVS)

Under ultrasound guidance, transabdominal (less commonly trans cervical) aspiration of placental villi is done, which provides viable cells from the trophoblastic layer of the placenta. This procedure is usually performed between 11 – 14 weeks of pregnancy. The sample obtained can be used for direct DNA analysis for a known mutation (e.g. in a previously affected child) or common aneuploidies by QF-PCR. A part of the sample is usually separated to set up culture (after cleaning of maternal decidua), which can then be used for complete karyotype analysis. The procedural risk of pregnancy loss is about 0.1 – 0.5%.[6,7] The primary advantage of CVS is that it can be performed earlier in pregnancy, thus providing an earlier diagnosis. But, chromosomal mosaicism can sometimes be encountered in the samples, which again requires amniotic fluid sampling to confirm true fetal karyotype.

### Preimplantation Genetic Diagnosis (PGD)

PGD involves the biopsy of an early embryo (produced through *in-vitro* fertilization) at the blastocyst stage (usually day five embryo) for genetic analysis. The choice of investigation depends upon the indication (chromosomal analysis or single gene testing). After the results, only the healthy (unaffected) embryos are transferred to the uterine cavity for implantation. This procedure helps at-risk couples to avoid possible termination of pregnancy. Since most techniques used in PGD use single-cell genomics, a chromosome confirmation by CVS or amniocentesis is also recommended. PGD is mainly requested by couples who wish to avoid possible termination of pregnancy following PND. Preimplantation genetic screening involves screening the embryos for chromosomal abnormalities to improve the pregnancy outcome among infertile couples of 35 years and over undergoing ART or having repeated IVF failures.[8] It is, however, currently not recommended by ACOG.

The standard prenatal screening tests, their diagnostic procedure, and their timing are listed in Table 25.2.

## VARIOUS GENOMIC TESTS

### Chromosomal Analysis

Conventional karyotyping is a widely available technique that detects structural and numerical (aneuploidy) chromosomal abnormalities at a resolution of 5–10 Mb. Heparinized blood is subjected to culturing and arresting dividing cells in metaphase, followed by Giemsa staining. A specific banding pattern for each chromosome helps in chromosomal identification.

QF-PCR is one of the commonly used rapid diagnostic tests that involve amplification and analysis of polymorphic markers on chromosomes to detect common aneuploidies. Other quick aneuploidy detection techniques such as quantitative fluorescent polymerase chain reaction (QF-PCR) or fluorescent *in situ* hybridization (FISH) for a specific chromosome such as 21, 18, 13 or a microdeletion syndrome (DiGeorge syndrome or Prader-Willi syndrome) are also used in a prenatal and neonatal setting for a rapid diagnosis in 24–48 hours. Such techniques are employed when one has "a priori" strong suspicion of a particular disorder.

### Chromosomal Microarray

Chromosomal microarray (CMA) detects chromosomal copy number changes. It uses thousands to millions of probes spread across the genome to detect regions of imbalance (deletions and duplications) compared to the reference genome. It offers higher resolution and sensitivity than the conventional karyotype and detects submicroscopic chromosomal imbalances, which cannot be seen in a standard karyotype. It is the first line of investigation for multiple congenital anomalies/malformations seen prenatally or postnatally, offering a diagnostic yield of 15–20%.[8]

### Multiplex Ligation-dependent Probe Amplification

Multiplex-ligation-dependent probe amplification (MLPA) is based on amplifying and detecting multiple known targets with

**Table 25.2: Prenatal screening tests, the diagnostic procedures, and their timing[1]**

| *Prenatal testing* | *Timings* | *Test for* | *Action* | *Detection rate# for Down syndrome (%)* |
|---|---|---|---|---|
| **Screening tests** | | | | |
| 1st trimester Ultrasonography | 10–$13^{+6}$ weeks (crown-rump length 45–84 mm) | Nuchal translucency (NT) and nasal bone | NT>99th centile (or >3.0 mm) and absent nasal bone require post-test counseling and diagnostic testing, e.g. amniocentesis | 64–70 |
| Dual marker (free-β-hCG + PAPP-A) | 10–$13^{+6}$ weeks (crown-rump length 45–84 mm) | Chromosomal aneuploidies (e.g. trisomy 21, 13, 18) | High risk requires post-test counseling and diagnostic testing, e.g. amniocentesis | 82–87 (when combined with NT/NB scan) |
| Quadruple marker (AFP, dimeric Inhibin-A, hCG, unconjugated estriol) | 15–22 weeks | Chromosomal aneuploidies, open neural tube defects | | 81 |
| NIPT | Ten weeks to term | Trisomy 21, 13, 18, Sex chromosome aneuploidies | | 99 |

*(Contd.)*

**Table 25.2: Prenatal screening tests, the diagnostic procedures, and their timing[1] (Contd.)**

| *Prenatal testing* | *Timings* | *Test for* | *Action* | *Detection rate[#] for Down syndrome (%)* |
|---|---|---|---|---|
| **Diagnostic tests** | | | | |
| CVS | 11–13 weeks (conventionally; but may be performed till later in gestation) | Fetal karyotype/enzyme assay /DNA analysis* | – | – |
| Amniocentesis | 15–20 weeks | Fetal karyotype/DNA analysis/ fetal infections* | – | – |
| Cordocentesis | 18–24 weeks | Fetal DNA analysis/ karyotype/ hematological studies (e.g. factor VIII assay)/ enzyme analysis* | – | – |
| PGD | Preimplantation (blastocyst stage—day 5–7 of embryo development) | Fetal DNA analysis | Confirmation with CVS or amniocentesis[8] | – |

*CVS:* Chorionic villus sampling; *hCG:* Human chorionic gonadotrophin; *PAPP-A:* Pregnancy-associated plasma protein-A; *NIPS:* Non-invasive prenatal screening; *PGD:* Preimplantation genetic diagnosis

**Test choice depends upon the indication, [#]% of affected individuals called screen-positive by the test*

a single primer pair. It detects deletions and duplications of small chromosomal segments/exons or whole genes. It is rapid and can detect aneuploidies, microdeletion syndromes, and exonic deletions, e.g. spinal muscular atrophy.

### *Methylation Specific MLPA (MS-MLPA)*

MS-MLPA, a variation of the MLPA technology, is used to detect the methylation profile at specific target regions. It is used in the diagnosis of diseases such as Prader-Willi syndrome, Russell-Silver syndrome, Beckwith-Weidemann syndrome, and transient neonatal diabetes due to maternal uniparental disomy of 6q24.2.

## Triplet Primed PCR (TP-PCR)

Triple-primed PCR is a method used to detect expanded alleles such as trinucleotide repeats. It helps diagnose expanded CTG repeats in DMPK in neonatal cases of congenital myotonic dystrophy.

## Sanger Sequencing

The technique requires di-deoxynucleotides to detect single nucleotide variants in the genes of interest. It can be used to sequence single genes when an apparent phenotype and common pathogenic variants suggest a particular disease, e.g. beta-thalassemia, cystic fibrosis, or Gaucher disease.

## Next-generation Sequencing (NGS)

It provides genome-wide coverage since massively parallel sequencing of multiple small DNA fragments is done using automated machines. The data is then analyzed based on the reference sequences, and variants are interpreted based on the phenotype. Variants are classified as pathogenic, likely pathogenic, benign, and presumably benign, and variants of uncertain significance (VUS) based on the guidelines provided by the American College of Medical Genetics and Genomics.[9]

- Whole exome sequencing (WES) sequences the exons of all the genes. This is an efficient testing method since the exome account for 1–2% of the genome but contains over 85% of deleterious variants. It includes the sequencing of the exon-intron junctions to identify splice site mutations. However, deep intronic variants cannot be identified.
- Clinical exome sequencing (CES): A gene panel test that includes 5000–6000 Online Mendelian Inheritance in Man

(OMIM) morbid genes known to be associated with clinical disease.

- By NGS technology, whole genome sequencing (WGS) includes sequencing of the entire genome, including exons, introns, intergenic regions, and the mitochondrial genome. The advantage of WGS over WES is that it can identify variants in the non-coding areas, such as deep intronic and promotor regions. It can also detect chromosomal abnormalities and trinucleotide repeats. However, big data's colossal cost and generation make its analysis tedious. Currently, WGS is mainly used in the research setting but is likely to become "one single test" in times to come. Table 25.3 compares the different genetic testing methods.

Table 25.3 lists the comparison between the different genetic tests, and Table 25.4 lists the type of blood sample that must be sent for a particular examination. Table 25.5 lists the genetic tests' typical clinical phenotype encountered in NICU.

**Table 25.3: Comparison between the different genetic tests**

| | *Conventional karyotype* | *Chromosomal microarray* | *Whole exome sequencing* | *Whole genome sequencing* |
|---|---|---|---|---|
| Resolution | Chromosomal abnormalities > 5 megabases (Mb) | 10–50 kilobases (kb) | Single nucleotide changes | Single nucleotide changes |
| Coverage | All chromosomes | Genome—depends on probe coverage | Exons of all the genes | All genes, introns, and intergenic regions |
| Turnaround time | 1–2 weeks | Two weeks | 4–6 weeks<br>Rapid exome 2 to 21 days | 6 weeks |
| Limitations | Requires viable cells. Only large abnormalities detected | It does not detect balanced translocations and inversions | Cannot detect deep intronic and intergenic variants<br>Limited ability to detect CNV | High cost<br>Difficulty in interpreting non-coding variants and novel genes |

**Table 25.4: Type of sample for genomic testing**

| *Test* | *Type of blood sample* |
|---|---|
| Karyotype, FISH | 2 ml heparin blood |
| Chromosomal microarray, QF-PCR, MLPA, NGS | EDTA blood*/Dried blood spot |

*FISH:* Fluorescence *in situ* hybridization; *QF-PCR:* Quantitative fluorescent polymerase chain reaction; *MLPA:* Multiplex ligation-dependent probe amplification; *NGS:* Next generation sequencing

**In case of a recent blood transfusion (less than two weeks), it is preferred to obtain any other tissue, such as a skin biopsy*

**Table 25.5: Genetic tests for common clinical phenotypes encountered in NICU**

| *Phenotype* | *Possible etiology* | *Test* |
|---|---|---|
| Congenital abnormalities, dysmorphism, growth retardation, skeletal dysplasia | Chromosomal abnormality | Karyotype, CMA |
| | Monogenic disorder | WES |
| Unexplained IUGR | Chromosomal abnormality | Karyotype, CMA |
| Nonspecific phenotypes and suspected monogenic<br>Large gene | Monogenic disorders | WES/WGS |

(Contd.)

**Table 25.5: Genetic tests for common clinical phenotypes encountered in NICU** *(Contd.)*

| *Phenotype* | *Possible etiology* | *Test* |
|---|---|---|
| Neuromuscular presentation: Floppiness, contractures, talipes with antenatal polyhydramnios | SMA | Targeted testing for SMN1 deletions using MLPA or RFLP |
| | Muscular dystrophy/myopathy | WES or NGS panel |
| | Myotonic dystrophy | Testing for triplet repeat expansion |
| Unexplained sepsis-like presentation, encephalopathy, seizures, jaundice, or cardiomyopathy<br>Any metabolic derangement—metabolic acidosis, hypoglycemia, high lactate, hyperammonemia, ketonuria | Inborn error of metabolism | WES or NGS panel + biochemical tests, e.g. blood TMS, urine GCMS |
| Ambiguous genitalia | Chromosomal and monogenic causes of Disorders of sex development | Karyotype, CMA, MLPA, and NGS-based methods for congenital adrenal hyperplasia |

*CMA:* Chromosomal microarray; *WES:* Whole exome sequencing; *WGS:* Whole genome sequencing; *MLPA:* Multiplex ligation-dependent probe amplification; *RFLP:* Restriction fragment length polymorphism; *TMS:* Tandem mass spectrometry; *GCMS:* Gas chromatography-mass spectrometry

## Which Test to Choose?

The choice of test depends on the

1. Clinical features and family—whether the infant's phenotype suggests a particular disorder or whether the patient has a nonspecific phenotype.
2. Cost and affordability.
3. Turnaround time.

Table 25.5 lists the genetic test for the typical clinical presentation in the NICU.

## Points to Remember While Ordering a Genomic Test

1. Appropriateness: Is this the proper test? For example, exome sequencing is not considered the first-line test to identify chromosomal abnormalities.
2. Interpretation may be difficult due to limited or nonspecific symptoms in the neonatal period.
3. Variants of unknown significance and inconclusive results may lead to difficulty in genetic counseling.
4. Turnaround time: The time to obtain the report is essential in the critical care setting.
5. The high cost of testing.
6. Identification of diseases for which there are no treatment available or late-onset conditions.
7. Psychosocial issues that require discussion in the presence of both parents who were expecting a normal pregnancy outcome.

## Newborn Screening Using Genomic Testing

Genomic testing has the potential in newborn screening programs. NGS has been used as a second-tier test for detecting immunodeficiencies and cystic fibrosis following expanded newborn screening.[10] The advantages of using genomic testing are:

1. Identify diseases not covered by biochemical screening.
2. Avoids confounders for biochemical screening tests such as gestation age, feeding state, and timing of sample collection. Challenges include high costs, technical feasibility, decisions on which genes to have, and difficulty interpreting the harmful effects of variants. Other essential factors are the age of onset of disease, correlation of disease severity and genotype, penetrance, and mode of inheritance.[11]

## NGS for Sick Newborns

Exome and genome sequencing are helpful in the diagnosis of a sick newborn with suspected monogenic disorders with clinical and genetic heterogeneity. Studies using WES and WGS have reported diagnostic yields between 20% to 50%.[12] A study from India reported a yield of 37.5% for clinical exome sequencing.[13]

In the last few years, rapid and ultrarapid exome or genome sequencing has gained attention as a first-line test in managing sick neonates. Improvements in technology have resulted in rapid and ultrarapid exome sequencing in which the results are reported within 2 to 21 days. Rapid exome or genome sequencing aims to deliver results within 21 days, whereas ultrarapid exome or genome sequencing reports results within five days.[14] A randomized control trial examining rapid WES versus rapid WGS demonstrated a similar time to results (median 11 vs. 11.2 days) and diagnostic yield (19 vs. 20%) between the two tests. Additionally, the study demonstrated that ultrarapid WGs (median 4.6 days) had a higher diagnostic yield (46%), thus demonstrating the utility of the test in first-line work-up critically ill neonates.[15]

Rapid exome facilitates a confirmatory diagnosis and often enables a change in management. Several recent studies have demonstrated the feasibility of implementing rapid WES or WGS in the clinical setting, with median turnaround times between 2 to 13 days and diagnostic yield between 24% and 60%. It is vital to save the DNA from the affected baby if the testing is opted for by the parents.

## Genetic Counseling

**Steps involved in genetic counseling:**

- **Gathering information and pedigree drawing:** Collecting the information by obtaining previous medical history (e.g. drug intake during pregnancy, recurrent abortions, previously affected child) and family history.
- **Risk assessment:** Based on the patterns of inheritance inferred from the pedigree analysis, or the genetic testing (of the proband in the family or the carrier), a precise risk estimate can be provided to the family, and testing is offered.
- A pre-test counseling session must provide information to the couple/parents regarding various screening and diagnostic tests available, their detection rates, costs, procedure, risks, turnaround time, and limitations. In the case of prenatal screening tests, the

patient should be informed that a prenatal diagnostic test would be required in case of a positive screen. Possible options after a positive diagnostic test should also be explained, e.g., termination of pregnancy, intrauterine intervention, or delivery at a tertiary hospital. Likely unexpected findings during the diagnostic tests, such as test failure, mosaicism, and detection of an incidental abnormality like a sex chromosome abnormality during testing for a particular chromosomal rearrangement, should also be discussed with the prospective parents.

- **Post-test counseling** after an abnormal diagnostic test should be done empathetically, including information about
  - The disease diagnosis and the underlying genetic basis.
  - The disease course and prognosis (including the life expectancy).
  - Available treatment options.
  - For prenatal cases: The option for termination of pregnancy and a fetal autopsy should be discussed.
- The goal of counseling should be to empower, encourage and enable the consult to make an informed decision best suited for their situation. One should never make decisions on the patient's behalf (non-directiveness), especially when decisions involve irreversible procedures such as reproductive decisions regarding medical termination of pregnancy, adoption or marriage, or undergoing prophylactic surgeries. As per the recent amendment in the PNDT Act, MTP is permissible for up to 24 weeks.[16] If the diagnosis is made after 24 weeks gestation, a medical board of various specialties helps make further decisions. Social and emotional distress arising due to the diagnosis of the baby should be addressed along with the introduction to a support group (if available).

## REFERENCES


1. Screening for Fetal Chromosomal Abnormalities. Obstetrics & Gynecology. 2020;136(4):859–867.
2. Alldred SK, Takwoingi Y, Guo B, Pennant M, Deeks JJ, Neilson JP, Alfirevic Z. First and second-trimester serum tests with and without first-trimester ultrasound tests for Down's syndrome screening. Cochrane Database Syst Rev. 2017 Mar 15;3(3): CD012599.
3. Driscoll D, Gross S. Screening for fetal aneuploidy and neural tube defects. Genetics in Medicine. 2009;11(11):818–821.
4. Salomon LJ, Alfirevic Z, Berghella V, Bilardo CM, Chalouhi GE, Da Silva Costa F, Hernandez-Andrade E, Malinger G, Munoz H, Paladini D, Prefumo F, Sotiriadis

A, Toi A, Lee W, on behalf of the ISUOG Clinical Standards Committee. ISUOG Practice Guidelines (updated): performance of the routine mid-trimester fetal ultrasound scan. Ultrasound Obstet Gynecol 2022; 59: 840–856.

5. Palomaki GE, Chiu RWK, Pertile MD, et al. International Society for Prenatal Diagnosis Position Statement: cell-free (cf)DNA screening for Down syndrome in multiple pregnancies [Online ahead of print]. Prenat Diagn. 2020. https://doi.org/10.1002/pd.5832.
6. Practice Bulletin No. 162: Prenatal Diagnostic Testing for Genetic Disorders. Obstet Gynecol. 2016 May;127(5):e108-e122.
7. Salomon LJ, Sotiriadis A, Wulff CB, Odibo A, Akolekar R. Risk of miscarriage following amniocentesis or chorionic villus sampling: a systematic review of the literature and updated meta-analysis. Ultrasound Obstet Gynecol. 2019 Oct;54(4):442-451. doi: 10.1002/uog.20353. Epub 2019 Sep 6. PMID: 31124209.
8. Preimplantation Genetic Testing: ACOG Committee Opinion, Number 799. Obstet Gynecol. 2020 Mar;135(3):e133-e137.
9. Richards S, Aziz N, Bale S, Bick D, Das S, Gastier-Foster J, et al. Standards and guidelines for interpreting sequence variants: a joint consensus recommendation of the American College of Medical Genetics and Genomics and the Association for Molecular Pathology. Genet Med [Internet]. 2015;17(5):405–23. Available from: https://doi.org/10.1038/gim.2015.30.
10. Smon A, Repic Lampret B, Groselj U, Zerjav Tansek M, Kovac J, Perko D, et al. Next-generation sequencing as a follow-up test in an expanded newborn screening program. Clin Biochem [Internet]. 2018;52:48–55. Available from: https://www.sciencedirect.com/science/article/pii/S0009912017305635.
11. Remec ZI, Trebusak Podkrajsek K, Repic Lampret B, Kovac J, Groselj U, Tesovnik T, et al. Next-Generation Sequencing in Newborn Screening: A Review of Current State. Front Genet. 2021;12(May).
12. Krantz ID, Medne L, Weatherly JM, Wild KT, Biswas S, Devkota B, et al. Effect of Whole-Genome Sequencing on the Clinical Management of Acutely Ill Infants with Suspected Genetic Disease: A Randomized Clinical Trial. JAMA Pediatr. 2021;92122(12):1218–26.
13. Anand V, Pournami F, Madhavilatha GK, Prabhakar J, Nandakumar A, Jain N. Genetic Testing in Neonatal Intensive Care: Experience from a Tertiary Care Unit. Indian J Pediatr. 2021;88(4):398–9.
14. Elliott AM, du Souich C, Lehman A, Guella I, Evans DM, Candido T, et al. RAPIDOMICS: rapid genome-wide sequencing in a neonatal intensive care unit—successes and challenges. Eur J Pediatr. 2019;178(8):1207–18.
15. Dimmock DP, Clark MM, Gaughran M, Cakici JA, Caylor SA, Clarke C, et al. An RCT of Rapid Genomic Sequencing among Seriously Ill Infants Results in High Clinical Utility, Changes in Management, and Low Perceived Harm. Am J Hum Genet. 2020;107(5):942–52.
16. Ministry of Law and Justice, Govt of India. The Medical Termination of Pregnancy (Amendment) Act 2021, no 8 of 2021. The Gazette of India. CG-DL-E-26032021-226130; 2021.

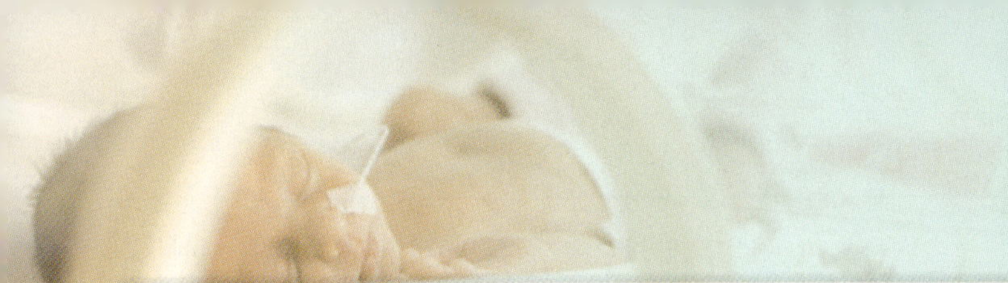

Section

10

# Therapeutic Modalities

CHAPTER

26

# Mechanical Ventilation

Mechanical ventilators are devices that support the patient's inadequate respiratory efforts until respiratory function improves either spontaneously or after an intervention.

Some common indications for mechanical ventilation are given below:[1]

| | *Condition* | *Manifestation or criteria* |
|---|---|---|
| 1. | Correction of hypoxemia | $FiO_2$ requirement > 40–60% or failure of non-invasive respiratory support |
| 2. | To reverse acute respiratory acidosis | pH <7.2 and $pCO_2$ >65 mm Hg |
| 3. | To relieve respiratory distress | Marked retractions, severe tachypnea (>80–100/min) |
| 4. | To treat apnea or poor respiratory efforts | Poor efforts or apnea requiring bag and mask ventilation |
| 5. | To prevent or treat lung atelectasis as in postoperative setting or neuromuscular disease | |
| 6. | To maintain a patent airway | Altered sensorium, sedation, anesthesia, neurological and neuromuscular illnesses |
| 7. | To decrease systemic or myocardial oxygen consumption as in shock | Septic shock, congestive cardiac failure, necrotizing enterocolitis, etc. |
| 8. | To reduce raised intracranial pressure through controlled hyperventilation | Cerebral edema, head injury and intracranial space occupying lesion |
| 9. | To stabilize chest wall | Flail chest, diaphragmatic palsy |

The goals of mechanical ventilation are to achieve acceptable gas exchange (alveolar ventilation and oxygenation) with minimum adverse effects and maximum patient comfort and to wean the patient off the ventilator support as soon as the underlying condition for initiating mechanical ventilation is no longer present.

The choice of ventilator modes for a neonate depends on various factors like equipment available in the NICU, underlying pathophysiology, and the physician's familiarity and comfort level with a particular mode. Although there cannot be a universal protocol for the use of mechanical ventilation in the neonatal unit, the availability of such a protocol that delineates a basic approach for initiation and weaning ensures uniformity in its application. Thus, it must be remembered that ventilation strategies and settings need to be modified as and when the disease process evolves.

**Modes of mechanical ventilation:** The different modes of ventilation and their relative advantages and disadvantages are listed in Table 26.1. Among the various modes, the patient-triggered ventilatory modes, namely SIMV, AC, or PSV, are preferred as they are associated with a reduction in air leaks and a shorter duration of ventilation.[2] There is some evidence that AC mode may be associated with a shorter duration of weaning as compared to SIMV.[2]

Based on the primary control variable, one can choose pressure-controlled ventilation (PCV), where inflation pressure is set, or volume-controlled ventilation (VCV), where preset tidal volume is set. Until recently, pressure-controlled, time-cycled, continuous-flow ventilation has been the standard of care in the NICU because delivering small tidal volumes was unsuccessful with older ventilators and significant endotracheal tube leaks in neonates. However, the advent of newer ventilators have made this possible, and studies have shown that VCV or volume guarantee ventilation may be more beneficial than PCV. Table 26.2 describes the various parameters that are either set or determined by the ventilator (V) in PCV, VCV, volume guarantee (VG), and pressure support ventilation (PSV).

**Evidence: Pressure controlled versus volume controlled or volume guarantee mode**

Two recent meta-analyses[3,4] have concluded that volume targeted/ guarantee mode is associated with a significant decrease in the combined outcome of death or bronchopulmonary dysplasia (BPD), lower rate of pneumothorax, less hypocarbia, decreased risk of severe intraventricular hemorrhage/ periventricular leukomalacia, and shorter duration of mechanical ventilation.

The preferred ventilator modes for various disease conditions that are followed in our unit are depicted in Table 26.3. We prefer assist control mode during the acute phase of ventilation and PSV

**Table 26.1: Modes of mechanical ventilation**

| *Mode* | *Description* | *Disadvantages* |
|---|---|---|
| Intermittent mandatory ventilation **(IMV)** | All breaths are mandatory.<br>Unloads the respiratory muscles. | Patient ventilator asynchrony. |
| Synchronized intermittent mandatory ventilation **(SIMV)** | Breaths are delivered in synchrony with the patient's spontaneous effort. Allows spontaneous breathing in between the mandatory breaths, which are unsupported.<br>Allows patient comfort and at the same time keeps respiratory muscles active. | Work of breathing can be high if spontaneous breaths are not supported adequately. Expiratory asynchrony can happen. |
| Assist control **(AC)** | All breaths are assisted and delivered in synchrony with the patient's spontaneous effort.<br>Unloads the respiratory muscles. Useful in acute phase of illness. | If the spontaneous respiratory rate is high, all breaths would still be assisted, and this can lead to hyperventilation and respiratory alkalosis. There is also a risk of patient-ventilator asynchrony and air trapping at higher rates.<br>When used for a long time, respiratory muscle wasting can occur. Expiratory asynchrony can happen. |
| Pressure support ventilation **(PSV)** | Patient controls the rate, inspiratory time, and flow rate. Eliminates expiratory asynchrony. Better patient comfort and less need for sedation. | Cannot be used in patients with poor respiratory drive or apnea.<br>Pressure support needs to be adjusted based on changing lung mechanics. |

**Table 26.2: Modalities of mechanical ventilation**

| *Modality* | *Description* | *Mode* | *Settings* | | | | | | *Remarks* |
|---|---|---|---|---|---|---|---|---|---|
| | | | *PIP* | $V_T$ | *PEEP* | *Ti* | *Rate* | *FiO₂* | |
| Pressure controlled ventilation (PCV) | Traditional neonatal ventilators are continuous flow, time-cycled, pressure-limited ventilators | IMV<br>SIMV<br>AC | ✓ | Variable | ✓ | ✓ | ✓ | ✓ | Simple design, easy to operate. Can ventilate despite a large ET leak.<br>The major disadvantage is that the $V_T$ varies with changes in lung compliance and excessively large $V_T$ can lead to inadvertent hyperventilation and lung injury from volutrauma. |
| Volume controlled ventilation (VCV) | Delivers a constant tidal volume | IMV<br>SIMV<br>AC | Variable | ✓ | ✓ | ✓ | ✓ | ✓ | The benefits of VCV include consistent $V_T$ delivery, less volutrauma (avoiding high $V_T$), less atelectotrauma (avoiding low VT), and more stable $PaCO_2$. |
| Volume guarantee (VG) | The operator sets a target expired $V_T$ and the ventilator adjusts the PIP for the next inflation based on the measurement of the expired $V_T$ of the previous breaths. | SIMV<br>AC<br>PSV | Set Pmax<br>✓ | ✓ | ✓ | ✓ | ✓ | ✓ | The set Pmax is different from the delivered PIP because the ventilator adjusts the delivered PIP to achieve the target $V_T$. The PIP max should be set high enough to allow fluctuations around the working PIP. |

*(Contd.)*

**Table 26.2: Modalities of mechanical ventilation (*Contd.*)**

| *Modality* | *Description* | *Mode* | *Settings* | | | | | | *Remarks* |
|---|---|---|---|---|---|---|---|---|---|
| | | | *PIP* | $V_T$ | *PEEP* | *Ti* | *Rate* | $FiO_2$ | |
| Pressure support ventilation (PSV) | Following detection of spontaneous patient effort, the ventilator delivers a breath that is flow-cycled but time limited. | | ✓ | | ✓ | For SIMV back up | For SIMV back up | ✓ | The clinician has control over the inspiratory pressure and time limit and the synchronized intermittent mandatory ventilation (SIMV) rate which provides a safety backup in case of apnea. Volume guarantee can be added to PSV mode. |

*PIP:* Peak inspiratory pressure; *PEEP:* Peak end expiratory pressure; *VT:* Tidal volume; *Ti:* Inspiratory time; $FiO_2$: Fractional inspired oxygen concentration

**Table 26.3: Preferred modes of ventilation in different lung conditions**

| *Underlying condition* | *Acute phase* | *Weaning* | *Comments* |
|---|---|---|---|
| Respiratory distress syndrome | A/C<br>Use the VG option to tailor PIP | *Choice 1:* PSV<br>*Choice 2:* SIMV+PSV | 1. Look for auto-triggering while using A/C or PSV modes (use SIMV if auto-triggering occurs).<br>2. Ensure that the leak is <30–40% while using VG. |
| Bronchopulmonary dysplasia | A/C or PSV<br>Use VG option to tailor PIP | *Choice 1:* PSV<br>*Choice 2:* SIMV+PSV | |

(*Contd.*)

**Table 26.3: Preferred modes of ventilation in different lung conditions** (*Contd.*)

| *Underlying condition* | *Acute phase* | *Weaning* | *Comments* |
|---|---|---|---|
| Meconium aspiration syndrome | A/C or SIMV | *Choice 1:* PSV<br>*Choice 2:* SIMV+PSV | Avoid using A/C if the baby's spontaneous breathing rate is >80 per minute. |
| Pneumonia | A/C or PSV | *Choice 1:* PSV<br>*Choice 2:* SIMV+PSV | |
| Transient tachypnea of newborn | A/C or PSV | *Choice 1:* PSV<br>*Choice 2:* SIMV+PSV | Avoid A/C if the baby's spontaneous rates are very high (> 80–90 per min) –expiratory time (Te) might get compromised; in these situations, use either PSV or SIMV. |
| Apnea/shock/asphyxia (conditions with normal lung or minimal lung disease) | SIMV (rates usually kept low) | SIMV | Avoid using A/C or PSV; chances of hypocarbia if the back-up rate is kept inadvertently high. |
| Failure of conventional ventilation, CDH, air-leaks | HFO | *Choice 1:* PSV<br>*Choice 2:* SIMV+PSV<br>*Choice 3:* Direct weaning to CPAP/oxygen by hood | Refer to HFV protocol |

***Note:*** *Choice 1 indicates the preferred mode of ventilation.*

while weaning the baby from the ventilator. Whenever possible, the volume guarantee (VG) option is used. However, VG is avoided if the leak displayed is >30–40%.

The usual settings on a mechanical ventilator are shown in Table 26.4. These settings are basic guides and need modification based on the disease condition and acuity of the illness.

Once mechanical ventilation is initiated, the settings must be tailored based on clinical evaluation supported by blood gases and/or chest X-rays as the disease condition evolves. Relying solely on blood gases alone may lead to late detection of worsening or delay in weaning, leading to lung injury. The various parameters that need to be monitored in a neonate on mechanical ventilation are listed in Table 26.5.

The suggested initial settings in common conditions are depicted in Table 26.6.

The subsequent ventilator adjustments should be tailored to meet adequate oxygenation and ventilation.

**Acute deterioration on mechanical ventilator:** Mechanically ventilated neonates can have episodes of acute deterioration manifesting as desaturation, apnea, bradycardia, or poor perfusion. This can be secondary to an acute event like endotracheal tube **D**isplacement or **O**bstruction, **P**neumothorax, **E**quipment failure (DOPE), worsening disease condition, or onset of a new pathophysiological process like PDA, sepsis, intraventricular hemorrhage, etc. (a useful mnemonic being *DOPE plus*).

Appropriate action would include quick clinical assessment, disconnection from the ventilator and manual bagging to rule out equipment failure, verifying ET position and patency, and a bedside trans-illumination of the chest if pneumothorax is suspected. Appropriate action would avert a potentially serious or life-threatening disaster. After initial stabilization, a chest radiograph, blood gas, and other ancillary tests can be done to diagnose worsening or new disease conditions.

**Weaning from a conventional mechanical ventilator:**[5] To decrease ventilator-induced lung injury and other adverse effects, the duration of ventilation should be as short as possible. Weaning should be attempted as soon as the underlying condition which mandated invasive ventilation begins to improve, the baby is clinically stable, and blood gases are acceptable. The various parameters that can be weaned in a ventilator are as follows.

**Table 26.4: Ventilatory parameters and their initial settings**

| *Parameter* | *Description* | *Setting* | *Remarks* |
|---|---|---|---|
| Tidal volume | This is the major determinant of alveolar ventilation. Alveolar ventilation = RR X ($V_T$—dead space). Increasing either will increase alveolar minute ventilation, but increasing $V_T$ has a greater impact than increasing rate, because of the effect of dead space. | 4–6 ml/kg<br>Maximum 8 ml/kg | Volutrauma if $V_T \geq 8$ ml/kg;<br>Atelectotrauma if tidal volume $\leq 3$ ml/kg |
| Peak inspiratory pressure (PIP) | The optimal PIP setting is one that results in adequate chest rise and audible breath sounds, and results in an adequate tidal volume delivery between 4 and 6 ml/kg. The PIP setting will also depend on the age and size of the infant and the underlying disease condition. | Start between 12–16 cm $H_2O$. Can increase to 20–25 in poorly compliant lungs as in severe RDS/ pneumonia, etc. | The exhaled $V_T$ for a set PIP in pressure-controlled ventilation and conversely, the PIP required to deliver a set $V_T$ in volume-controlled ventilation should be constantly evaluated and monitored. |
| Peak end expiratory pressure (PEEP) | PEEP is an important determinant of mean airway pressure and therefore the adequacy of oxygenation. Optimum PEEP ensures that the lung's functional residual capacity (FRC) is maintained. | The initial PEEP setting depends on the underlying lung condition. PEEP of 5 to 6 cm $H_2O$ is reasonable in diseases with poor lung compliance, while in diseases with risk of air trapping like meconium aspiration syndrome, 3–4 cm $H_2O$ should be adequate. PEEP can be titrated upward if $FiO_2$ remains above 40%. | Inadvertently high PEEP or failure to reduce PEEP as lung compliance improves leads to overdistension of the lung, hypercarbia, increased pulmonary vascular resistance, impairment of venous return, and decreased cardiac output. |

(*Contd.*)

**Table 26.4: Ventilatory parameters and their initial settings** *(Contd.)*

| *Parameter* | *Description* | *Setting* | *Remarks* |
|---|---|---|---|
| Inspiratory time (Ti) | Ti depends on the time constant of the respiratory system which in turn depends on the size of the infant and underlying lung condition. Smaller infants have shorter time constants and diseases with poor lung compliance like RDS have shorter time constants compared to diseases with higher airway resistance like BPD and MAS.<br>In flow cycled modes like PSV, Ti is patient determined and inflation is terminated when inspiratory flow declines to a preset value, usually 15% of peak flow. Here, the set Ti value is only an upper limit that into play when flow cycling fails to occur. | Ti is set around 0.4 to 0.5 second for term infants and 0.25 to 0.35 second for a preterm infant. | The flow time scalar graph is a useful adjunct to adjust this parameter. Ti should be sufficient to allow completion of inspiratory flow before the ventilator cycles off into expiration and avoid a significant inspiratory hold that increases patient–ventilator asynchrony. |
| Rate | Depends on the lung condition and infant. | 40 (range of 30–60 per min) | In RDS, with shorter time constants, a higher rate is preferred. In MAS, a lower rate with adequate Ti and Te is preferred. |
| Expiratory time (Te) | Disease conditions with greater airway resistance need adequate Te to allow complete emptying of lungs during exhalation. Te can be either directly set or altered using Ti and rate. | | Insufficient TE is depicted in the flow time scalar as failure of the expiratory flow to return to zero before the next inflation |

*(Contd.)*

**Table 26.4: Ventilatory parameters and their initial settings** *(Contd.)*

| *Parameter* | *Description* | *Setting* | *Remarks* |
|---|---|---|---|
| $FiO_2$ | $FiO_2$ should be adjusted to achieve a $SpO_2$ target of 90–95% by optimizing lung volume. This may include increasing the PEEP in increments of 0.5–1 cm $H_2O$ until $FiO_2$ is below 30%. | Begin at 30–50% and optimize based on $SpO_2$ and underlying condition. | Excessive oxygen can lead to oxygen toxicity. If $FiO_2 > 60\%$, rule out PPHN or inadequate MAP. |
| Trigger sensitivity | Trigger sensitivity helps to optimize patient–ventilator interaction. | Trigger should be set at the most sensitive value to provide a rapid ventilator response and minimize workload to trigger an inflation. With *Babylog 8000 plus*, this is an arbitrary scale from 1–10 and 1 represents the most sensitive setting corresponding to a flow trigger at 0.2 L /min. | Auto triggering (leading to tachypnea) can occur if there is ET tube leak or water condensate in the circuit. |

**Table 26.5: Parameters that are monitored in ventilated neonates**

| | |
|---|---|
| **Clinical Parameters** | • Patient comfort and synchrony. Presence of respiratory distress such as chest retractions, head bobbing, tachypnea even in presence of normal saturations and blood gases may indicate inadequate ventilatory support. Such situations may need increase in ventilator setting.<br>• Color, perfusion, and capillary refill<br>• Chest rise with spontaneous breaths and ventilator inflations<br>• Respiratory rate including spontaneous breaths.<br>• Retractions or work of breathing<br>• Breath sounds audible symmetrically to all lung areas, adventitial sounds, and ET leak<br>• Heart sounds and murmur<br>• Others: Sensorium (activity), blood pressure, and urine output<br>(*agitation or patient-ventilator asynchrony often reflects inadequate ventilator support rather than lack of sedation*) |
| **Ventilatory parameters** | • Exhaled tidal volume for a set PIP in pressure-controlled ventilation and measured PIP for a set VT in volume-controlled ventilation.<br>• Spontaneous respiratory rate.<br>• Minute ventilation (200 to 300 ml/kg/min) usually indicates adequate ventilation.<br>• Mean airway pressure.<br>• Percentage ET leak.<br>• Flow-time scalar to evaluate the adequacy of inspiratory and expiratory time, inspiratory hold. |
| **Pulse oximetry** | Oxygen saturation between 90–95%. |
| **Blood gas analysis** | Blood gases are usually indicated 30 minutes after the initiation of mechanical ventilation and 30 minutes after making *significant* changes in the setting. Blood gases may be needed frequently (6–8 hourly) during acute illness and less often (12 hourly or once in 24 to 48 hours) in chronically ventilated neonates. The usual targets are: |

(*Contd.*)

**Table 26.5: Parameters that are monitored in ventilated neonates (*Contd.*)**

| | |
|---|---|
| | PH ≥ 7.25<br>$PCO_2$ 45–55 mmHg<br>$PaO_2$ 50–70 mmHg<br>Base excess between (–5 to +5) and $HCO_3$ in the normal range |
| **Chest radiograph** | After the first intubation, a chest radiograph should always be performed to confirm the position of the ET tube and to evaluate lung expansion. Flattening of the diaphragm and greater than 8 posterior rib spaces on CXR indicates over-expansion of lungs. Adequacy of PEEP is best determined based on oxygen requirement rather than lung expansion on CXR. |

**Table 26.6: Initial ventilator settings in common conditions**

| *Condition* | *Suggested initial settings* |
|---|---|
| **Respiratory distress syndrome—poorly compliant low volume lungs with shorter time constants** | Early and aggressive use of non-invasive ventilation and early use of surfactant by INSURE technique decreases the need for invasive ventilation.<br>Initial settings:<br>• PIP 14–16 cm $H_2O$ or VT of 5–6 ml/kg<br>• PEEP 5–6 cm $H_2O$<br>• Rate 40–60/min<br>• Ti 0.35 seconds |

(*Contd.*)

**Table 26.6: Initial ventilator settings in common conditions** (*Contd.*)

| *Condition* | *Suggested initial settings* |
|---|---|
| **Transient tachypnea of newborn (TTN)** | Rarely, TTN may require invasive ventilation.<br>Initial settings:<br>• PIP 12–16 cm $H_2O$ or $V_T$ of 4–5 ml/kg<br>• PEEP 4 to 5 cm $H_2O$<br>• Rate 40–60/min<br>• Ti 0.35–0.45 seconds |
| **Apnea of prematurity (AoP)**<br>**Asphyxia** | AoP that is unresponsive to caffeine and non-invasive respiratory support may need invasive ventilation. As the lungs are essentially normal, it needs minimal settings:<br>• PIP 12–14 cm $H_2O$ or $V_T$ of 4–5 ml/kg<br>• PEEP 4 cm $H_2O$<br>• Rate 20–30/min<br>• Ti 0.4 seconds |
| **Meconium aspiration syndrome** | The clinical features of MAS may be quite variable depending on the predominant pathophysiology—surfactant inactivation and chemical pneumonitis leading to atelectasis versus airway obstruction. The choice of ventilator setting depends on the above, which can be understood based on clinical findings and chest radiograph in a majority.<br>Use lower PEEP 3.5–4 if risk of air leak is high.<br>Target $SpO_2$ 91–95% to avoid PPHN.<br>$V_T$ 5–6 ml/kg or PIP adjusted to achieve $V_T$ of 5–6 ml/kg<br>Rate ≤30<br>Ti 0.35–0.50 seconds<br>PEEP 4–7 cm $H_2O$ if atelectatic picture and lower if air trapping is suspected.<br>If PPHN is severe, adequate lung requirement can be achieved using high frequency ventilation before beginning inhaled nitric oxide. |

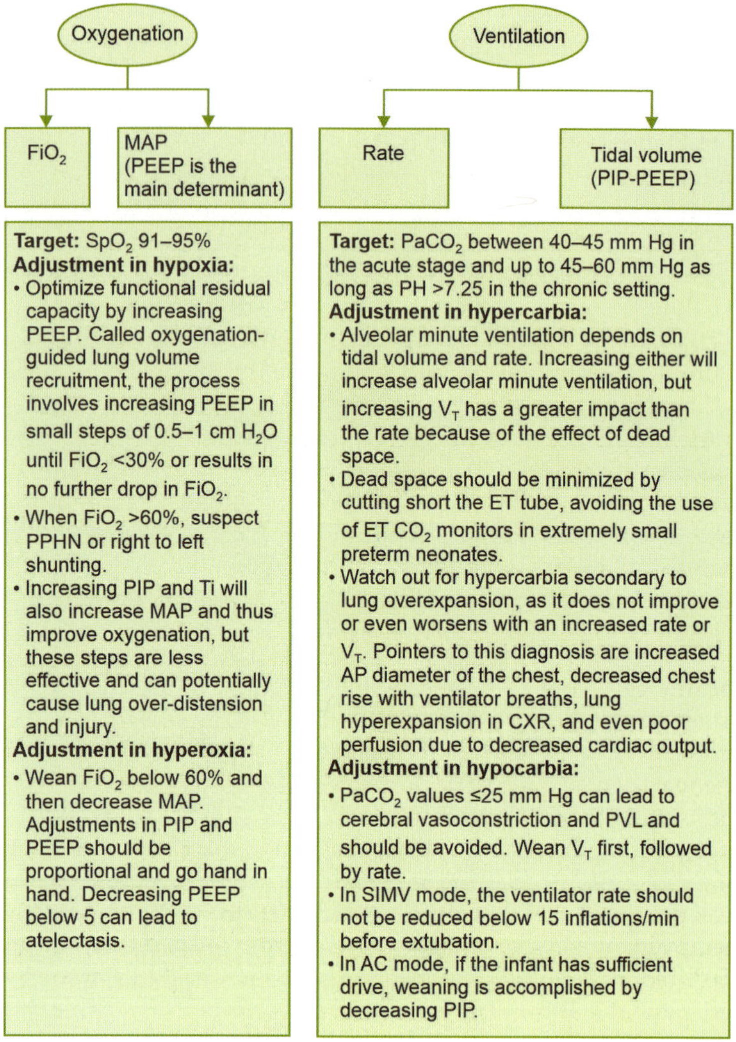


**Fig. 26.1:** Oxygenation and ventilation in mechanical ventilation

1. **Tidal volume:** Wean $V_T$ in volume-controlled mode to maintain $pCO_2$ <50 mm Hg. Dropping $V_T$ <4 ml/kg will lead to atelectasis and should be avoided.
2. **Peak inspiratory pressure (PIP):** Wean PIP based on delivered tidal volumes. PIP can be dropped gradually as compliance improves, reflected in higher VT for the same set PIP. In volume guarantee mode, the PIP is automatically weaned as compliance improves.

3. **PEEP:** Wean as indicated when $FiO_2$ <30%. Oxygenation is the best guide to wean PEEP rather than lung inflation on CXR. In conditions with a high risk of air trapping, one can lower PEEP while accepting higher $FiO_2$. Generally, weaning PEEP < 5 cm $H_2O$ should be avoided to maintain FRC and prevent atelectasis.
4. **Rate:** Wean as tolerated for $pCO_2$ <50 mm Hg. Generally, the rate is weaned once PIP or $V_T$ has been weaned. Weaning rates when PIP is high (example ≥ 18–20 cm $H_2O$) can lead to increased work of breathing. In SIMV mode, rates should not be dropped below 15–20 bpm as it can lead to excessive work of breathing. In PSV and AC modes, the set rate represents the backup rate, and dropping rates does not lead to weaning. Typically, Ti (inspiratory time) is not altered in most neonates.

Although there is no fixed protocol for weaning, some considerations should be kept in mind—most potentially harmful parameters should be weaned first, weaning should occur in small decrements with one parameter at a time to avoid flip-flop, all changes should be documented and ensure adequate support to decrease work of breathing during the weaning process.

**Extubation from mechanical ventilation:** Once ventilatory parameters have been decreased sufficiently, the underlying condition is resolved, and the infant has adequate spontaneous efforts, they can be considered ready for extubation. For example, a neonate ventilated for RDS in the pressure-controlled SIMV mode with settings of PIP ≤ 16 cm $H_2O$, PEEP ≤ 5 cm $H_2O$, rate 20, and $FiO_2 \leq 0.30$ can be considered ready to be extubated to CPAP. Older infants ventilated for chronic conditions can be extubated from peak pressures or tidal volume. As adjuncts to extubation, caffeine therapy in preterm neonates <32 weeks' gestation is associated with a 50% reduction in extubation failure.[6] This can be initiated early or peri-extubationally in the same doses as recommended for apnea of prematurity. CPAP applied immediately after extubation reduces the incidence of respiratory failure and the need for re-intubation in very preterm infants.[7]

Despite successful extubation, up to one-third of neonates can require re-intubation. The reasons for re-intubation may be significant apnea, hypoxia, acidosis or hypercarbia, upper airway obstruction due to edema or stenosis, or excessive work of breathing. While it is challenging to predict failures, some risk factors are listed as follows.

**Risk factors for extubation failure**

- Lower GA (<26 weeks).
- Prolonged ventilation (>10–14 days).
- History of previous extubation failure.
- Use of sedatives (e.g. morphine, fentanyl).
- Multiple reintubations: Upper airway problem.
- Evidence of residual lung injury: BPD, pulmonary interstitial emphysema.
- Extubation from high ventilatory settings or high $FiO_2$.
- Hemodynamically significant PDA.
- Hemodynamic instability, sepsis, NEC.

## REFERENCES

1. Slutsky AS. Mechanical ventilation. American College of Chest Physicians' Consensus Conference. Chest. 1993;104(6):1833–59.
2. Greenough A, Rossor TE, Sundaresan A, Murthy V, Milner AD. Synchronized mechanical ventilation for respiratory support in newborn infants. Cochrane Database Syst Rev. 2016;9:CD000456.
3. Peng W, Zhu H, Shi H, Liu E. Volume-targeted ventilation is more suitable than pressure-limited ventilation for preterm infants: a systematic review and meta-analysis. Arch Dis Child Fetal Neonatal Ed. 2014;99(2):F158–65.
4. Wheeler K, Klingenberg C, McCallion N, Morley CJ, Davis PG. Volume-targeted versus pressure-limited ventilation in the neonate. Cochrane Database Syst Rev. 2010(11):CD003666.
5. Sinha SK, Donn SM. Weaning newborns from mechanical ventilation. Semin Neonatol. 2002;7(5):421–8.
6. Henderson-Smart DJ, Davis PG. Prophylactic methylxanthines for endotracheal extubation in preterm infants. Cochrane Database Syst Rev. 2010(12):CD000139.
7. Davis PG, Henderson-Smart DJ. Nasal continuous positive airways pressure immediately after extubation for preventing morbidity in preterm infants. Cochrane Database Syst Rev. 2003(2):CD000143.

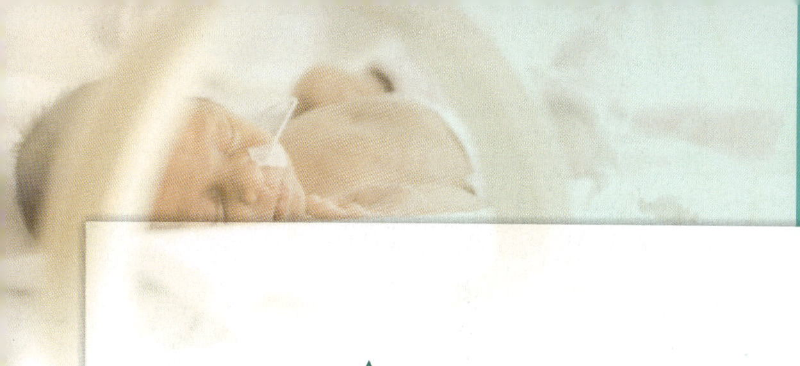

# Annexures

1. Drugs in Pregnancy and Breastfeeding
2. Filling out the International Death Certificate
3. Important ICD-10 Codes for Assigning Causes of Neonatal Deaths
4. Genetic Diagnostic Algorithms for Common Neonatal Nursery Scenarios with Suspected Genetic Etiology

ANNEXURE 1

# Drugs in Pregnancy and Breastfeeding

| Table A1.1: Drugs in pregnancy and breastfeeding | | | |
|---|---|---|---|
| *Drugs during pregnancy: Risk to the fetus (FDA)* | | *Drugs during breastfeeding-risk to infant (AAP)* | |
| *Category* | *Risk* | *Category* | *Risk* |
| A | None | L1 | Safest; no risk |
| B | Possibly none (animal studies but no human studies) | L2 | Safer; remote risk |
| C | Possibly yes. Use if benefits outweigh risks. | L3 | Moderately safe. Use if benefits outweigh risks. |
| D | Yes. Use if benefits outweigh risks. | L4 | |
| | Possibly hazardous; use in life-threatening or serious conditions not having any safer option. | | |
| X | Definitive risk. Avoid the drug. | L5 | Contraindicated |
| NR | Not reviewed | | |

| *Group* | *Name* | *Pregnancy* | *Lactation* |
|---|---|---|---|
| Analgesics and NSAID | Acetaminophen | B | L1 |
| | Ibuprofen | B (T2)<br>D (T1, T3) | L1 |
| | Indomethacin | B (T2)<br>D (T1, T3) | L3 |
| | Ketorolac | B (T2)<br>D (T1, T3) | L2 |
| | Mefenamic acid | D (T1, T3) | L2 |
| | Naproxen | D (T1, T3) | L3 |
| | Piroxicam | C | L1 |

*(Contd.)*

*(Contd.)*

| *Group* | *Name* | *Pregnancy* | *Lactation* |
|---|---|---|---|
| Narcotic analgesics | Codeine | C | L4 |
| | Fentanyl | C | L1 |
| | Methadone | C | L3 |
| | Morphine | C | L4 |
| | Propoxyphene | C | L2 |
| Non-narcotic | Propofol | B | L2 |
| | Midazolam | B | L2 |
| | Tramadol | C | L4 |
| Anesthetics | Halothane | B | L2 |
| | Lidocaine | A | L2 |
| | Methohexital | A | L3 |
| | Thiopental | C | L3 |
| Gastrointestinal | Cisapride | C | L2 |
| | Domperidone | – | L1 |
| | Diphenoxylate | B | L4 |
| | Metoclopramide | B | L2 |
| | Ondansetron | C | L2 |
| | Promethazine | A | L2 |
| | Ranitidine | B | L2 |
| | Sucralfate | A | L2 |
| Antibiotics | Amoxicillin | C (T1, T3) | L1 |
| | Azithromycin | A | L2 |
| | Aztreonam | B | L2 |
| | Cephalosporins | B | L1 |
| | Ciprofloxacin | D | L4 |
| | Clindamycin | B | L2 |
| | Erythromycin | B | L2 |
| | Gentamicin | C | L2 |
| | Nitrofurantoin | C (T3) | L2 |
| | Ofloxacin | D | L2 |
| | Penicillin | A | L1 |

*(Contd.)*

(*Contd.*)

| Group | Name | Pregnancy | Lactation |
|---|---|---|---|
| | Streptomycin | D | L1 |
| | Sulbactam | A | L1 |
| | Sulfisoxazole | C | L2 |
| | Tetracycline | D (T2, T3) | L2 |
| | Ticarcillin | A | L1 |
| | Trimethoprim/ sulfamethoxazole | C | L2 |
| Anticoagulants | Bishydroxycoumarin (dicumarol) | | NR |
| | Warfarin | D | L2 |
| Anticonvulsants | Carbamazepine | B | L2 |
| | Ethosuximide | C | L2 |
| | Phenytoin | C | L2 |
| | Valproic acid | C | L4 |
| | Gabapentin | B | L2 |
| | Lamotrigine | B | L4 |
| | Phenobarbitone | D | L4 |
| Antifungals | Fluconazole | C | L2 |
| | Ketoconazole | B | L2 |
| Antihistamines | Fexofenadine | B | L2 |
| | Loratadine | B | L1 |
| Antivirals | Acyclovir | B | L2 |
| | Interferon-alpha | C | L2 |
| Asthma | Terbutaline | B | L2 |
| | Theophylline | A | L1 |
| | Beclomethasone | C | L2 |
| | Budesonide | C | L2 |
| | Monteleukast | B | L3 |
| Contraceptives, Hormones | Estradiol | X | L1 |
| | Clogestone | – | NR |
| | Contraceptive pill with estrogen/progesterone | X | L3 (may interfere with milk production) |

(*Contd.*)

(*Contd.*)

| *Group* | *Name* | *Pregnancy* | *Lactation* |
|---|---|---|---|
| | Levonorgestrel | X | L2 |
| | Medroxyprogesterone | X | L1 |
| | Norethynodrel | X | L2 |
| | Progesterone | – | L3 |
| Cough | Codeine | C | L3 |
| | Noscapine | – | NR |
| Decongestants | Pseudoephedrine | C | L3 (acute use)<br>L4 (chronic use) |
| Anti-diabetic drugs | Insulin | B | L1 |
| | Tolbutamide | D (T3) | L4 |
| | Rosiglitazone | C | L3 |
| Diarrhea medications | Loperamide | B | L2 |
| Diuretics | Acetazolamide | C | L2 |
| | Chlorothiazide | A | L1 |
| | Spironolactone | C | L2 |
| Antiarrhythmics, Antihypertensives | Disopyramide | C | L2 |
| | Flecainide | C | L3 |
| | Mexiletine | B | L2 |
| | Procainamide | C | L3 |
| | Quinidine | C | L2 |
| | Captopril | C (T2, T3) | L1 |
| | Diltiazem | C | |
| | Enalapril | C (T1)<br>D (T2, T3) | L2 |
| | Hydralazine | C (T3) | L2 |
| | Labetalol | C | L2 |
| | Methyldopa | A | L2 |
| | Metoprolol | C (T2, T3) | L4 |
| | Minoxidil | C | L2 (topical)<br>L3 (oral) |
| | Nifedipine | C | L2 |
| | Propranolol | C (T2, T3) | L4 |

(*Contd.*)

(*Contd.*)

| *Group* | *Name* | *Pregnancy* | *Lactation* |
|---|---|---|---|
| | Verapamil | C | L2 |
| | Digoxin | B | L2 |
| Antimalarials | Chloroquine | B | L2 |
| | Hydroxychloroquine | B | L2 |
| | Pyrimethamine | B | L3 |
| | Quinine | D | L2 |
| | Mefloquine | C | L2 |
| Medications for diagnostic studies | Diatrizoate | – | NR |
| | Fluorescein | B | L4 |
| | Gadolinium | C | L2 |
| | Iohexol | B | L2 |
| | Iopanoic acid | B | L2 |
| | Metrizamide | B | L2 |
| | Metrizoate | B | L2 |
| Migraine | Sumatriptan | C | L3 |
| Sedatives | Zolpidem | B | L3 |
| Steroids | Methylprednisolone<br>Prednisolone<br>Prednisone | C | L2 |
| Thyroid medications | Carbimazole,<br>Methimazole | D | L3 |
| Anti-tubercular agents | Rifampicin | C | L3 |
| | Pyrizinamide | C | L3 |
| | Ethambutol | B | L2 |
| | Isoniazid | B | L2 |
| Anti-depressants | Amitriptyline | C | L2 |
| | Bupropion | B | L3 |
| | Citalopram | C | L4 |
| | Fluoxetine | C | L2 |
| | Mirtazapine | C | L4 |
| | Sertraline | B | L4 |
| | Venlafaxine | C | L3 |

(*Contd.*)

(*Contd.*)

| *Group* | *Name* | *Pregnancy* | *Lactation* |
|---|---|---|---|
| Influenza | Oseltamivir | C | L2 |
| | Amantadine | C | L3 |
| Anti-rheumatoid | Azathioprine | D (T3) | L3 |
| | Cyclophosphamide | D | L5 |
| | Infliximab | C | L2 |
| | Sulfasalazine | B | L4 |
| Antipsychotic | Haloperidol | C | L4 |
| Hypercholestero-lemia | Cholestyramine | B | L1 |
| | Clofibrate | C | L3 |
| | Gemfibrozil | C | L3 |
| | Niacin | A | L3 |
| | Statins | X | L3 |
| Hypothyroidism | Levothyroxine | A | L1 |
| Hyperthyroidism | Sodium iodide ($I^{31}$) | X | L4 |
| | Propylthiouracil | B | L2 |

ANNEXURE

2

# Filling out the International Death Certificate

A death certificate (DC) has two parts: **Part 1** deals with direct cause and **Part 2** deals with contributory cause of death (Fig. A2.1)

| **Cause of Death** | | |
|---|---|---|
| **I**<br>Disease or condition directly leading to death*<br><br>***Antecedent causes***<br>Morbid conditions giving rise to the above cause, stating the underlying condition last | (a) ____________<br>due to or as a consequence of<br>(b) ____________<br>due to or as a consequence of<br>(c) ____________<br>due to or as a consequence of<br>(d) ____________ | **Approximate interval between onset and death**<br>____________<br>____________<br>____________ |
| **II**<br>Other significant conditions contributing to the death, but not related to the disease or condition causing it<br>____________<br>____________<br>____________<br>**This does not mean the mode of dying e.g. heart failure, respiratory failure. It means the disease, injury or complication that caused death.* | | ____________<br>____________<br>____________ |

**Fig. A2.1:** International death certificate

**Part I**

a. Write the disease or condition that directly caused the death.

b. Write any intermediate cause of death.

c. Write the underlying cause of death on the last line.

If the disease or condition leading directly to death (1a) and the underlying cause of death (1c) happen to be the same—fill in only line I(a). If death is due to an external cause such as a fall—give details of the external cause as the underlying cause of death.

**Part II**

Write in this part, some other condition or disease that contributed to the death, but which is not part of the sequence that led to death. If there is none, keep it blank

**Example:** A term baby weighing 2200 gm born through meconium stained liquor developed meconium aspiration syndrome (MAS) and PPHN and required ventilation for 60 hours. The baby also developed features of HIE stage 2.

On day 5 of life, the baby developed sepsis which progressed to septic shock and acute renal failure. The baby died of hyperkalemia on day 6 of life.

**The chain of event:** Septic shock→acute renal failure→hyperkalemia

It does not appear that either of MAS, PPHN or HIE contributed to death—as the baby had reasonably recovered from all of that.

Therefore, (a) hyperkalemia, (b) acute renal failure and (c) septic shock would be filled out in Part 1 and Part 2 would be left blank. In addition, time interval between its onset and death would be entered for each condition.

# Important ICD-10 Codes for Assigning Causes of Neonatal Deaths

| *ICD 10 code* | *Cause of death* | *Criteria* |
|---|---|---|
| **Infectious and parasitic diseases** | | |
| A09 | Diarrhoea | Frequent/liquid/watery loose or soft stools |
| | | Possibly with fontanelle depressed OR eyes sunken OR urine volume low |
| A33/ A34 | Neonatal Tetanus | Baby able to suck after birth AND stopped sucking after 3 days AND baby's body became rigid with or without convulsions |
| | | Possibly with umbilical cord inflammation OR fever |
| **Diseases of the respiratory system** | | |
| J22 | Acute lower respiratory tract infection | Cough OR fever AND rapid breathing OR difficult breathing with indrawing of chest (often local term) |
| **Certain conditions originating in the perinatal period** | | |
| P05 | Low birth weight (full term pregnancy) | Smaller than average size baby. If weighted, birth weight below 2.5 kilograms AND no other obvious causes of death AND full term pregnancy |
| | | Possibly with poor sucking after birth OR death at 3–7 days |
| P07 | Prematurity (not full term) | Born between 28 and 36 but before 37 weeks of gestation AND no other obvious causes of death |
| P10 | Birth trauma | Bruises at birth, or elongation/swelling/blood clots over skull OR any limb broken at birth OR convulsions first 72 hours of birth |
| | | Possibly with instrument delivery or complicated delivery |

*(Contd.)*

(Contd.)

| ICD 10 code | Cause of death | Criteria |
|---|---|---|
| P21 | Asphyxia at birth | Delayed or poor breathing or no breathing at birth OR delayed or no cry at birth AND<br>Any sign of life at birth (i.e. exclude stillbirths) OR convulsions in 72 hours |
| | | Possibly with prolonged or difficult labour OR death at 3–7 days OR cold to touch |
| P36 | Bacterial sepsis of newborn | Fever AND<br>No other obvious causes of death (like ARI, diarrhoea) |
| | | Possibly with cord infection OR poor sucking OR limp and lethargic, coma |
| P80 | Hypothermia | Central part of the body felt cold AND Lethargic AND stopped feeding |
| | | Possibly with exposure to cold |
| **Other** | | |
| Q89 | Congenital malformations | Abnormality of head (small, flat, swelling), spine, body, arms or legs reported at birth<br>For specific diagnoses refer to codes Q65–Q88 |
| P96 | Ill-defined/ unspecified | |

**Ref:** SRS collaborators: Registrar General of India/Centre for Global Health Research Prospective Study of 6 Million Indians. Technical document No5b (available at www.cghr.org), University of Toronto, 2003

ANNEXURE

# Genetic Diagnostic Algorithms for Common Neonatal Nursery Scenarios with Suspected Genetic Etiology 4

1. Infant with skeletal dysplasia
2. Pre-conceptional counselling for β-thalassemia
3. Diagnosis and prenatal counselling of Down syndrome
4. Workup of an infant with multiple congenital anomalies
5. Neonate with microcephaly (congenital microcephaly)
6. Non-immune hydrops
7. Floppy neonate
8. Infant with congenital heart disease (genetic approach only)

## 1. Infant with Skeletal Dysplasia

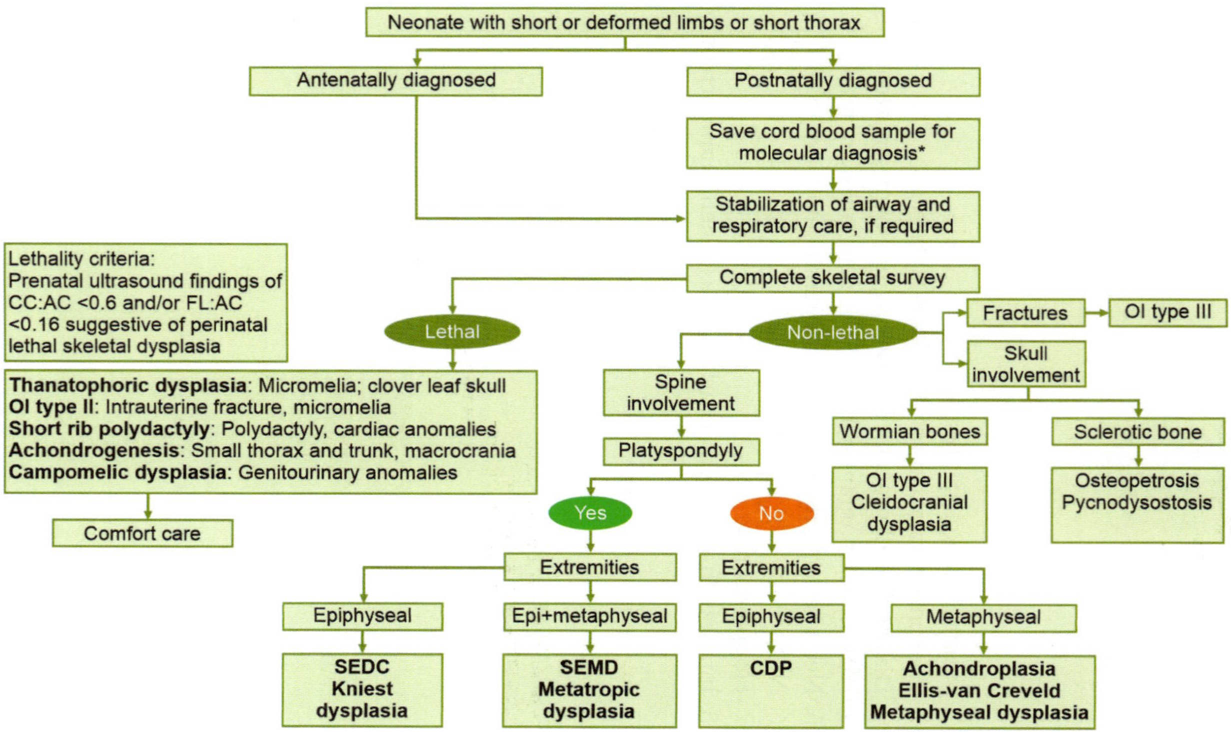

**Footnote:**

*SEDC:* Spondyloepiphyseal dysplasia congenita; *OI:* Osteogenesis imperfecta; *CDP:* Chondrodysplasia punctata; *SEMD:* Spondylometaphyseal dysplasia

*__Molecular diagnosis (Sanger sequencing or whole exome sequencing based on the clinical suspicion):__ Most skeletal dysplasias are monogenic disorders with commonly involved genes like COL2A1 gene (type II collagen disorders, achondrogenesis, stickler dysplasia); COL1A1, COL1A2 gene (osteogenesis imperfecta; SOX9 gene: Campomelic dysplasia); FGFR3 gene (achondroplasia, thanatophoric dysplasia; PTHR1 gene: Jansen metaphyseal chondrodysplasia); DYNC2H1 gene (asphyxiating thoracic dystrophy); EVC 1,2 gene (LIMBIN) (Ellis-van Creveld syndrome); Unknown cases: Whole exome sequencing

## REFERENCES

1. Krakow D. Skeletal dysplasias. Clin Perinatol. 2015 Jun;42(2):301–19, viii. doi: 10.1016/j.clp.2015.03.003. Epub 2015 Apr 8. PMID: 26042906; PMCID: PMC4456691.
2. Panda A, Gamanagatti S, Jana M, Gupta AK. Skeletal dysplasias: A radiographic approach and review of common non-lethal skeletal dysplasias. World J Radiol. 2014 Oct 28;6(10):808–25. doi: 10.4329/wjr.v6.i10.808. PMID: 25349664; PMCID: PMC4209426.

## 2. Pre-conceptional Counselling for β-Thalassemia

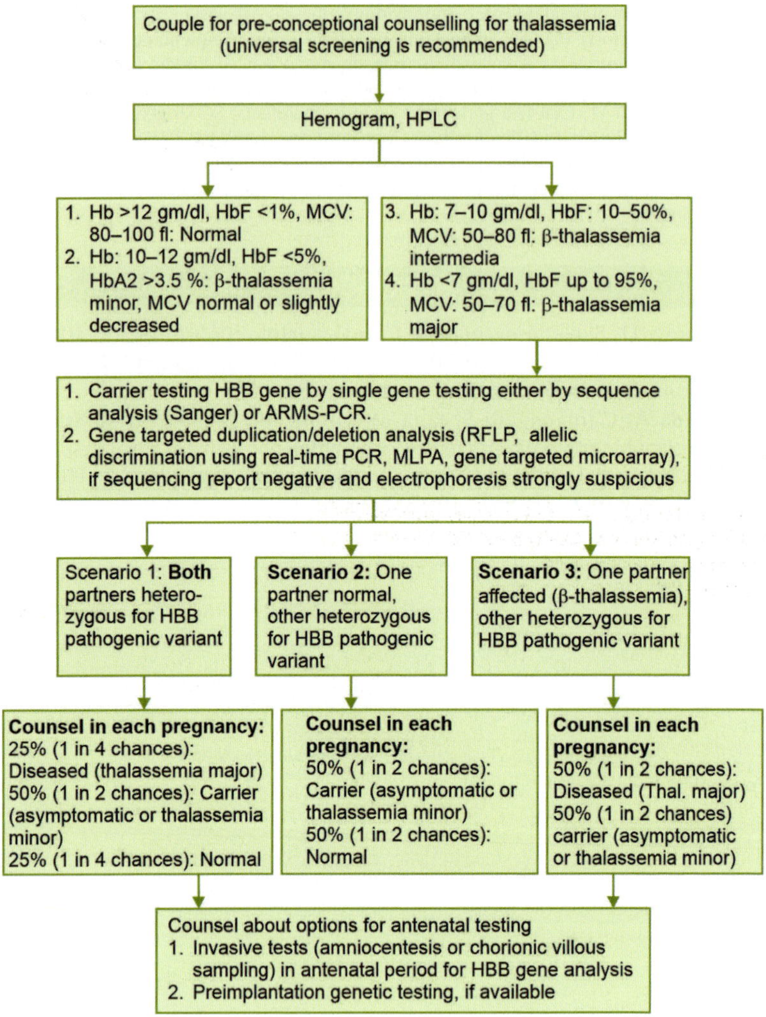


## REFERENCE

1. National health mission guidelines on hemoglobinopathy in India; 2016.

## 3. Diagnosis and Prenatal Counselling of Down Syndrome

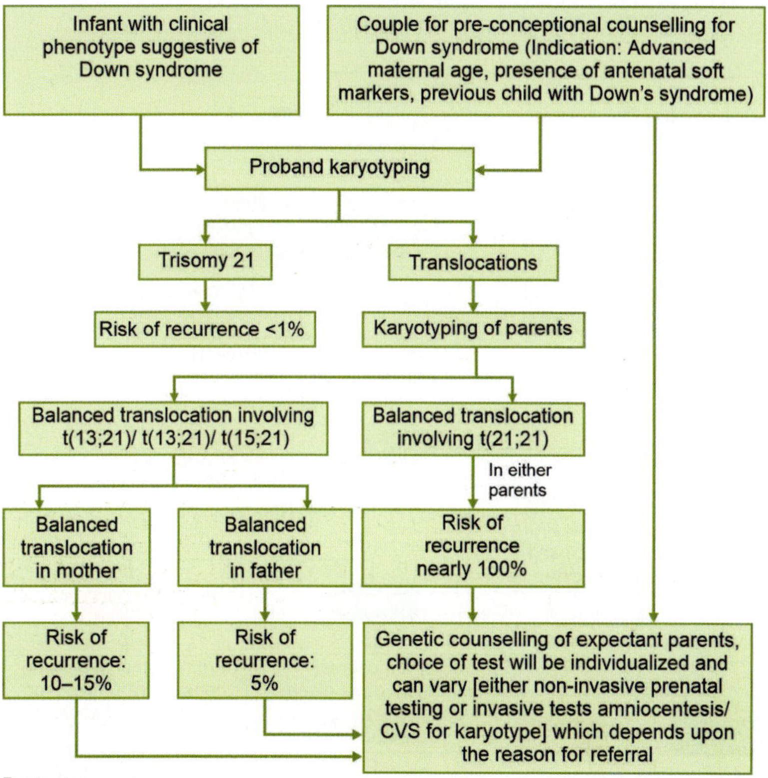


**Footnote:**

*Other supportive investigations at birth/diagnosis:*

**Complete blood count** for transient abnormal myelopoiesis, polycythemia, **thyroid profile** for congenital hypothyroidism, **echocardiography** for screening of congenital heart disease, **ophthalmologic evaluation** for strabismus, cataract, nystagmus, **hearing screening** (ABR/OAE) for congenital hearing loss, monitor for growth and development, start early stimulation therapies

## REFERENCE

1. Marilyn J. Bull, Tracy Trotter, Stephanie L. Santoro, Celanie Christensen, Randall W. Grout, the council on genetics; Health Supervision for Children and Adolescents With Down Syndrome. *Pediatrics* May 2022; 149 (5): e2022057010. 10.1542/peds.2022-057010.

## 4. Workup of an Infant with Multiple Congenital Anomalies

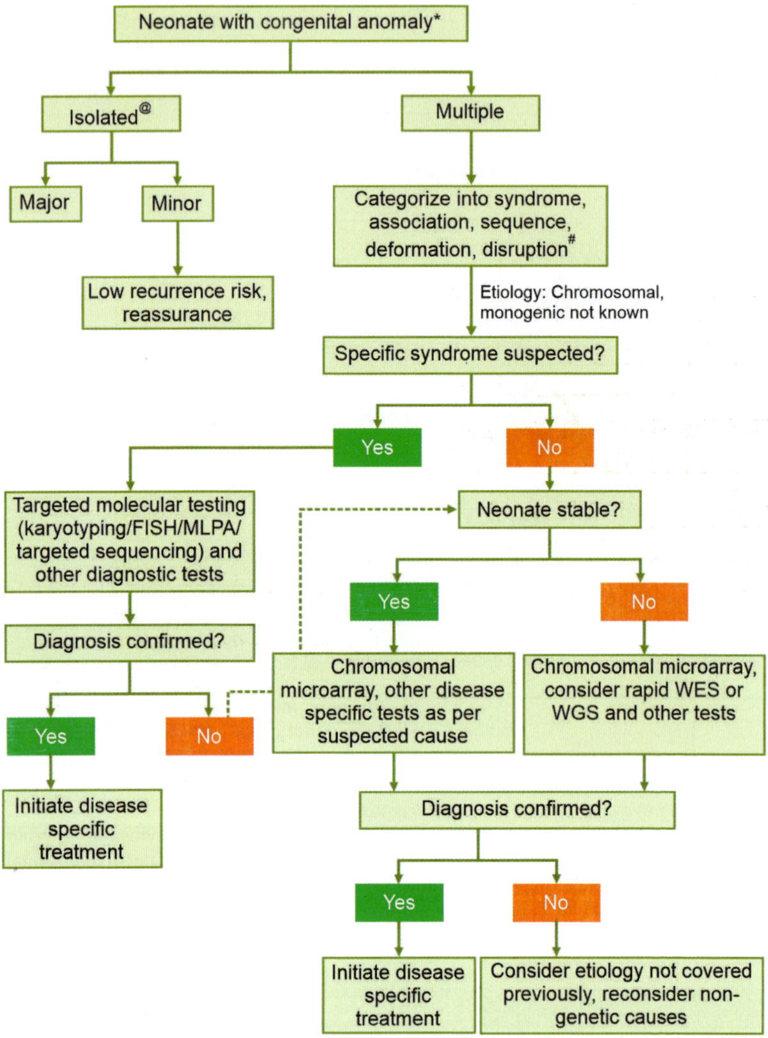


**Footnote:**

****Supportive investigations:*** Infantogram, USG genitourinary system and echocardiogram

***Abbreviations:*** *FISH:* Fluorescence *in-situ* hybridization; *MLPA:* Multiplex ligation-dependent probe amplification; *WES:* Whole exome sequencing, *WGS:* Whole genome sequencing

@In polygenic cases risk of recurrence 2–5%

**#Definitions**

***Malformation:*** A structural defect arising from a localized error in morphogenesis that results in abnormal formation of a tissue or organ

***Syndrome:*** Appearance of multiple malformations in unrelated tissues that have a known unifying cause
***Association:*** A group of malformations that occur together more than would be expected by chance alone
***Sequence:*** A pattern of malformations and deformations which is a consequence of a single malformation
***Deformation:*** Mechanical (extrinsic) force causing alteration of structure of intrinsically normal tissue
***Disruption:*** *In utero* tissue destruction after a period of normal morphogenesis
***Dysplasia:*** Atypical organization of cells into tissue or organ

## 5. Neonate with Microcephaly (Congenital Microcephaly)

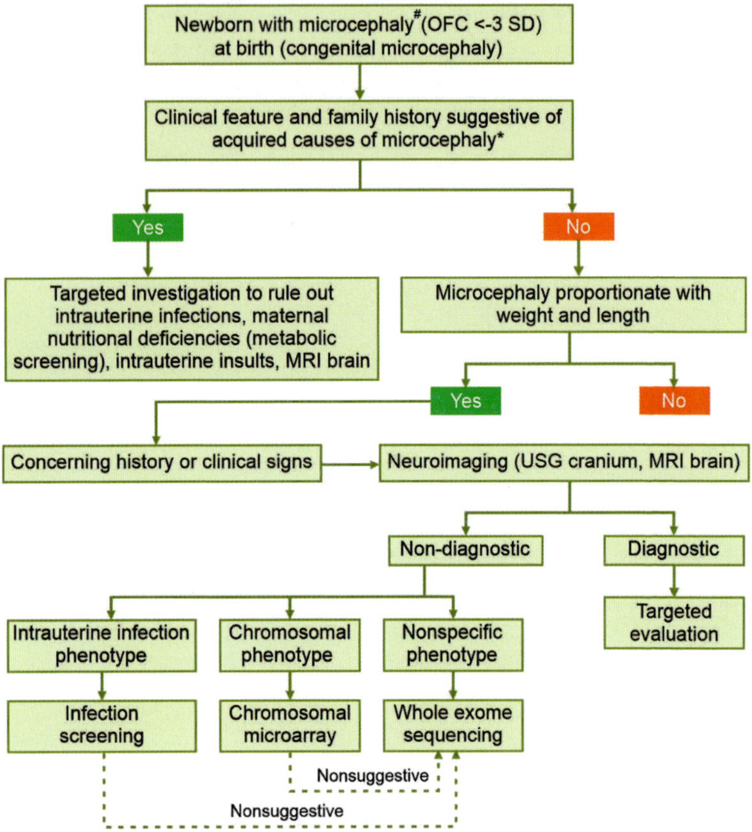


#Various studies have defined microcephaly as head size <–2 SD or <–3 SD as per gestation, gender. However, etiological yield of investigations (including genetic) for isolated border line microcephaly (–2 to –3 SD) usually low in majority of cases.

*Acquired causes:

1. Disruptive intrauterine insults (death of monozygotic co-twin), ischemic stroke, hemorrhagic stroke)
2. Intrauterine infections (TORCHes groups, HIV, Zika), teratogen exposure in pregnancy (maternal alcoholism, phenylketonuria, uncontrolled DM)
3. Deficiency of micronutrient and macronutrient in pregnancy: Maternal hypothyroidism, folate deficiency, malnutrition, placental insufficiency

**Genetic causes:** Any severe microcephaly (OFC <–5 SD), mostly suggestive of genetic etiology

1. Isolated: AR, AD, X-linked, rarely chromosomal
2. Syndromic
   a. Chromosomal: Trisomy 21,13,18, unbalanced rearrangement
   b. Contiguous gene deletions: Deletions in 4p, 5p, 7q11.23, 22q11 regions
   c. Single gene defect: Cornelia de Lange syndrome, holoprosencephaly, Smith-Lemli-Opitz syndrome, etc.

## REFERENCES

1. Becerra-Solano LE, Mateos-Sánchez L, López-Muñoz E. Microcephaly, an etiopathogenic vision. Pediatrics & Neonatology. 2021 Jul;62(4):354–60.
2. Microcephaly Diagnostic Guidelines [Internet]. [cited 2023 Oct 12]. Available from: https://starship.org.nz/guidelines/microcephaly-diagnostic-guidelines/

## 6. Non-immune Hydrops

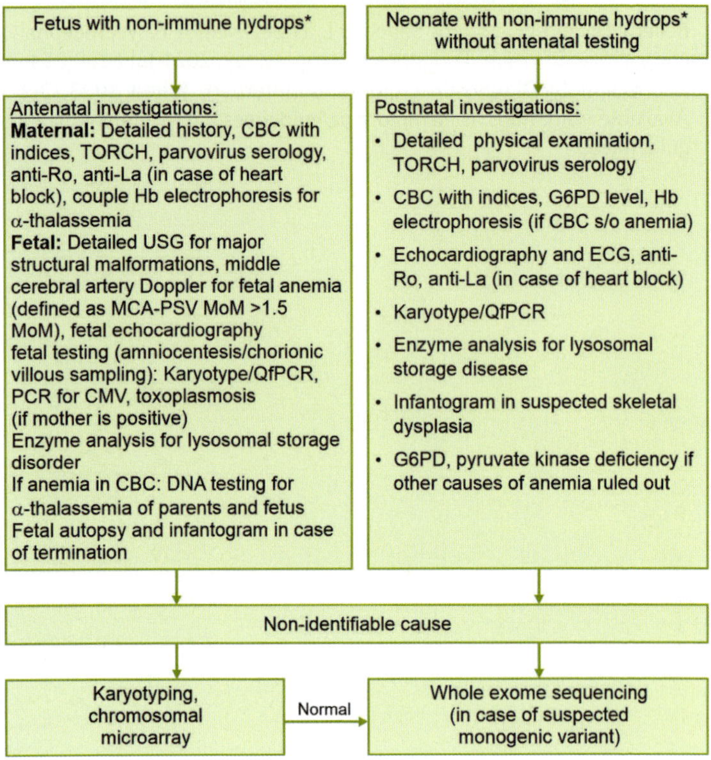


**Footnote:**

***Abbreviations used:*** *QfPCR:* Quantitative fluorescent PCR; *CBC:* Complete blood count

***Aetiology for Non-immune hydrops fetalis with relative percentages[2]:***

Idiopathic: 29.4%, cardiovascular: 11.8%, chromosomal: 2.9%, genetic and metabolic cause: 8.8%, hematological: 8.8%, infection: 2.9%, lymphatic dysplasia: 23.6%, others:11.8%

*Non-immune hydrops is characterised fluid accumulation in at least two extra vascular space out of the following: 1. Skin edema 2. Ascitis, 3. Pleural effusion, 4. Pericardial effusion along with ICT negativity

## REFERENCES

1. Norton ME, Chauhan SP, Dashe JS. Society for Maternal-Fetal Medicine (SMFM) Clinical Guideline #7: nonimmune hydrops fetalis. American Journal of Obstetrics and Gynecology. 2015 Feb;212(2):127–39.
2. Takci S, Gharibzadeh M, Yurdakok M, Ozyuncu O, Korkmaz A, Akcoren A, et al. Etiology and outcome of hydrops fetalis: report of 62 cases. Pediatr Neonatol. 2014;55:108–13.

## 7. Floppy Neonate

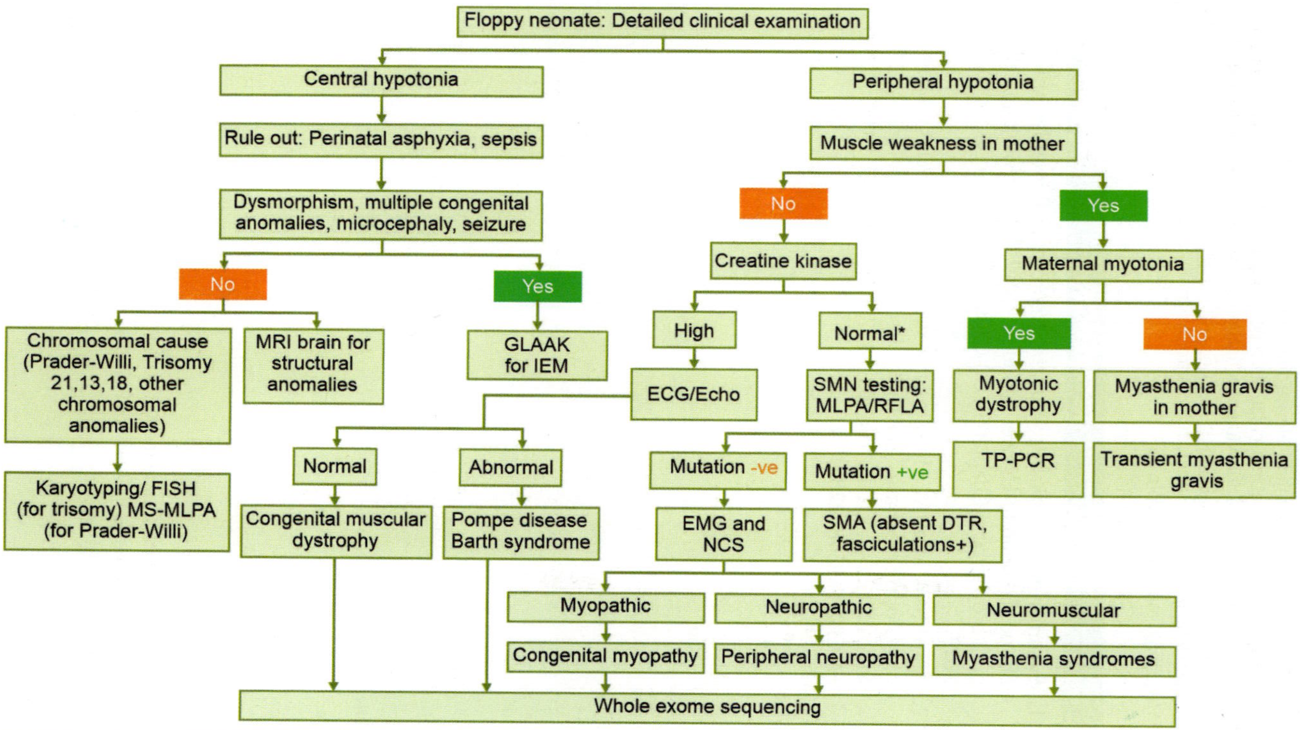

**Footnote:**
*Creatine kinase might be mildly elevated in spinal muscular atrophy
***Abbreviations:*** *SMA:* Spinal muscular atrophy; *FISH:* Fluorescent *in-situ* hybridization; *MS-MLPA:* Methylation specific-Multiplex ligation probe amplification; *GLAAK:* Glucose, lactate, acidosis, ammonia, ketones; *TP-PCR:* Triplet repeat primed PCR; *RFLA:* Restriction fragment length polymorphism; *EMG:* Electromyography; *NCS:* Nerve conduction studies; *SMA:* Spinal muscular atrophy

## REFERENCES

1. Swaiman KF. *Swaiman's Pediatric Neurology:* Principles and Practice. 5th ed. Edinburgh: Elsevier Saunders; 2012. http://www.clinicalkey.com/dura/browse/bookChapter/3-s2.0-C20091593902. Accessed October 12, 2023.
2. Ahmed MI, Iqbal M, Hussain N. A structured approach to the assessment of a floppy neonate. Journal of Pediatric Neurosciences. 2016 Jan–Mar;11(1):2–6. DOI: 10.4103/1817-1745.181250. PMID: 27195025; PMCID: PMC4862282.

## 8. Infant with Congenital Heart Disease (Genetic Approach Only)

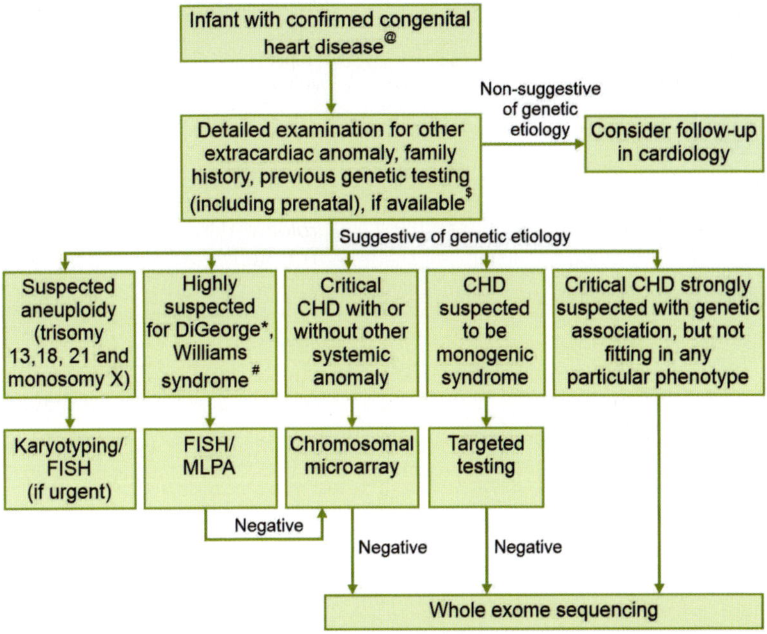


**Footnote:**

$Congenital heart disease not requiring detailed genetic evaluation: Isolated ASD, VSD, PDA (in preterms)

*In presence of conotruncal lesions like interrupted aortic arch, truncus arteriosus, tetralogy of Fallot and ventricular septal along with characteristic phenotype (facial features, hypocalcemia, absence of thymus: Investigate for 22q11.2 deletion)

#In presence of supravalvular aortic stenosis and peripheral pulmonary stenosis along with other characteristic phenotype: Investigate for 7q11.23

@Genetic counselling of parents: Except for monogenic syndromic causes most CHD are multifactorial with recurrence risk <1%, if previous 1 sibling or parent is affected: 2–6%, ≥ 2: up to 20–30%

## REFERENCE


1. Marian AJ, Watkins H, Seidman C. Genetics of Congenital Heart Disease. Circulation research. 2013;(Feb):707–20.

# Index